RESPIRATORY FUNCTION IN SPEECH AND SONG

50000120

Respiratory Function in Speech and Song

Thomas J. Hixon, Ph.D.
University of Arizona

and

Collaborators
Harvard School of Public Health
University of Wisconsin
Hine Veterans Administration Medical Center
University of Arizona

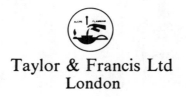

Taylor & Francis Ltd
London

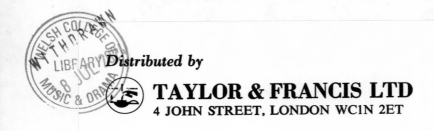

Distributed by

TAYLOR & FRANCIS LTD
4 JOHN STREET, LONDON WC1N 2ET

College-Hill Press
A Division of
Little, Brown and Company (Inc.)
34 Beacon Street
Boston, Massachusetts 02108

© 1987 by Little, Brown and Company (Inc.)

Library of Congress Cataloging in Publication Data
Main entry under title:

Hixon, Thomas J.
   Respiratory function in speech and song.

Includes indexes.
   1. Respiration. 2. Speech—Physiological aspects.
3. Singing—Physiological aspects. I. Title.
[DNLM: 1. Respiratory System—physiology. 2. Speech—
physiology. WF 102 H676r]
QP121.H66 1987   612'.21   86-14787
ISBN 0-316-36528-9

British Library Cataloging in Publication Data

Hixon, Thomas J.
Respiratory Function in Speech and Song.
1. Voice
I. Title
612'.78 QP306
ISBN 0-85066-655-4

ISBN 0-316-36528-9

Printed in the United States of America

For
Kala Singh
In Memory of Her Gentle Countenance
With Hope for Peace

CONTENTS

FOREWORD

Dr. Thomas Hixon is a pioneer in spirit and in fact. He marches to the dictates of lucid thinking, which means that one rarely finds Dr. Hixon following a beaten path. His grasp of speech production systems and their functions is awesome.

   Dr. Hixon's investigations of respiratory function characterize his scholarship. The extent to which scientifically credible information is known about breathing for speech and singing is directly attributable, in large part, to the work of Thomas Hixon and his colleagues. He not only blazed much of the trail of modern research about breathing for speech and singing, he then built the settlements along the frontiers of this research with some of the investigations included in this remarkable volume.

William H. Perkins, Ph.D.
University of Southern California

PREFACE

This book is a collection of 12 manuscripts from my laboratory having to do with the behavior of the respiratory apparatus in the generation of speech and song. Many of these manuscripts have been published previously as articles in scholarly journals or as chapters in books, but they have been edited heavily for this book to provide for consistency in style and terminology.

More than a decade of work on normal and abnormal function is spanned by the manuscripts included here. Over this time, I have been fortunate to have been associated with a group of dedicated colleagues and students, many of whom are coauthors on the manuscripts selected for inclusion here. I am indebted to all of these individuals, but especially to Dr. Jere Mead, who took me under his wing for two years as a National Institutes of Health Special Research Fellow in the Department of Physiology at the Harvard School of Public Health. I also am indebted to the National Institute of Neurological and Communicative Disorders and Stroke for its continuous support of my research over the years.

When I agreed to put this book together, I had no idea how many pleasant memories the process would evoke. For many of these memories, I again am indebted to my colleagues and students, and, as well, to many subjects and clients.

Finally, I wish to acknowledge the careful work of Ms. Susan Altman, who managed the editorial production of the book and quietly endured my incessant galley marginalia.

Thomas J. Hixon
Tucson, Arizona

COLLABORATORS

Linda L. Forner, Ph.D. Department of Speech Pathology and Audiology, University of Cincinnati, Cincinnati, Ohio

Michael D. Goldman, M.D. Department of Pulmonary Medicine, University of Utah Medical Center, Salt Lake City, Utah

Jeannette D. Hoit, M.A. Department of Speech and Hearing Sciences, University of Arizona, Tucson, Arizona

Mary Z. Maher, Ph.D. Department of Drama, University of Arizona, Tucson, Arizona

Jere Mead, M.D. Department of Physiology, Harvard School of Public Health, Boston, Massachusetts

Anne H. B. Putnam, Ph.D. Department of Speech Pathology and Audiology, University of Alberta, Edmonton, Alberta

John T. Sharp, M.D. Department of Cardiopulmonary Medicine, Veterans Administration Medical Center, Hines, Illinois

Peter J. Watson, M.S. Department of Speech and Hearing Sciences, University of Arizona, Tucson, Arizona

CHAPTER 1

Respiratory Function in Speech

Thomas J. Hixon

W hatever the task performed by the respiratory (breathing) apparatus, several important factors must be considered if the basic functioning of the apparatus is to be understood mechanically. Foremost among these factors are the structure of the respiratory pump, the forces applied to and by its various parts, and the movements of those parts as manifested geometrically and through volume and flow events. This chapter considers each of these factors as it relates to the adult respiratory apparatus in two important behaviors; namely, respiration for life purposes and respiration for speech purposes. Although function for life purposes is of secondary interest in this book, it is necessary to consider such function in detail because the principles involved form a basis for understanding the mechanics of speech respiration.

Reprinted by permission of the publisher from *Normal Aspects of Speech, Hearing, and Language*, F. Minifie, T. Hixon, and F. Williams (Eds.), pp. 75–125, © 1973, Prentice-Hall, Englewood Cliffs, NJ.

RESPIRATION FOR LIFE PURPOSES

For life purposes, the main function of respiration is to provide oxygen to the cells of the body and to remove carbon dioxide from them. This requires movement of air to and from special gas-exchange surfaces within the body, this movement being accomplished by a remarkably engineered biological pump. This pump includes an energy source, passive elements that couple this source to the air it moves, the air itself, and the passageways through which the air is moved (Mead and Milic-Emili, 1964). Of interest in this section are the structure of this pump and a simple analysis of its behavior as a machine.

Structure of the Respiratory Apparatus

Figure 1–1 depicts a cut-away front view of the body trunk or *torso*, which houses most of the important structures of the respiratory apparatus. The torso consists mainly of skeletal framework and muscular tissue and is divided into upper and lower cavities by a dome-shaped partition called the *diaphragm*. The upper cavity, known as the *thorax*, or chest, is almost totally filled with the heart and various structures of the *pulmonary system* (respiratory airways and lungs), whereas the lower cavity, the *abdomen* or belly, contains much of the digestive system along with various other organs and glands. Because both the thorax and abdomen participate importantly in respiratory function, it is essential that the structure of each be examined closely. Two other aspects warranting close examination are the principal features of the pulmonary system and the unitary nature of the lungs and thorax.

Thorax

Figure 1–2 illustrates the skeletal framework of the torso, the thoracic portion of which is, perhaps, best described as a barrel-shaped cage of bone and cartilage. At the back of the torso a series of 34 irregularly shaped *vertebrae* form the *vertebral column* or backbone, as it is referred to commonly. The uppermost seven vertebrae are termed *cervical* (neck); the next lower 12, *thoracic* (chest); and the next three lower groups of five, *lumbar, sacral,* and *coccygeal* (collectively abdominal), respectively. The thoracic segment of the column forms only a small portion of the total cage, most of it being formed by the *ribs,* which are 12 flat, arch-shaped bones found on each side of the body. These bones attach to thoracic vertebrae, from which they slope downward and around the sides of the thorax, giving roundness to the cage and forming its lateral walls. At the front, most of the ribs attach to bars of *costal cartilage* (rib cartilage), which in turn are connected to a long flat bone, the *sternum*, or breastbone, that serves as a front post for the thorax. Typical architecture for the thoracic cage finds the upper pairs of ribs attached to the

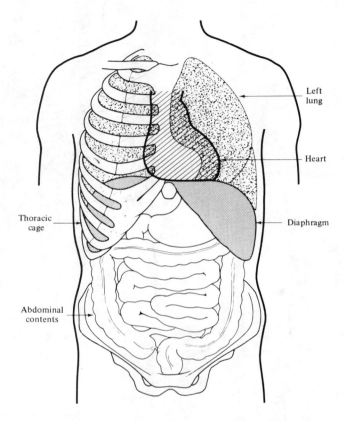

FIGURE 1-1. Cut-away front view of the adult torso, illustrating some important structures of the respiratory apparatus. The external wall of the entire apparatus is removed together with the muscles from the right side of the thoracic cage. The left side of the thoracic cage is not shown.

sternum by their own costal cartilages, the lower ribs on each side sharing cartilages variously, and the lowermost two on each side "floating" without front attachments.

Completing the thoracic skeleton is the *pectoral girdle* (shoulder girdle), which is situated around the top of the barrel-shaped cage. The front of this girdle is formed by the two *clavicles* (collar bones), each of which is a bony strut running from the upper sternum over the first rib toward the side and back of the thorax. At the back, the clavicles attach to two triangularly shaped bony plates, the *scapulae* (shoulder blades), which complete the girdle and cover much of the upper back portion of the cage.

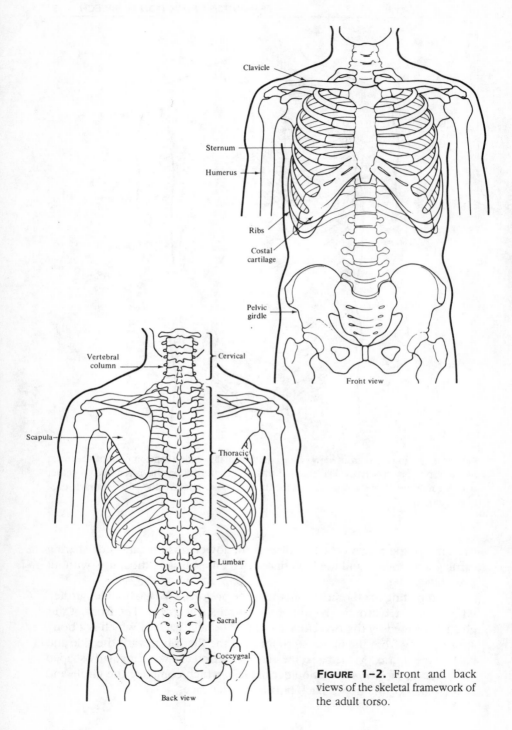

Clavicle

Sternum

Humerus

Ribs

Costal
cartilage

Pelvic
girdle

Front view

Vertebral
column

Cervical

Scapula

Thoracic

Lumbar

Sacral

Coccygeal

Back view

FIGURE 1–2. Front and back views of the skeletal framework of the adult torso.

4

Both muscular and nonmuscular tissues serve to complete the vertical walls of the thorax by filling the spaces between the ribs and covering the inner and outer surfaces of the cage. The muscular tissues are especially important in respiratory function and are considered later, as is the previously mentioned diaphragm, which doubles as the convex floor of the thorax and the concave roof of the abdomen.

Abdomen

The shape of the abdomen is not amenable to simple description by its skeletal structure as is the barrel-shaped cage of the thorax. The only skeletal structure included in the somewhat oblong-shaped abdominal cavity is the lower portion of the vertebral column at the back, and two large, irregularly shaped *coxal bones* (hip bones) at the base. These two bones, together with the sacral and coccygeal vertebrae, form the *pelvic girdle* (bony pelvis). For the most part, the abdomen is constructed of two broad, complex sheets of connective tissue and a number of very large muscles. The two connective sheets cover the front and back walls of the abdomen and are referred to, respectively, as the *abdominal aponeurosis* and the *lumbodorsal fascia*. The muscles of concern are found on all sides of the abdomen, with those situated on the front and side walls combining with the abdominal aponeurosis to form a belly girdle that completely encloses and, in part, supports the abdominal contents. Like the muscles of the thorax, those of the abdomen are important in respiration and are discussed subsequently in this chapter.

Pulmonary System

The major features of the pulmonary system are shown in Figure 1–3. In terms of gross structure, this system consists of two components, the *respiratory airways* and the *lungs* (organs of respiration). The former is a highly complex and variable tract with a number of subdivisions and branches through which air can be moved to and from the lungs. The cavities of the nose, mouth, and throat (together called the *upper airway*) are included in this tract along with the *larynx*, which functions as an airway valve. Discussion here is limited to the structure of the *lower airway* (the air passageway below the larynx).

Situated immediately beneath the larynx and running downward into the thorax is the *trachea* or windpipe. This is a semirigid tube composed of 16 to 20 C-shaped cartilages interconnected by fibrous tissue and muscle. The open ends of these cartilages face posteriorly where the tube is completed by a flexible wall shared with the *esophagus* (a muscular tube leading to the stomach). At its lower end, the trachea divides into two smaller semirigid tubes, the left and right *main-stem bronchi*. Each of these divides into *lobar bronchi*, and each of these in turn divides, and so on through more than 20 generations.

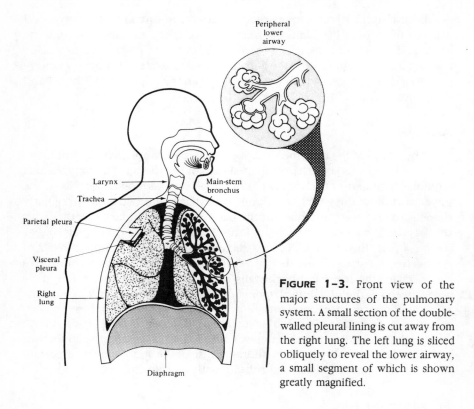

FIGURE 1–3. Front view of the major structures of the pulmonary system. A small section of the double-walled pleural lining is cut away from the right lung. The left lung is sliced obliquely to reveal the lower airway, a small segment of which is shown greatly magnified.

Approaching the periphery of the lung, the system finally arborizes into *terminal bronchioles, respiratory bronchioles, alveolar ducts, alveolar sacs,* and multitudes of very tiny *alveoli,* the last being the site where oxygen and carbon dioxide are exchanged during the respiratory process.

The lungs themselves are most simply described as cone-shaped structures that are of a porous, spongy texture and that possess an abundance of resilient elastic fibers. Although it represents a gross oversimplification of their structure, there is merit in thinking of the lungs as large air-filled elastic sacs that can change size and shape. Both lungs rest on the top surface of the diaphragm, from which they extend upward, one on each side, to almost fill the lateral chambers of the thoracic cavity. The outer surfaces of the lungs are covered with a delicate air-tight membrane called the *visceral pleura,* while a similar membrane, the *parietal pleura,* lines the inner surface of the thoracic walls and the top of the diaphragm. Together these membranes form a double-walled sac that completely encases the lungs. Both walls of this sac are covered with a thin layer of lubricating fluid that permits them to move easily on one another, and that also serves the important function of *linking* the two pleural surfaces together in much the same manner that a film of water holds two glass plates together (Comroe, 1965).

Lungs-Thorax Unit

Although the lungs and thorax normally operate together as a unit, it is important to realize that their natural resting positions in the intact unit are different from their individual resting positions when the two are separated. For example, with the lungs removed from the thorax, their resting position is a collapsed state in which they contain almost no air. By contrast, the resting position of the thorax with the lungs removed is a more expanded state (greater volume). With the lungs and thorax held together as a unit by *pleural linkage*, the respiratory apparatus assumes a natural resting position between these two separate positions such that the lungs are somewhat expanded and the thorax is somewhat compressed. The springs pictured in Figure 1–4 illustrate this relationship by analogy (Comroe, Forster, DuBois, Briscoe, and Carlsen, 1962). In this figure, the lungs and thorax are represented by separate springs, each in its resting position and unaffected by the other. The right side of the schema shows a different resting position for each spring when the two are held together as in pleural linkage. The net result is a stretching of the "lungs spring" and a compression of the "thoracic spring." This coupled resting position is analogous to that designated as the *resting expiratory level* in the human respiratory apparatus. At this level the respiratory pump is in a mechanically neutral or balanced position, at which the force of the lungs to collapse is opposed by an equal and opposite force of the thorax (including the diaphragm and abdomen) to expand.

At this juncture it is well to distinguish three important pressures within the respiratory pump: two within the thorax and one within the abdomen. The pressure within the lungs is referred to as *alveolar pressure*. That within the thorax but outside the lungs (i.e., between the two pleural walls) is designated as *pleural pressure*. Finally, the pressure within the abdomen is termed *abdominal pressure*.

Mechanics of Respiration

This section discusses the elements of normal respiration from the standpoints of dynamic performance and static properties of the respiratory pump, assuming the reader has knowledge of respiratory structure. It is convenient to consider these elements under four headings: inspiration, expiration, the pulmonary subdivisions, and the volume-pressure relationships of the respiratory pump. The discussion under each heading is limited to respiratory function in the upright position in normal individuals.

Inspiration

The phase of respiration during which air flows into the lungs is referred to as *inspiration* or *inhalation*. Aspects of this process that warrant attention include various aerodynamic events, the nature of thoracic enlargement, and the forces involved.

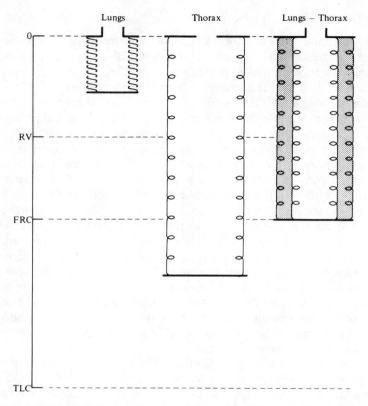

FIGURE 1–4. Spring analogy depicting the volumes (i.e., spring lengths) assumed by the lungs and the thorax when each is independent of the other and when the two are linked together by pleural linkage. The horizontal dashed lines represent lung volume levels (see Fig. 1–13) appropriate to the spring lengths. (After Comroe, J., Jr., et al.: *The lung: Clinical physiology and pulmonary function tests.* © 1962 Year Book Medical Publishers, Inc. Used by permission.)

AERODYNAMIC EVENTS. Basic to understanding inspiration, or air movement of any type, is the principle that *air flows from regions of higher pressure to regions of lower pressure.* With the airways open and the respiratory pump in its neutral position at the resting expiratory level, the pressure within the lungs (alveolar pressure) equals that outside the body (atmospheric pressure). To accomplish inspiration, alveolar pressure must be decreased sufficiently below atmospheric that a pressure gradient will exist in favor of inward flow. This gradient is created in the human respiratory apparatus by muscular forces that increase the size of the thorax. Because, as a result of pleural linkage, the lungs and thorax move as a unit, any increase in thoracic volume leads to a stretching of the lungs, an expansion of alveolar air, and a decrease in alveolar pressure.[1]

Figure 1–5 is a simplified illustration of selected volume, flow, and pressure changes that occur during a normal breathing cycle initiated from the resting expiratory level. In this figure the relationships may be seen among (1) the amount of air within the lungs (lung volume), (2) the rate of change of lung volume (flow), and (3) the alveolar pressure. For now, only the inspiratory portion of the cycle is of concern. As illustrated, there are two moments during this phase when alveolar pressure is atmospheric: at the beginning and end of inspiration (zero and 2 seconds on the horizontal axis). Because no pressure gradient exists at these two moments, flow also is zero. During inspiration alveolar pressure drops below atmospheric magnitude (to −1 centimeter of water [cm H_2O]), the extent of its drop and the shape of the pressure curve depending, for the most part, on the rapidity and extent of lung enlargement and the degree to which the respiratory airways are open. Because flow is proportional to the pressure difference between the lungs and atmosphere, changes in flow follow those in alveolar pressure. The specific relationship between flow and pressure depends, of course, on the type of flow being generated.[2] As can be seen in Figure 1–5, the most rapid negative (inspiratory) flow during the cycle is about −0.5 liter per second (LPS) and occurs when alveolar pressure is lowest (i.e., when the pressure difference between the lungs and atmosphere is greatest). Throughout inspiration, the volume of air within the lungs is continuously increasing, until by the end of a normal inspiration, the lung volume is about 0.5 liter (L) greater than it was at the resting expiratory level.

---

[1]Air molecules within the lungs provide pressure (force per unit area) by colliding with one another and with the structures of the lungs. When the volume of air within the lungs is expanded, the molecules are less crowded, so they are involved in fewer collisions and the pressure is lower. Conversely, when the volume is decreased, collisions are more frequent and the pressure is greater. Specifically, volume and pressure are inversely related, provided that temperature remains constant and that the respiratory airways are closed to the outside. Under such circumstances, doubling the volume halves the pressure and halving the volume doubles the pressure.

[2]The two flows most commonly recognized are laminar and turbulent. Laminar flow is smooth or streamline with its driving pressure being directly related to flow. Turbulent flow, by contrast, is erratic in both direction and magnitude, its driving pressure being proportional to the square of flow. Turbulence can occur at high flows in smooth straight tubes, or at low flows in tubes containing irregularities, such as the partial closure of the respiratory airways by the larynx. Both laminar and turbulent flow may exist in different portions of the respiratory airways at the same time. During normal respiration, flow is mostly laminar, whereas at higher than usual flows it becomes predominantly turbulent. For additional information refer to Comroe (1965) and Rouse and Howe (1953).

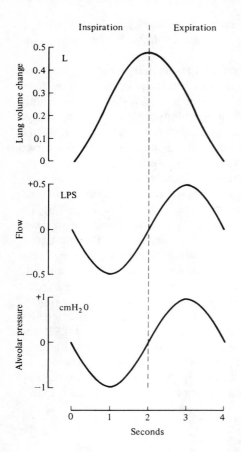

FIGURE 1-5. Simplified illustration of lung volume (L), flow (LPS), and alveolar pressure (cmH_2O) changes during a quiet breathing cycle. Actually, expiration is longer than inspiration, and waves for the two phases of the breathing cycle are asymmetrical. (After Comroe, J., Jr.: *Physiology of respiration.* © 1965 Year Book Medical Publishers, Inc. Used by permission.)

CHANGES IN THORACIC VOLUME. With an awareness that thoracic enlargement leads to inspiratory flow, it is relevant to examine the nature of changes in thoracic volume during inspiration. This is done most simply by considering the three dimensions in which the size of the thorax increases—vertical, anteroposterior, and transverse. Vertical enlargement is easiest to explain in that it results primarily from lowering the base of the thorax (diaphragm), as shown schematically in Figure 1–6. The anteroposterior and transverse increases, illustrated in Figure 1–7, are the result of somewhat more complex thoracic changes involving movements of the ribs and sternum. Recall that the ribs attach to the vertebral column posteriorly, from which they slope downward and forward toward the front of the thoracic cage. Upon elevation, the ribs go through two types of movement, one likened to the raising of a pump handle, the other likened to the raising of a bucket handle. In the pump-handle movement the front ends of the ribs move upward and forward along

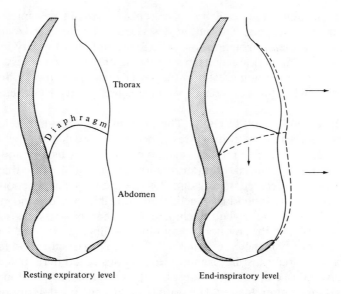

FIGURE 1-6. Resting and end-inspiratory positions of various respiratory structures during quiet breathing. Vertical increase in the thorax is caused mainly by footward displacement of the diaphragm, which in turn increases abdominal pressure and drives the abdominal wall outward.

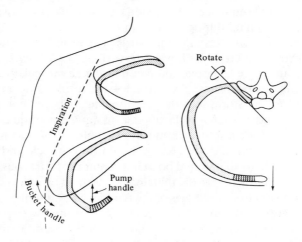

FIGURE 1-7. Front and top views of ribs, illustrating the pump-handle and bucket-handle motions responsible for anteroposterior and transverse diameter changes in the thorax. (After Cherniack, R., and Cherniack, L.: *Respiration in health and disease.* Philadelphia: W. B. Saunders Company, 1961. Used by permission.)

with the sternum, the result being an enlargement in the anteroposterior diameter of the thorax. The action described as bucket handle amounts to an outward *eversion* (rotation) of each rib around an imaginary line joining its two ends. This action results in a widening of the thorax transversely, the extent of increase being greater in the lower than upper thorax because the lower ribs swing through arcs of larger imaginary circles (Siebens, 1966).

FORCES OF INSPIRATION. The muscular energy expended during inspiration serves to overcome (1) resistance to air flow through the respiratory airways, (2) resistance to the deformation of respiratory tissues, and (3) elastic recoil of the lungs-thorax unit (Mead and Martin, 1968). More than a dozen muscles may be involved in providing this energy at one time or another during inspiration. Their individual mechanical contributions depend on various factors, the most important including (1) other muscles that are active simultaneously, (2) the amount of air within the lungs, and (3) the forcefulness of the respiratory maneuver (Campbell, 1958). The structure and function of the most important inspiratory muscles are considered here, this discussion being divided to consider separately the forces of quiet inspiration and those of forced inspiration. It should be borne in mind that the descriptions offered for individual muscle behaviors are based on the assumption that only the muscle under consideration is active, a convenient but in most instances an unrealistic assumption. Also, where controversy surrounds the function of certain muscles, the descriptions given are based on what is judged to be the most compelling experimental evidence. All of the statements that follow concerning the consequences of individual muscle activities assume that the muscles are shortening during contraction.

Quiet inspiration. Resting individuals take air into their lungs a dozen or more times a minute. This inward flow of air, called *quiet inspiration*, usually goes unnoticed, despite the fact that *active* muscular contraction is needed to enlarge the thorax. Two muscles, the diaphragm and the external intercostals, are most responsible for thoracic enlargement under these circumstances and as such are classified as the muscles of quiet inspiration. Figure 1–8 depicts their structure and shows their location within the body.

The *diaphragm* is a dome-shaped structure of muscle and tendon that bears resemblance to an inverted bowl. Its centermost part consists of a thin, flat, *central tendon*, whereas the remainder is formed by a rim of muscle that radiates downward from the edges of the tendon. The bottom of this muscular rim attaches around the internal circumference of the lower portion of the thorax; these attachments include the bottom of the sternum, the lower ribs and their cartilages, and the first three or four lumbar vertebrae. When the muscular rim contracts, the diaphragm is pulled downward and slightly forward, thus increasing the thoracic cavity in a vertical direction. Contraction of the diaphragm also increases the circumference of the thorax through eleva-

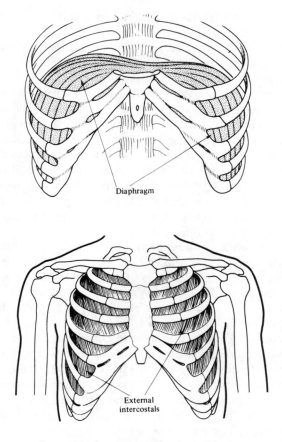

FIGURE 1–8. Muscles of quiet inspiration.

tion of the lower ribs. The combined action of lowering the base of the thorax and expanding its circumference is sufficient to account for most of the change in thoracic volume during quiet inspiration. In association with this volume change, the component of diaphragmatic activity that is resolved into footward displacement of the structure causes an increase in abdominal pressure and a driving outward of the abdominal wall (see Figure 1–6).

The *external intercostal* muscles are 11 relatively thin layers of muscular tissue that completely fill the rib interspaces. Each runs between the lower edge of one rib and the upper edge of the rib immediately below, the individual fibers oriented forward and downward. Although structurally inaccurate, it is useful to think of the external intercostals, from a mechanical viewpoint, as a large sheet of muscle linking other ribs to the fixated first rib, the cervical vertebrae, and the base of the skull (Draper, Ladefoged, and Whitteridge, 1959). When the external intercostals shorten during contraction, each elevates the rib below, thus increasing the anteroposterior and transverse dimensions of the thorax. Also, they tense the tissue-filled rib interspaces, preventing them from being sucked inward during inspiration.[3]

As mentioned earlier, most of the change in thoracic volume during quiet breathing is accounted for by diaphragmatic activity. It should be understood, however, that there exists a substantial capability for independence of motion between the thoracic cage and the diaphragm-abdomen unit (Konno and Mead, 1967). Witness to this is the ability to inspire mainly with either the thoracic muscles or the diaphragm. A further example is the ability to produce paradoxical movements of the thorax and diaphragm-abdomen during breathing. The main point to be made is that it is possible to move air both in and out of the lungs through a wide variety of relative displacements of the thoracic cage and diaphragm-abdomen.

Forced inspiration. Inspiration of a more vigorous nature than that of the resting individual is called *forced inspiration*. Innumerable gradations of forced inspiration may occur in terms of both the volume of air inspired and the effort exerted during the inspiratory maneuver. During these more vigorous intakes of air, *accessory muscles* are employed to help the diaphragm and external intercostals increase thoracic volume. These muscles, shown in Figures 1–9 and 1–10, warrant individual consideration.

The *sternocleidomastoid* is a relatively large muscle located on the side of the neck, its fibers originating from the bony skull behind the ear and passing downward in two divisions. One division inserts into the top surface of the clavicle whereas the other attaches to the top portion of the front of the sternum. With the head held in a fixed position, contraction of the sternocleidomastoid raises the sternum, and because of their attachments thereto, the ribs are elevated.

The *scalenus muscle group* includes three muscles found on the side of the neck: the *scalenus anterior, medius,* and *posterior*. The anterior originates as four tiny muscular tabs from the third through sixth cervical vertebrae. These tabs converge into a relatively thick muscle bundle that runs downward and laterally to insert along the inner border of the top surface of the first rib. The medius arises as tiny tabs from the lower six cervical vertebrae. Fibers descend along the side of the vertebral column and, like the anterior segment, merge into a single bundle, this one inserting along the upper border of the first rib just behind the scalenus anterior. The final member of the group, the posterior, is located behind the medius. The fibers of the posterior muscle

---

[3]The intercartilaginous (between the costal cartilages) segment of the *internal intercostal* muscles is so arranged that the internal intercostals also exert inspiratory force on the thoracic cage (Taylor, 1960). Their main function is expiratory, however, and they are discussed as such in the section on expiratory forces.

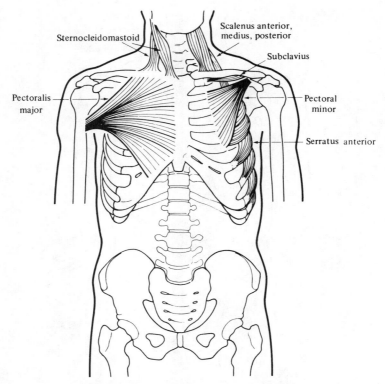

FIGURE 1–9. Accessory muscles of inspiration.

arise from the lower two or three cervical vertebrae as muscular tabs that converge as they pass downward and laterally to attach to the outer surface of the second rib. Upon contraction of the scalenus group, the first two ribs are elevated.

The *subclavius* is a relatively small, narrow muscle originating on the undersurface of the clavicle and running slightly downward and toward the midline, where it attaches to the junction of the first rib and its cartilage. Contraction of the subclavius brings about an elevation of the first rib, provided that the clavicle is braced.

The *pectoralis major* is a large, fan-shaped muscle found on the upper front wall of the thorax. It arises from the *humerus* (the major bone of the upper arm) and fans out widely across the thorax, having a complex insertion that includes the front surfaces of the upper costal cartilages, the sternum, and the inner half of the clavicle. When the upper arm is held in a fixed position, contraction of the pectoralis major draws the sternum and ribs upward.

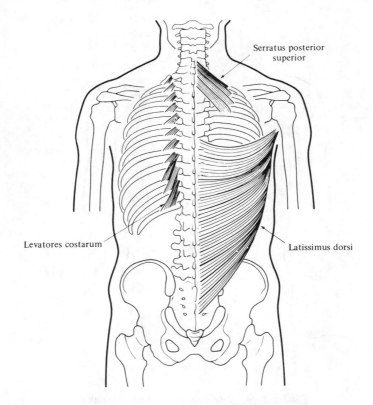

FIGURE 1–10. Accessory muscles of inspiration.

The *pectoralis minor* is a relatively large, thin muscle situated underneath the pectoralis major. It originates from the front surface of the scapula and radiates downward toward the midline, where its fibers insert into the outer surfaces of the second through fifth ribs near their cartilages. If the scapula is anchored, the pull of the pectoralis minor will lift ribs two through five.

The *serratus anterior* is a large, thin muscle located on the side wall of the thorax. It arises from the front surface of the scapula and passes forward around the side of the thoracic cage, where it diverges into a number of thin, finger-like muscular tabs. These insert into the outer surfaces of the upper eight or nine ribs. If the scapula is secured in position, action of the serratus anterior will raise the upper ribs.

The *levatores costarum* (rib raisers) are 12 small muscles located on the back of the thoracic cage. These originate from the seventh cervical and upper 11 thoracic vertebrae with each muscle extending downward and slightly outward to the back surface of the rib immediately below the vertebra of origin. In the lower thorax, some muscle fibers also extend to the second rib below. When the levatores costarum contract, they raise the ribs.

The *serratus posterior superior* muscle is located on the upper back portion of the thorax. It is a flat, thin muscle originating from the back of the vertebral column; points of origin include the seventh cervical and the first three or four thoracic vertebrae. Fibers of the serratus posterior superior slant downward across the back of the thorax to insert as muscular tabs into the second through fifth ribs. This muscle serves to elevate the ribs to which it attaches.

The *latissimus dorsi* is a large muscle located on the back of the body, its fibers originating from the humerus and fanning out to run downward across the back of the lower thorax. This muscle has a complex insertion into the lower portion of the vertebral column and lower ribs. Attachments include the lower six thoracic, the lumbar, and the sacral vertebrae, as well as the posterior surfaces of the lower three or four ribs. When the humerus is braced, contraction of the fibers inserted into the lower ribs will elevate them.

Expiration

Air flow from the lungs is termed *expiration* or *exhalation*. As with inspiration, features of expiration that warrant consideration here are the aerodynamic behavior of the respiratory pump and the forces applied to and by its various parts. ·

AERODYNAMIC EVENTS. Remember that alveolar pressure is equal to atmospheric pressure at the end of inspiration. Air will flow out of the lungs if alveolar pressure is made to exceed that of the atmosphere by an amount sufficient to overcome resistance—that is, if a pressure gradient is established in favor of outward flow. In the human respiratory pump this is accomplished at times by nonmuscular forces, and at other times by both muscular and nonmuscular forces, which reduce the size of the lungs-thorax unit, thereby compressing the alveolar air and raising its pressure above atmospheric.

Consideration already has been given to volume, flow, and pressure changes associated with the inspiratory phase of the quiet breathing cycle. In the right half of Figure 1-5, these same aerodynamic events are illustrated for a *quiet expiration*. There alveolar pressure is seen to be equal to atmospheric pressure at both the beginning and the end of expiration (2 and 4 seconds on the abscissa), rising to +1 cm H_2O in between. As pressure fluctuates, flow increases from zero to approximately +0.5 LPS and then decreases to zero, the maximum flow coinciding with maximum alveolar pressure. The shapes of the pressure and flow curves during quiet expiration are determined mainly by the recoil forces of the lungs and thorax (including the diaphragm and abdomen) and the resistance to flow through the airways. The 0.5 L or so of air taken into the lungs during inspiration is expelled as expiration proceeds, until the normal volume at the resting expiratory level is attained.

FORCES OF EXPIRATION.   As with inspiration, the forces exerted during expiration serve to move air and nonelastic tissues and to overcome the elastic recoil of the lungs-thorax unit. Two types of expiration, passive and active, are employed in meeting the various demands for expelling air from the lungs. In the case of the latter, the mechanical contributions of the muscles involved are dependent on the same factors as discussed previously for the inspiratory muscles.

Passive expiration. Expiration above the resting expiratory level usually is *passive.* As such, it is accomplished not by muscular effort, but by nonmuscular forces that return the lungs and thorax to their usual volumes at the resting expiratory level. During *quiet* inspiration, potential energy is created by the contraction of inspiratory muscles and stored in the stretched elastic fabric (tissues) of the lungs. When the inspiratory muscles are relaxed, the external force (muscular effort) distending the lungs no longer exists. Consequently, the stored energy is released and the lungs recoil toward a smaller volume—like a stretched spring recoils when released. Being linked to the thorax, the recoiling lungs pull inward on the thoracic walls and upward on the diaphragm. This action causes the thoracic cavity to decrease in size along the dimensions in which it expanded during inspiration; namely, vertically, anteroposteriorly, and transversely. The total force of lung recoil at any instant depends only in part on the recoil force of the actual elastic fabric of the lungs. Other factors contribute, the most important of which is a very special surface film found within the lungs. This film coats the inside of each of the tiny alveoli, forming a liquid-air interface (boundary) whose surface tension causes it to recoil like a tiny bubble. The combined recoil force of the 300 million or so alveolar surfaces is responsible for as much or more of the total lung recoil as the actual elastic fabric of the lungs. This is clearly demonstrated by the fact that it requires less than half the pressure to fully inflate a lung when liquid-filled than when air-filled (Radford, 1964). The basis for this difference is that in the liquid-filled lung the normal liquid-air interface of each alveolus is replaced by a liquid-liquid interface whose surface tension is negligible (Comroe, 1965).

Unlike quiet inspiration, deep inspiration[4] involves the storage of potential expiratory energy within the elastic tissues of the lungs *and* thorax

---

[4]Deep inspiration in this context is defined as any inspiration in which the thorax is expanded beyond its own resting position (lungs removed). In the spring analogy of Figure 1–4, deep inspiration would involve a stretching of the thoracic spring to a length greater than that shown for the normal resting position of the thorax alone.

(including the diaphragm and abdominal structures). Therefore, following deep inspiration *both* the lungs and thorax recoil toward smaller volumes with the sum of their recoil forces determining the total force of passive expiration. It is important to realize that the thorax contributes to the development of positive passive expiratory forces *only* at relatively high lung volumes (above 55% of the vital capacity) at which it is expanded beyond its own resting position, and therefore, tends to recoil to a smaller size. Otherwise, and as is the case in quiet expiration, the forces of the thorax and lungs are in opposition, with the lungs attempting to reduce their size and the thorax attempting to increase its size (i.e., the two springs are working against one another).

Lest this be misunderstood from previous discussion, the inspiratory muscles do not cease their activity the instant flow changes direction between inspiration and passive expiration (Agostoni, 1964). They actually continue their activity into the early part of expiration (beyond the 2 second point in Figure 1–5) with the force they exert gradually decreasing and acting as a releasing brake against the lung recoil forces just described. Thus, although the term passive expiration characterizes most expirations above the resting expiratory level, such expirations are only truly passive (i.e., involve no muscular effort) after the inspiratory muscles have ceased their activity.

Active expiration. Although most expirations are passive, countless degrees of *active* expiration are possible in which muscular forces are employed to reduce the volumes of the lungs and thorax. The term "active expiration" has two meanings as it is used in this chapter: one relative to the use of muscular effort above the resting expiratory level and the other for expirations below that level. Above the resting level, active expiration is accomplished by using expiratory muscles to decrease the size of the thorax with greater force than the decrease caused by passive (nonmuscular) forces alone. By analogy, this amounts to a forcing of the stretched lungs-thorax spring unit back to its resting position rather than permitting it to return there of its own accord. In the respiratory pump this action results in a more rapid than usual reduction in lung volume and a substantial increase in both alveolar pressure and flow. As for expirations below the resting level, the term "active expiration" always applies. This is because any decrease in thoracic volume from the resting level, like any increase from that level, requires the use of muscular force, regardless of the depth or forcefulness with which the expiration occurs.

It should be apparent by this juncture that whereas expirations above the resting level can be either passive or active, those below the resting level must be active. Knowing this, it is relevant to examine the muscles responsible for active reduction of thoracic size under the conditions just described. Each of the muscles of concern has one or both of two important mechanical functions: (1) it lowers the ribs or sternum, or both, to decrease the anteroposterior and transverse dimensions of the thorax; and (2) it raises the abdominal pressure and forces the diaphragm upward, thus decreasing the vertical dimension of the thorax. Figures 1–11 and 1–12 show the expiratory muscles, each of which warrants consideration with reference to its structure and function.

The *internal intercostals* are 11 thin muscles situated within the rib interspaces underneath the external intercostals. They extend from around the sides of the thorax to the sternum but do not fill the interspaces at the back of the thoracic cage. The fibers of the internal intercostals run upward and forward from the upper border of one rib to the lower border of the rib immediately above, their course being at approximately right angles to the fibers of the external intercostals. From a mechanical viewpoint it is useful to think of the internal intercostals as a sheet of muscle linking the ribs to the pelvic girdle through a number of other muscles, principally those of the abdomen. On contraction, the internal intercostals pull the ribs downward and stiffen the rib interspaces.

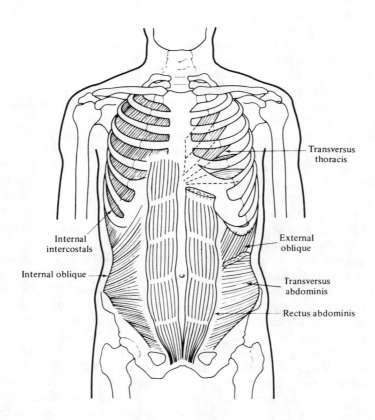

FIGURE 1–11. Muscles of expiration.

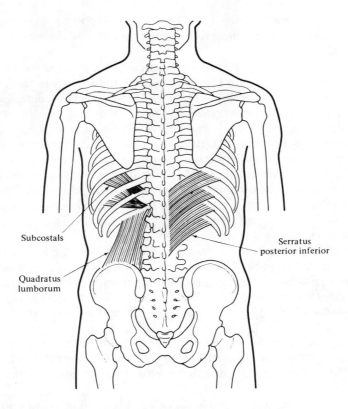

FIGURE 1-12. Muscles of expiration.

The *transversus thoracis* is a thin, fan-shaped muscle found on the inside, front wall of the thorax. It originates at the midline on the inner surface of the lower sternum and the fourth or fifth through seventh costal cartilages. From this broad origin it fans out across the thorax and divides into a number of muscular tabs that insert variously into the inner surface of the costal cartilages and bony ends of ribs two through six. The upper fibers run nearly vertically, whereas the intermediate and lower fibers run obliquely and horizontally, respectively. When the transversus thoracis contracts, it exerts a downward pull on the ribs to which it attaches.

The *subcostal* muscles are located on the inside back wall of the thorax. These vary considerably in number from person to person, being most often located and best developed in the lower portion of the rib cage. The subcostals originate close to the vertebral column on the inner surfaces of ribs, from which their fibers extend upward and laterally, inserting into the inner surface of the rib immediately above the rib of origin, or skipping a rib or two in their course and inserting into higher ribs. Upon contraction, the subcostals act to depress the ribs.

The *serratus posterior inferior* muscle is located on the lower back portion of the thorax. This thin, flat muscle originates from the lower two thoracic and upper two or three lumbar vertebrae. Its fibers slant upward across the back of the thorax diverging into four flat muscular tabs that insert into the lower borders of the last four ribs on the back of the cage. When the serratus posterior inferior contracts, it pulls down on the lower ribs.

The *quadratus lumborum* is a flat sheet of muscle located on the back wall of the abdominal cavity. It arises from the top of the coxal bone and its fibers run upward and slightly toward the midline, diverging into several muscular tabs. These insert into the first four lumbar vertebrae and the lower border of the inner half of the lowest rib. Contraction of the quadratus lumborum depresses the lowest rib.

The *latissimus dorsi* was discussed earlier in this chapter as a muscle of inspiration. Although the fibers attached to the lower three or four ribs are capable of raising them during inspiration, contraction of the muscle as a whole compresses the lower portion of the thoracic cage. Therefore, it is not contradictory to view the latissimus dorsi as a muscle of both inspiration and expiration.

The next four muscles usually are regarded as the most important muscles of active expiration. They are referred to collectively as the abdominal muscles, and include the rectus abdominis, external oblique, internal oblique, and transversus abdominis.

The *rectus abdominis* is a long, ribbon-like muscle found on the front of the abdominal cavity. It originates from the upper front edge of the coxal bone and runs upward, parallel to the midline, to insert into the fifth, sixth, and seventh costal cartilages and lower sternum. The rectus abdominis is encased in a fibrous sheath or sleeve that is formed by the complex abdominal aponeurosis. Together with the rectus, this sheath forms a front post for the abdomen which can be viewed as a continuation of the sternal post of the thoracic cage. When the rectus abdominis contracts, it draws the lower ribs and sternum downward and forces the abdominal contents inward.

The *external oblique* is a very broad, flat muscle that is situated on the side and front portions of the lower thorax and abdomen. This muscle arises as a number of tabs from the outer surface of the lower eight ribs and its fibers run downward across the abdomen at various angles. Fibers toward the back of the body descend nearly vertically to insert into the upper surface of the top portion of the coxal bone, whereas others run obliquely downward and toward the front of the abdomen to attach to the abdominal aponeurosis near the midline. When it contracts, the external oblique draws the lower ribs downward and displaces the contents of the abdomen inward, thus raising the abdominal pressure.

The *internal oblique* is a large, flat muscle located on the side and front walls of the abdominal cavity. It lies under the external oblique and has a rather extensive origin, which includes much of the upper surface of the coxal bone and the lumbodorsal fascia. The fibers of the internal oblique fan out across the abdomen to insert into the abdominal aponeurosis and the costal cartilages of the lower three or four ribs. Upon contraction, this muscle drives the abdominal wall inward and draws the lower ribs downward.

The *transversus abdominis* is a flat, broad muscle located on the front and side of the abdomen under the internal oblique. It has a complex origin which includes the upper surface of the coxal bone, the lumbodorsal fascia, and the inner surfaces of the costal cartilages of ribs seven through twelve. The fibers of the transversus abdominis run horizontally around the abdomen where, at the front, they attach to the abdominal aponeurosis. When the transversus abdominis contracts, it displaces the abdominal wall inward, thereby elevating abdominal pressure.

Pulmonary Subdivisions

The pulmonary system is capable of holding various amounts of air. This air can be measured with a number of different simple devices, some of which trace out a permanent record of air volume changes called a *spirogram*. Figure 1–13 shows an example of such a tracing and illustrates in principle the various *lung volumes* and *capacities* (Pappenheimer et al., 1950).

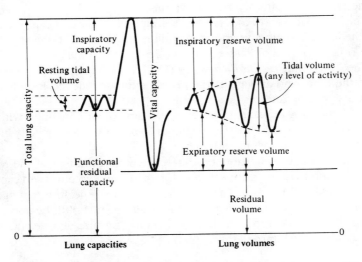

FIGURE 1–13. Spirogram illustration of lung volumes and lung capacities. (After Pappenheimer, J., et al.: Standardization of definitions and symbols in respiratory physiology. *Federation Proceedings, 9,* 602–605, 1950. Used by permission.)

LUNG VOLUMES. The primary lung volumes are four in number and mutually exclusive (i.e., they do not overlap).

The *tidal volume* (TV) is the amount of air inspired or expired during a respiratory cycle. Under usual conditions, its magnitude is dictated by the oxygen needs of the body. In the resting individual it is termed *quiet tidal breathing* and its magnitude may be determined from a single respiratory cycle or from the average volume of a series of quiet breaths.

The *inspiratory reserve volume* (IRV) is the maximum amount of air that can be taken into the lungs and airways from the *end-inspiratory level* (i.e., the peak of each tidal volume cycle).

The *expiratory reserve volume* (ERV) is the greatest volume of air that can be expired from the resting expiratory level.

The *residual volume* (RV) is the amount of air that remains in the lungs and airways at the end of a maximum expiration. Of the four primary lung volumes the RV is the only one that cannot be measured directly, because no matter how forceful the expiration, the pulmonary system cannot be emptied. It is possible, however, to estimate indirectly the residual volume through the use of special respiratory tests (Mead and Milic-Emili, 1964).

LUNG CAPACITIES. Like the primary lung volumes, the lung capacities also are four in number. Each capacity includes two or more of the lung volumes just discussed.

The *inspiratory capacity* (IC) is the maximum volume of air that can be inspired from the resting expiratory level. This capacity is the sum of the tidal volume and the inspiratory reserve volume.

The *vital capacity* (VC) is the greatest amount of air that can be expelled from the lungs and airways after a maximum inspiration. It encompasses all of the primary lung volumes except the residual volume.

The *functional residual capacity* (FRC) is the volume of air contained within the lungs and airways at the resting expiratory level. It includes the expiratory reserve and residual volumes.

The *total lung capacity* (TLC) is the volume of air contained within the lungs and airways at the end of a maximum inspiration. This capacity includes all four of the primary lung volumes.

To give some indication of the relative magnitudes of the various pulmonary subdivisions, sample values for all the lung volumes and capacities are presented in Table 1–1. The data shown are for a healthy, young, adult male, breathing at sea level in a standing position. It should be appreciated that these values vary with many factors, including posture, age, height, weight, sex, and altitude (Comroe et al., 1962).

Volume-Pressure Relationships

Much of the discussion to this point can be integrated into a single graph, a knowledge of which serves as an important basis for understanding the

RESPIRATORY FUNCTION IN SPEECH

Table 1-1. *Values (L) for the Various Pulmonary Subdivisions of a Healthy, Young, Adult Male, Breathing at Sea Level in a Standing Position*

Lung Volume or Capacity	Magnitude (L)
Tidal Volume	0.5
Inspiratory Reserve Volume	2.5
Expiratory Reserve Volume	2.0
Residual Volume	2.0
Inspiratory Capacity	3.0
Vital Capacity	5.0
Functional Residual Capacity	4.0
Total Lung Capacity	7.0

discussions on speech breathing to follow. Such a graph, known as a volume-pressure diagram (Campbell, 1958, 1968; Rahn, Otis, Chadwick, and Fenn, 1946), is of analytical value in relating the nonmuscular and muscular forces of respiration to each other, to the alveolar pressure, and to the various levels of the lung volume. One form of the volume-pressure diagram is illustrated in Figure 1–14. There the amount of air within the lungs (expressed as a percentage of the vital capacity) is displayed on the vertical axis, with alveolar pressure on the horizontal axis. Points to the right of zero (atmospheric pressure) represent pressures greater than atmospheric; those to the left are subatmospheric. The three curves shown represent the volume-pressure relations during (1) relaxation, (2) maximum expiration, and (3) maximum inspiration.

RELAXATION PRESSURE. The pressure produced entirely by nonmuscular forces of the respiratory apparatus is termed the *relaxation pressure*. This pressure, developed in the lungs and airways when the respiratory muscles are relaxed, varies in magnitude depending on how much the lungs are inflated or deflated from the resting expiratory level. At lung volumes above the resting position, relaxation results in passive expiration through generation of a positive pressure (above atmospheric). This pressure decreases as the lungs are deflated from the total lung capacity to the resting expiratory level. Relaxation at lung volumes below the resting level results in subatmospheric alveolar pressure, with the magnitude of this pressure increasing (i.e., becoming less subatmospheric) as the lungs inflate from the residual volume to the resting expiratory level.[5] In the midvolume range,

---

[5]Up to now inspiration has been considered an active process. Following expiration below the resting expiratory level, however, inspiration may be passive. This can be demonstrated by the simple experiment of expiring to the residual volume and then relaxing. On relaxation, the respiratory pump recoils back to its resting level without the aid of muscular effort. For an analogy, consider the action of a compressed spring when it is released.

relaxation pressure changes nearly in direct proportion to volume, whereas at the extremes of lung volume, pressure changes more abruptly. The basis for the differences at the volume extremes is the relative stiffness of the lungs and thorax, the lungs being stiffer at high lung volumes and the thorax being stiffer at low volumes.[6]

Departures from relaxation pressure can be achieved at any lung volume through the use of muscular effort (Mead, Bouhuys, and Proctor, 1968). Pressures less than the relaxation pressure (i.e., to the left of the curve) require that a "net" *inspiratory* muscle effort be added to the relaxation pressure. Those pressures that exceed the relaxation pressure (i.e., those to the right of the curve) require that a "net" *expiratory* muscle effort be added to the relaxation pressure. It is important to specify "net" in such descriptions because although pressures less than relaxation can be produced solely through inspiratory effort and pressures more than relaxation can be produced solely through expiratory effort, it is possible to depart from the relaxation pressure curve with both inspiratory and expiratory forces operating simultaneously but with one or the other being predominant. Furthermore, it is possible to stay on the relaxation pressure curve during muscular effort (i.e., to produce a pressure equal to the relaxation pressure at any lung volume) by exerting inspiratory and expiratory forces that are equal and opposite and thus cancelling. It follows that pressure equal to the relaxation pressure at a given lung volume cannot be used as evidence for a lack of muscular effort.

MAXIMUM PRESSURES. The curves labeled *maximum expiration* and *maximum inspiration* in Figure 1–14 show, respectively, the greatest positive and negative pressures that can be developed through the use of muscular effort. As such, these curves define the limits within which respiratory function must occur, or to which it is possible to depart from the relaxation pressure at each lung volume. As with relaxation pressure, pressures developed during maximum efforts depend on lung volume. The maximum expiratory pressure, for example, decreases as the lungs deflate from the total lung capacity to the residual volume. Maximum inspiratory pressure, on the other hand, increases (i.e., becomes less subatmospheric) as the lungs are inflated from the residual volume to the total lung capacity. Maximum expiratory pressures are greater at higher lung volumes because the relaxation pressure is greater and because the expiratory muscles are stretched to more optimum lengths for generating tensions (Siebens, 1966). Along similar lines, greater negative pressures can be produced at lower volumes because the respiratory pump recoils toward a larger volume with greater force, and because the inspiratory muscles are operating under more favorable length-tension conditons.

---

[6]Although it is beyond the scope of this chapter, it should be mentioned that the relaxation pressure for the total respiratory apparatus can be analyzed into several components. Most commonly partitioned are the pressure caused by recoil of the lungs and the pressure due to recoil of the thorax (including the diaphragm and abdomen). For a detailed account of the various components, see Agostoni and Mead (1964) and Konno and Mead (1968). Refer also to Chapter 4.

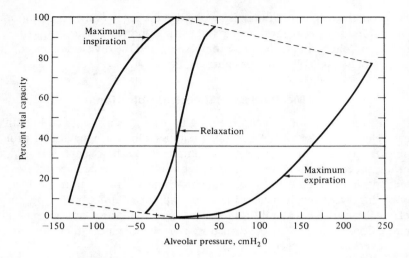

FIGURE 1-14. Lung volume-alveolar pressure relations during relaxation, maximum expiration and maximum inspiration. (After Agostoni, E., and Mead, J.: Statics of the respiratory system. *In* W. Fenn and H. Rahn [Eds.]: *Handbook of physiology.* Washington, DC: American Physiological Society, 1964. Used by permission.)

RESPIRATION FOR SPEECH PURPOSES

Now that the elements of normal respiration have been considered, attention is directed toward respiratory function in speech. This calls for discussion of the task facing the respiratory pump as well as examination of how that task is accomplished by the body machinery.

Role of the Respiratory Pump in Speech

The ease with which breathing occurs in speech gives little hint as to the important role the respiratory pump plays in the human's ability to communicate orally. Viewed broadly, that role is to provide the driving forces necessary for the generation of sounds, those forces being supplied in the form of pressures and flows that act on and interact with various structures within the head and neck. To be more specific, the respiratory pump participates in speech by displacing structures, creating pressures behind valves, and generating flows through constrictions within the larynx and upper airway. These activities, in association with intricate and rapid maneuvers of other parts of the speech apparatus, create the disturbances of air that constitute speech at the acoustical level. Because respiratory forces provide the basic energy source for all speech and voice production in the English language, the events of speech breathing are of fundamental importance in any account of oral communication. Within the broad spectrum of physiological function in speech, the respiratory pump is involved in the regulation of such important parameters as speech and voice intensity (loudness), vocal fundamental frequency (pitch), linguistic stress (emphasis), and the division of speech into various units (syllables, words, phrases, etc.).

Mechanics of Speech Respiration

Most accounts of speech breathing portray it as a simple and relatively featureless behavior of the speech apparatus, albeit a behavior of primary importance. Actually, there is great complexity in the events of respiration during speech, complexity that equals and in many respects surpasses that of events in other parts of the speaking machinery. This section considers the more important mechanical aspects of respiratory function in speech and relates these to the general problem that speech imposes on the respiratory pump. Considered first are the demands of steady utterances, then the demands of conversational speech.

Demands of Steady Utterances

The simplest mechanical problem facing the respiratory pump in speech is one in which the utterance requires relatively constant average pressure, flow, and resistance of the upper airway. Speech activities meeting these criteria are the focus of this section, being a useful starting point for the study of speech breathing physiology. The discussion offered here deals with the aerodynamic events associated with such utterances as well as the forces provided by the respiratory pump.

AERODYNAMIC EVENTS. Figure 1–15 illustrates in simplified form the nature of volume, flow, and pressure events associated with a prolonged utterance produced throughout most of the vital capacity. The speech activity in this instance consists of an isolated sustained vowel produced at constant normal loudness and pitch levels. The data are representative of *average values*[7] for a variety of utterances consisting mainly of equally stressed syllables as when repeating a single syllable, counting, reciting the alphabet, and so forth (Bouhuys, Proctor, and Mead, 1966; Draper et al., 1959). The

---

[7]The recordings shown are simplified in several ways. For example, they do not portray rapid variations associated with vocal fold vibration or the heartbeat. Although they represent the average values for a variety of utterances, the particular example shown is for a prolonged vowel and therefore gives no indication of the nature of rapid changes in pressure, flow, and volume that occur during syllable utterances. In effect, the tracings of Figure 1–15 have high frequency information (rapidly changing events) "filtered off" them. It is assumed that the alveolar pressure recording approximates that which would be obtained just below the larynx (i.e., subglottal or tracheal pressure). Actually, alveolar and subglottal pressures differ by a small amount during speech because of a resistive pressure loss between the alveoli and the larynx, this loss increasing slightly with decreasing lung volume (Bouhuys et al., 1966).

top tracing in Figure 1–15 shows lung volume decreasing at a constant rate during the speech activity, from near the total lung capacity to near the residual volume. Flow and alveolar pressure show abrupt increases at the onset of speech activity, maintenance at constant values during the utterance, and abrupt decreases at the end of speech. Because both pressure and flow are constant during the utterance, it follows that the average resistance (i.e., pressure/flow) offered by the larynx and upper airway also is constant.

RESPIRATORY FORCES. Both muscular and nonmuscular forces are involved in the regulation of respiratory behavior for utterances like that illustrated in Figure 1–15. The general problem of combining such forces to achieve a desired alveolar pressure is the concern of the next four sections, which consider, respectively, the total force provided, the activity of specific muscles involved in providing this total force, the special role played by hydraulic events within the abdomen, and the effect of changing body position within a gravity field.

Muscular pressures. Recall that the relaxation pressure curve portrays the nonmuscular forces of respiration, with the magnitude of the pressure developed during relaxation depending on how much air is contained within the lungs. It is useful to think of the relaxation pressure as a spring-like

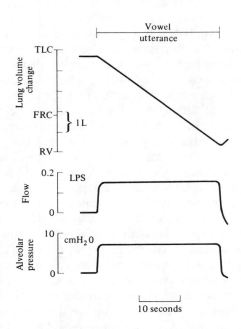

FIGURE 1–15. Lung volume change (L), flow (LPS) and alveolar pressure (cm H_2O) during an isolated vowel utterance produced throughout most of the vital capacity.

background force that is expiratory at lung volumes above the resting expiratory level and inspiratory at lung volumes below that level. Recall further that departures from relaxation pressure can be achieved at any lung volume through the use of muscular effort, with (1) pressures less than the relaxation pressure resulting from "net" or solely inspiratory efforts, (2) pressures greater than the relaxation pressure resulting from "net" or solely expiratory efforts, and (3) pressures equal to the relaxation pressure indicating either no muscular effort (i.e., muscular relaxation) or equal and simultaneous inspiratory and expiratory efforts. By viewing the relaxation pressure and departures from it in these terms, it is possible to use the volume-pressure diagram to determine graphically the sign and magnitude of muscular force that must be added to the spring-like background force to achieve the alveolar pressure required for any utterance (Hixon, Siebens, and Ewanowski, 1968; Mead et al., 1968). The main point to keep in mind for any such analysis is that *the amount of muscular pressure required at a given instant during speech depends on the alveolar pressure needed and the relaxation pressure available at the prevailing lung volume.*

Figure 1–16 presents an example of the application of the type of analysis just described. The alveolar pressure from the normal-loudness utterance of Figure 1–15 is replotted in the upper half of the figure (this time against lung volume) together with the relaxation volume-pressure characteristic of the respiratory apparatus (illustrated earlier in Figure 1–14). Note that the needed alveolar pressure of 7 cm H_2O is less than the relaxation pressure during the early part of the utterance (throughout the high lung volumes), equal to it at one point (where the curves intersect), and greater than it during the latter part of the utterance (throughout the low lung volumes). Because the difference between the alveolar pressure and relaxation pressure represents the muscular pressure, the horizontal distance (i.e., the hatched area) between the speech curve and the relaxation pressure curve indicates the muscular pressure that must be added to the relaxation pressure to achieve the alveolar pressure needed at each lung volume for speech. For convenience this pressure difference is plotted in the lower half of Figure 1–16. The horizontal axis depicts muscular pressure, with negative and positive values representing net inspiratory and net expiratory forces, respectively. Examination of the muscular pressure graph reveals that at high lung volumes a net inspiratory force is added to the relaxation pressure, the magnitude of this force decreasing as speech proceeds and air leaves the lungs. Near 50% of the vital capacity the net force is zero, whereas below that level a positive muscular pressure is required in increasing amounts as lung volume continues to decrease. For this particular utterance, then, where a constant alveolar pressure of 7 cm H_2O is required, the sign of the muscular pressure provided at high lung volumes is opposite to that of alveolar pressure and flow. In other words, a situation exists in which inspiratory effort is exerted during an expiratory task, namely, speech production. This is not unlike the situation discussed earlier, in which the activity of the inspiratory muscles during quiet breathing persists

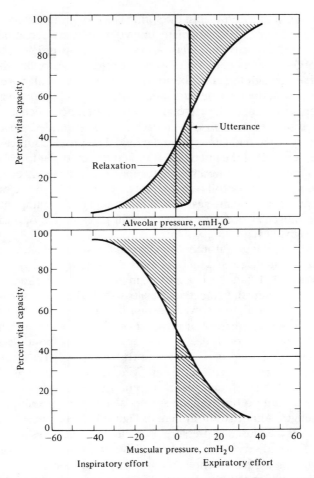

FIGURE 1–16. Upper: Lung volume-alveolar pressure relations during relaxation and during an isolated vowel utterance of normal loudness produced throughout most of the vital capacity. (Relaxation curve after Agostoni, E., and Mead, J.: Statics of the respiratory system. *In* W. Fenn and H. Rahn [Eds.]: *Handbook of physiology.* Washington, DC: American Physiological Society, 1964. Used by permission.) Hatched area between the curves shows the muscular pressure required for the utterance. Lower: Lung volume-muscular pressure relations replotted from data of the upper graph. Negative values represent net inspiratory forces and positive values represent net expiratory forces.

into expiration. In the present situation, inspiratory effort is employed at high lung volumes to counteract the full force of the spring-like recoil of the respiratory pump, a recoil that would provide more pressure than needed were the relaxation pressure not opposed to some extent at high lung volumes (Bouhuys et al., 1966). The negative muscular work done in opposing the excessive relaxation pressure in this circumstance may be thought of as a braking or checking action against the spring-like background force. In contrast to high lung volumes, at intermediate lung volumes (between about 50% and 35% of the vital capacity) the relaxation pressure is insufficient to meet the demands of the utterance. It is necessary, therefore, to supplement the background force through the contribution of a positive muscular pressure. This means that within the intermediate range of lung volumes the relaxation and muscular pressures are of the same sign for this utterance. Such is not the case below the resting level because the muscular pressure added must overcome the inspiratory recoil of the pump and, beyond that, provide sufficient pressure to meet the demands of the utterance. It should be noted that for this seemingly simple utterance of sustaining a vowel, the muscular pressure needed is initially opposite in sign to the recoil pressure of the pump, then in the same sign as that of the pump, and finally again opposite in sign to the pump, but the signs of both the muscular pressure and the recoil pressure are opposite to their respective signs at high lung volumes.

Some may find it useful at this juncture to consider the muscular pressure problem in analogous terms, such as apply to the simple mechanical system shown in Figure 1–17. In this illustration, in place of the respiratory apparatus is a hand bellows, which, in functional analogy to the human respiratory pump, has (1) a mechanism (hand power) to pull its handles apart, corresponding to negative muscular pressure or inspiratory effort, (2) a countermechanism (again hand power) to push its handles together, corresponding to positive muscular pressure or expiratory effort, and (3) a spring between the handles, corresponding to the relaxation pressure provided by the lungs-thorax unit, which will exert varying degrees of inspiratory or expiratory force on the handles depending on how far the spring is stretched or compressed from its resting length. Although the system of Figure 1–17 has general application to all aspects of the muscular pressure problem, two examples of its functional equivalence should serve sufficiently to illustrate the usefulness of reasoning by analogy. For a first example, consider the functional analogy of the mechanical system to the checking action of the human pump. Suppose the handles of the bellows were maximally spread apart (i.e., the total lung capacity of the bellows) and then released. If the pressure created within the bellows chamber by the recoiling spring exceeded that desired, this pressure could be reduced to a specified level by the simple opposing maneuver of pulling with appropriate force on the handles of the system. As a second example, consider the application of the analogue to a situation in which a positive muscular pressure is needed, as would be the case if it were a requirement that a steady chamber pressure be maintained below resting spring length (i.e., the resting expiratory level). In such a circumstance it would be necessary to compress the system by pushing on the handles of the bellows with an appropriately increasing force that would overcome the inspiratory recoil of the spring and add an amount of pressure equal to the desired chamber pressure.

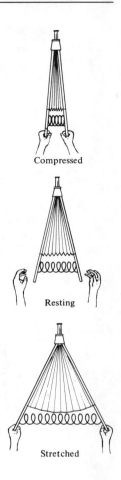

Compressed

Resting

Stretched

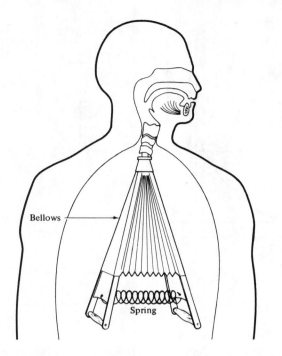

Bellows

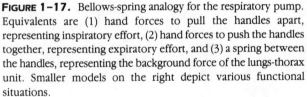

Spring

FIGURE 1–17. Bellows-spring analogy for the respiratory pump. Equivalents are (1) hand forces to pull the handles apart, representing inspiratory effort, (2) hand forces to push the handles together, representing expiratory effort, and (3) a spring between the handles, representing the background force of the lungs-thorax unit. Smaller models on the right depict various functional situations.

Because alveolar pressure demands differ for different utterances, speech activities requiring pressures other than the 7 cm H_2O considered in Figure 1–16 require different muscular pressures at each lung volume. This is illustrated in Figure 1–18, where the alveolar and muscular pressures for a soft and a very loud utterance are constrasted with a normal-loudness utterance. It is clear in Figure 1–18 that an even greater negative muscular pressure must be used to counteract the relaxation pressure at high lung volumes for the soft than for the normal-loudness utterance. In addition, this counteraction must continue to a lower lung volume for the softer of the two utterances. In terms of the preceding analogy, these events would require that the recoil of the stretched lungs-thorax spring be opposed more and to shorter spring lengths to achieve a lower chamber pressure for the less demanding pressure maneuver. Continuing with the soft-normal contrast, less positive muscular pressure needs to be added to the relaxation pressure at low lung volumes

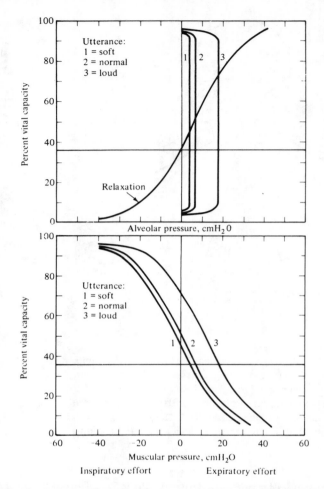

FIGURE 1-18. Upper: Lung volume-alveolar pressure relations during relaxation and during three isolated vowel utterances of different loudnesses produced throughout most of the vital capacity. (Relaxation curve after Agostoni, E., and Mead, J.: Statics of the respiratory system. *In* W. Fenn and H. Rahn [Eds.]: *Handbook of physiology.* Washington, DC: American Physiological Society, 1964. Used by permission.) Lower: Lung volume-muscular pressure relations replotted from data of the upper graph. Negative values represent net inspiratory forces and positive values indicate net expiratory forces.

for the soft than for the normal-loudness condition, a situation that by analogy requires less forceful pushing on the bellows handles for the condition requiring lower pressure. When the alveolar pressure demand is great, such as for the very loud utterance depicted in Figure 1-18, a positive muscular pressure is required throughout most of the vital capacity. This is because the relaxation pressure does not exceed the needed alveolar pressure over most of the lung volume range. A compression of the bellows system would be required at nearly every spring position were this task subjected to analogue treatment.

By this point it should be obvious that with knowledge of the relaxation pressure characteristic, the alveolar pressure developed during speech, and the lung volume at which speech is produced, it is possible to specify the muscular pressure that is required at every instant. Thus, the respiratory pump accomplishes the task that speech imposes on it by adding, at each instant, a muscular pressure that is precisely equal to the difference between the alveolar pressure desired and the relaxation pressure available. The important implication of this statement is that *each alveolar pressure produced in speech demands a different muscular pressure at each lung volume.*

Electromyographic activity. Once informed of the magnitude and sign of the total muscular pressure applied during speech, it is relevant to examine the specific muscles involved in the active regulation of this pressure. This requires consideration of the time course of muscle activity and how that activity relates to the mechanical properties of the respiratory pump as well as the demands placed on it. Beginning with an utterance of normal loudness, Figure 1–19 presents an account of several of the more important muscles involved. The upper part of that figure is a duplication of the lower half of Figure 1–16, whereas the lower part of the figure is a diagrammatic representation of the temporal activity[8] of six muscles that play a part in generating the muscular pressures depicted in the upper graph (Draper et al., 1959; Ladefoged, 1967). Of the muscles considered, previous description has characterized the diaphragm and external intercostals as inspiratory, the internal intercostals, external oblique, and rectus abdominis as expiratory, and the latissiumus dorsi as potentially inspiratory or expiratory. During a deep inspiration, such as that preceding speech intitiated at near the total lung capacity, the diaphragm, external intercostals, and accessory muscles are active. As shown in Figure 1–19, the diaphragm and external intercostals remain active as speech begins despite the fact that expiration is occurring. This observation is consistent with the negative muscular pressure requirement shown in the

---

[8]This activity is determined through study of the voltage variations associated with muscle activity. The technique used is termed *electromyography* and involves the sensing of electrical activity of muscles through metal electrodes placed on the body surface over muscles or inserted directly into muscles through the skin. Electrical changes occur when a muscle is active under three circumstances: (1) miometric contraction, in which the muscle shortens, (2) isometric contraction, in which its length does not change, and (3) pliometric contraction, in which it lengthens under the influence of other forces acting on it (Agostoni, 1964). There is no way to differentiate unequivocally among these three types of activity in the respiratory muscles during speech. Inferences must be made about the type of activity on the basis of the mechanical behaviors of various parts of the respiratory pump and on the pressure changes associated with their actions. Figure 1–19 amounts to a binary statement of the activity of each muscle considered. It indicates only when a muscle is, or is not, active electrically and says nothing about the tensions created by the different muscles at different times.

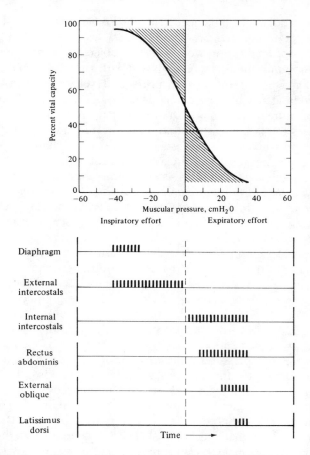

FIGURE 1–19. Upper: Lung volume-muscular pressure relations during an isolated vowel utterance of normal loudness produced throughout most of the vital capacity (see Figure 1–16). Negative values represent net inspiratory forces and positive values represent net expiratory forces. Lower: Diagrammatic representation of the temporal activity of six muscles involved in generating the muscular pressures depicted in the upper graph. (Lower graph after Draper, M., et al.: Respiratory muscles in speech. *Journal of Speech and Hearing Research, 2*, 16–27, 1959. Used by permission.)

upper part of the figure. There is reason to believe that other inspiratory muscles may participate in this counteraction behavior (Eblen, 1963); however, insufficient research has been done to determine this unequivocally. In any event, the activity of the chief muscle of inspiration, the diaphragm, is seen to cease early in the utterance despite the fact that the relaxation pressure exceeds the needed alveolar pressure (i.e., the muscular pressure is negative).

The activity of the external intercostal muscles proceeds well into the utterance and, although not determinable from Figure 1–19, it diminishes gradually until the muscular pressure demand is zero. This recall, is the instant when the available relaxation pressure is equal to the alveolar pressure demanded for the utterance. For the utterance to continue below the lung volume corresponding to the instant of zero muscular pressure it is necessary that a positive muscular pressure be added to the relaxation forces of the pump. This pressure is provided initially by the internal intercostal muscles, which are activated the moment a positive muscular pressure is needed and which increase their level of activity as the lung volume reduces further. As the pump passes through the resting expiratory level and is faced with the problem of overcoming its inspiratory recoil, abdominal muscles (i.e., the external oblique and rectus abdominis) are brought into play to supplement the contribution of the internal intercostals. Finally, at the lower extreme of the lung volume (near RV) the latissimus dorsi becomes active. Assuming its activity to be expiratory, at least four muscles are implicated as expiratory participants in speech near the end of the utterance, when the negative recoil of the respiratory apparatus is maximal. There is reason to suspect that other expiratory muscles may be involved in respiratory regulation at low lung volumes (Hixon, Minifie, Peyrot, and Siebens, 1968); however, as with the inspiratory muscles at high lung volumes, experimental information is incomplete.

It is important to mention that the account just offered is not universal among speakers or to repeated utterances by the same individual. Although it represents the usual pattern of activity for normal speakers who do not use their diaphragms, it is possible to depart from this pattern consciously. Although many combinations of muscle activity could achieve the same end result (i.e., the desired alveolar pressure), certain combinations undoubtedly are more efficient than others from the viewpoint of function of the body machinery. With regard to this point, it is interesting to note and tempting to ascribe significance to the fact that there is no antagonistic muscle activity (i.e., no simultaneous inspiratory and expiratory activity) at any point throughout the utterance depicted in Figure 1–19. If the activities of the muscles portrayed are representative of other muscles with similar functions, the muscular pressure values shown are related solely to inspiratory activity at high lung volumes and solely to expiratory activity at low lung volumes. This again is not meant to imply that the muscles function in this fashion under all circumstances. Indeed, there is evidence (Draper et al., 1959) that some individuals occasionally use inspiratory and expiratory muscles simultaneously during speech.

Because each alveolar pressure produced in speech demands a different muscular pressure at each lung volume, it would be expected that muscular activity would likewise be different for different alveolar pressures at different lung volumes. This is evident in Figure 1–20 which portrays the dependence

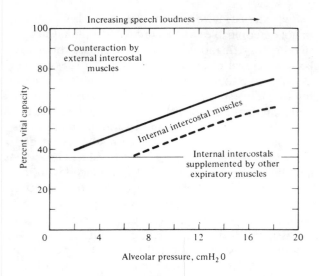

FIGURE 1-20. Graph illustrating which muscles or groups of muscles are active at different lung volumes and alveolar pressures (or loudnesses) during speech when the diaphragm is inactive. (After Draper, M., et al.: Respiratory muscles in speech. *Journal of Speech and Hearing Research, 2*, 16–27, 1959. Used by permission.)

of muscular activity on alveolar pressure and lung volume graphically. From Figure 1–20 predictions can be made as to which muscles or groups of muscles will be active at different lung volumes and alveolar pressures during speech when the diaphragm is inactive (Draper et al., 1959; Ladefoged, 1967). The vertical axis in the figure represents lung volume; the horizontal dimension represents alveolar pressure.[9] Assuming a relatively steady alveolar pressure with decreasing lung volume, the pattern of muscular activity when speaking at a given alveolar pressure can be determined by following any vertical line downward. For example, when speaking from near the total lung capacity with an alveolar pressure of 10 cm H_2O, the external intercostal muscles cease their activity at about 58% of the vital capacity, the internal intercostals take over from there to approximately the 44% level and thereafter the internals are supplemented by other expiratory muscles. The significant point

---

[9]Figure 1–20 is redrawn from the work of Draper and colleagues (1959). Their study used esophageal pressure measurements, which were assumed to be the equivalent of tracheal or alveolar pressures. Esophageal and alveolar pressures actually differ by an amount equal to the volume-dependent recoil pressure developed by the stretched lungs (Bouhuys et al., 1966; Ladefoged, 1967, 1968). Unfortunately, lung recoil data were not obtained for the subjects studied by Draper and colleagues (1959); hence, the original version of Figure 1–20 cannot be adjusted with great precision. A good approximation to the truth has been provided in Figure 1–20, however, by correcting the original pressure data on the basis of predicted static recoil pressures for the lungs of healthy normal subjects (Agostoni and Mead, 1964).

to be made in conjunction with Figure 1–20 is that speech using relatively high alveolar pressures involves less "checking" on the part of the external intercostals and earlier and greater activity of the internal intercostals and other expiratory muscles than speech requiring low alveolar pressures. Furthermore, the determinants of the activities of specific muscles are largely those discussed earlier relating to the muscular pressure problem—namely, the alveolar pressure required and the recoil force contributed by the lungs-thorax unit.

Abdominal hydraulics. Despite the diaphragm's status as the most important muscle of inspiration, it has been noted above that this structure ceases its electrical activity at high lung volumes in most speakers, although there is a continuing need for negative muscular pressures for certain types of utterances. The generation of such pressures without recourse to the diaphragm is made possible in the upright position because of the influence of gravity on the abdominal contents (Bouhuys et al., 1966). From a mechanical viewpoint, the abdomen may be likened to a liquid-filled container (Fig. 1–21) in which its top (the diaphragm) and part of its lateral wall (the abdominal wall) are distensible (Agostoni and Mead, 1964). The weight of the abdominal contents is supported in part by the wall of the abdomen and in part by pleural pressure. The latter manifests itself as an upward force pulling on the relaxed diaphragm, this pull being transmitted to the abdominal contents to support them in a manner somewhat analogous to the support of a water column by suction in a drinking straw. Through various respiratory maneuvers the relative support of the abdominal contents can be shifted in favor of either the abdominal wall or the negative pleural pressure, support in favor of the latter being of foremost importance to the generation of negative muscular pressure at high lung volumes during speech. As shown previously, a low alveolar pressure demand at high lung volume finds the external intercostal muscles active even in the absence of diaphragmatic activity. These muscles, and possibly other inspiratory muscles acting on the walls of the thorax, elevate the rib cage and expand it to a size greater than it would assume during relaxation at the same lung volume (Hixon, Mead, and Goldman, 1970; Konno and Mead, 1967). An elevated rib cage in combination with a relaxed abdominal wall and a relaxed diaphragm causes most of the support of the abdominal contents to be shifted to the pleural pressure (Mead et al., 1968). During such a maneuver the relaxed diaphragm is sucked upward, the abdominal pressure becomes more negative than its value during relaxation at the same lung volume, and the abdominal wall is sucked inward. With a pressure more negative than usual acting on the abdominal side of the diaphragm, a downward pull is placed on the structure, this pull balancing that of the negative pleural pressure. Were it not for the hydraulic properties of the abdomen in the upright position, the rib cage muscles would be relatively ineffective in lowering pleural pressure without active contraction of the diaphragm. The next section examines a circumstance under which the abdomen does not exert this important influence.

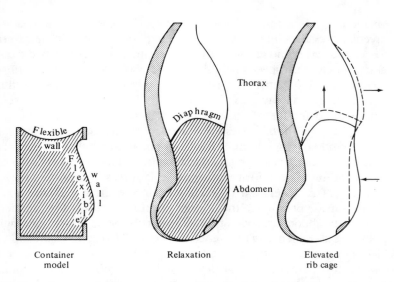

FIGURE 1-21. Container model of the diaphragm-abdomen system, together with illustrations of the resting and elevated rib cage positions of various respiratory structures. During relaxation the abdominal contents are supported against gravity by the wall of the abdomen and by lung recoil acting to elevate the diaphragm. Elevation of the rib cage through muscular effort causes it to expand, the diaphragm to be sucked upward, and the abdominal wall to be sucked inward. (After Agostoni, E., and Mead, J.: Statics of the respiratory system. *In* W. Fenn and H. Rahn [Eds.]: *Handbook of physiology.* Washington, DC: American Physiological Society, 1964. Used by permission.)

Effects of position. Departures from the upright position have marked effects on the behaviors and interactions of various respiratory parts, these effects being related mainly to the influence of gravity. As an illustration of the complexity of events involved, the more important contrasts of function in the upright and supine (i.e., lying on the back) positions are considered here. In the upright position, gravity acts in an expiratory direction on the rib cage and in an inspiratory direction on the abdomen (Fig. 1–22). The effect is mainly on the abdomen, being greater at low than at high lung volumes because the height of the abdomen is greater and its wall less stiff in the former situation (Agostoni and Mead, 1964). As discussed in the previous section, the abdominal contents are supported against gravity by the abdominal wall and the upward lifting force of the negative pleural pressure. In shifting from the upright to supine position, a new mechanical situation exists wherein the gravitational effect is expiratory on both the rib cage and abdomen. Compared to the upright position there is less gravitational effect with changes in lung volume in the supine position because the height of the abdomen is less (Agostoni and Mead, 1964). A significant feature of shifting to the supine

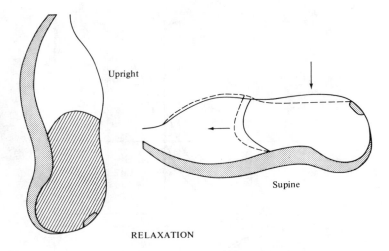

FIGURE 1–22. Resting positions of various respiratory structures during relaxation in the upright and supine positions. Gravity acts in the expiratory direction on the rib cage and in the inspiratory direction on the abdomen in the upright position. In the supine position, gravity acts in the expiratory direction on both the rib cage and abdomen. The diaphragm is displaced headward in the supine position and the forces of the abdomen which act to distend the diaphragm are balanced by the diaphragm's own elastic force. (After Agostoni, E., and Mead, J.: Statics of the respiratory system. *In* W. Fenn and H. Rahn [Eds.]: *Handbook of physiology.* Washington, DC: American Physiological Society, 1964. Used by permission.)

position is that pleural pressure no longer has a major role in supporting the abdominal contents. With gravity acting on the relaxed abdomen, the diaphragm is displaced into the rib cage until the forces acting to distend it are balanced by its own elastic force. As a consequence of this headward displacement of the diaphragm, the resting expiratory level of the pump changes from its upright value of approximately 35% of the vital capacity to a supine value of about 20%. An important outcome of this total set of events is a change in the relaxation volume-pressure characteristic of the apparatus. Figure 1–23 shows the relaxation pressure curves for both the upright and supine positions. The two curves differ in slope and shape, with the supine curve being displaced to the right (i.e., the spring-like background force is greater at corresponding lung volumes in the supine than upright position). The lower half of Figure 1–23 shows the muscular pressures needed for the production of the normal-loudness utterance depicted in the upper part of the figure. A greater negative muscular pressure is required throughout the high lung volumes for the supine than upright position, this negativity continuing to a lower lung volume in the supine than in the upright position. At low lung volumes, less positive muscular pressure is needed in the supine

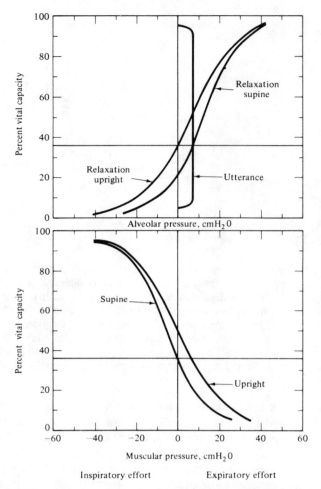

FIGURE 1-23. Upper: Lung volume-alveolar pressure relations during relaxation in the upright and supine positions and during an isolated vowel utterance of normal loudness produced throughout most of the vital capacity. (Relaxation curve after Agostoni, E., and Mead, J.: Statics of the respiratory system. *In* W. Fenn and H. Rahn [Eds.]: *Handbook of physiology.* Washington, DC: American Physiological Society, 1964. Used by permission.) Lower: Lung volume-muscular pressure relations replotted from data of the upper graph. Negative values represent net inspiratory forces and positive values represent net expiratory forces.

than in the upright position for the same utterance. On first consideration it seems a simple problem of adding somewhat different muscular pressures to the relaxation pressure at each lung volume for the two positions. The pump is operating under very different mechanical conditions, however, a principal difference being the function of the diaphragm in the two positions. Although abdominal hydraulics enable a footward pull to be placed on the relaxed diaphragm in the upright position, they do not enable such a circumstance to exist in the supine position (Hixon et al., 1970). Consequently, conditions requiring a negative muscular pressure at high lung volumes in the supine position require that the diaphragm be active. In effect this activity is needed to overcome the influence of gravity on the abdominal contents, an influence that causes the diaphragm to be displaced headward.

Although only two positions have been considered here, it should be realized that every positional change requires a different solution to the mechanical problem of providing a given alveolar pressure. Indeed, the complexity of respiratory function in speech becomes staggering when consideration is given to the innumerable positions in which the body is oriented and reoriented with respect to gravity. In this regard it should be noted that whereas the influence of gravity is manifested in other parts of the speech apparatus with positional change, the functional adjustments that must be made by the respiratory pump far exceed those required in other parts of the speaking machinery.

Demands of Conversational Speech

The mechanical problem facing the respiratory pump in conversational speech is far more complex than that imposed by steady utterances. This section deals with some important features of that problem by considering selected aspects of three general topics: aerodynamic events, forces provided by the respiratory pump, and neurophysiological mechanisms that govern in part the actions of the respiratory machinery. Unless otherwise indicated, discussion of each topic is limited to function in the upright position.

AERODYNAMIC EVENTS. For the speech activities discussed thus far, the task of the respiratory pump is that of providing steady average pressures, flows, and resistances during single expirations throughout most of the vital capacity. Conversational speech is not characterized by aerodynamic events of this nature (except for brief durations), nor is it often produced on expirations encompassing a great deal of the vital capacity. As for the pressures, flows, and resistances, they are in nearly constant states of change during conversational speech, these changes often being rapid and of substantial magnitude. The specific nature of such changes depends on a host of factors, which can be categorized broadly into the following: (1) at what location within the total speech apparatus the aerodynamic events are examined (e.g., alveolar pressure, nasal flow, laryngeal resistance, etc.), (2) what phonetic factors are involved (e.g., specific sounds produced, serial ordering of sounds, etc.), and (3) what prosodic features are operating (e.g., variations in speaking rate, vocal pitch, stress, etc.). Although the entire topic of aerodynamic events is within the province of speech breathing mechanics, the specific details of pressure, flow, and resistance changes have been judged to be more appropriately considered within the broader contexts of speech physiology; specifically in contexts concerning the dynamics of laryngeal and articulatory valving mechanisms. This leaves as the major area for discussion here the lung volume variations in conversational speech.

Lung volume changes. In breathing for life purposes, approximately 0.5 L of air is exchanged during each quiet tidal breath. By definition, breathing of this type occurs between the resting expiratory level and the tidal end-inspiratory position, the range between these covering approximately 10% of the vital capacity. Although it is possible to consciously restrict speech to this limited range of lung volumes or to produce it within nearly any segment of the vital capacity, there are roughly defined lung volume limits within which certain types of utterances typically occur (Hixon et al., 1970). For example, as is illustrated in Figure 1–24, in the upright position most conversational speech of normal loudness is produced within the midrange through volumes encompassing approximately 60% to 35% of the vital capacity. Deeper breaths are taken for speech of this nature than during normal quiet tidal breathing. Indeed, seldom are running speech phrases on new breaths initiated from lung volumes at or below the quiet end-inspiratory level. Of the many factors influencing the depth of inspiration during conversational utterances, the most important is the alveolar pressure demanded for the ensuing utterance. Witness to this pressure influence is very loud speech, which demands high alveolar pressures and usually is initiated from higher lung volumes (e.g., 80% to 60% VC) than speech of normal loudness. As a further example, very soft speech, which demands low alveolar pressures, frequently is initiated at lower lung volumes than speech of normal loudness—still from volumes generally above the tidal end-inspiratory level, however. In the upright position, breathing phrases usually are terminated slightly above or at the resting expiratory level (around 40% to 35% VC) during conversational utterances of normal loudness, with occasional phrases encroaching modestly on the expiratory reserve volume. These latter instances most often result from the speaker's desire to complete a continuing utterance without inspiratory interruption to the communication process. Soft speech finds expiratory phrases ending near the same lung volumes as speech of normal loudness, whereas loud utterances frequently are terminated at lung volumes above the resting expiratory level, sometimes appreciably above.

The lung volumes used for conversational speech in other positions differ from those in the upright position (Hixon et al., 1970). In the supine position, for example, volume events occur at lower levels of the vital capacity than in the upright position. Remember that in shifting from the upright to supine position, the resting level of the respiratory pump decreases from approximately 35% VC to about 20% VC. As with the upright position, the supine speaker uses lung volumes above his or her resting expiratory level

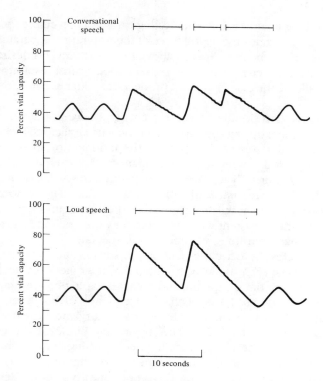

FIGURE 1–24. Lung volume changes characteristic of conversational and loud speech in the upright position. Utterance is during the bracketed time segments shown above each of the tracings.

(20% VC) with the inspirations in preparation for speech involving deeper breaths than for quiet breathing. For speech of normal loudness most events occur between 45% and 20% VC in the supine position, with soft speech being initiated from somewhat lower lung volumes and loud speech being initiated from higher levels (e.g., 60% to 50% VC). As with the upright position, relatively few expirations during speech in the supine position extend below the resting level of the respiratory pump. In further similarity to the upright position, the supine speaker's loud speech phrases are more likely to end at higher lung volumes than speech of normal loudness or soft speech.

Mechanical factors are in part responsible for the use of the midvolume range of the vital capacity for speech and for the utterance of most speech above the resting expiratory level. Use of the midvolume range is more desirable than use of either the upper or lower end of the vital capacity, because at these extremes the respiratory apparatus is stiffer and, therefore, mechanically more costly to control with muscular forces. By restricting utterances to lung volumes above the resting expiratory level, the speaker can take advantage of the positive recoil force of the respiratory apparatus to help drive the speech mechanism. Speech above the resting level is desirable also because no muscular energy needs to be expended against inspiratory recoil forces, as would be the case for speech produced at volumes below the resting level.

The relative partitioning of volume change between the rib cage and abdomen-diaphragm during speech depends on various factors, including the regulatory idiosyncrasies of the speaker, the loudness of speech, and the phonetic and prosodic content of the utterances (Hixon et al., 1970). Some speakers use predominantly rib cage motion to displace volume during speech, whereas others use predominantly abdominal motion. The reasons for the choice of one motion over the other by a given speaker are uncertain; however, speakers are highly consistent with respect to how their rib cage and abdomen interact with changes in lung volume during speech.

Of final interest here are the temporal aspects of lung volume changes in conversational speech. It has been noted that the quiet breathing cycle is repeated 12 or more times a minute and involves expirations that are slightly longer than inspirations. For speech, the frequency of breathing typically decreases and the relative durations of the inspiratory and expiratory phases change considerably (Fig. 1–24). The inspiratory phase of the cycle, for example, usually is more abrupt than in quiet breathing because the speaker inspires rapidly during speech to minimize interruption to the speaking situation. The expiratory phase, on the other hand, typically is lengthened for speech because air leaves the lungs more slowly due to the high resistances in the upper airway. The result is an expiratory phase that is many times longer than the expiratory phase of quiet breathing and many times longer than the inspirations associated with either speech or quiet breathing. It is difficult to characterize the temporal aspects of volume events during speech in any quantifiable manner. Perhaps the most useful summary statement on temporal aspects is that whereas life respiration is highly regular in rate and rhythm, a hallmark of the volume events of conversational speech is the irregularity of the breathing cycle.

RESPIRATORY FORCES. As with steady utterances, both muscular and nonmuscular forces are involved in the regulation of the respiratory pump for conversational speech. These are considered in the next two subsections.

Muscular pressures. The muscular pressure problem in conversational speech can be viewed in the same terms and subjected to the same type of graphical volume-pressure solution as the problem for steady utterances. Recall that the muscular pressure required at a given instant during speech depends on the alveolar pressure demanded and the relaxation pressure available. As noted previously, the lung volumes used in conversational speech are for the most part in the midrange of the vital capacity (i.e., about 60% to 35% VC). Referring to the volume-pressure diagram of Figure 1–14, it can be seen that the relaxation pressure available within those lung volume limits ranges between 10 and 0 cm H_2O. If 7 cm H_2O is taken as the average alveolar pressure required for conversational speech of normal loudness, the relaxation pressure throughout most of the midrange of volumes is less than that demanded of the respiratory pump. Accordingly, a positive muscular pressure must be added to the relaxation pressure. This muscular pressure must be increased gradually so as to compensate for the decreasing recoil force of the respiratory pump with reducing lung volume. This aspect of the muscular pressure problem for conversational speech is solved in a manner identical to that discussed earlier for sustained utterances. In the present instance, however, positive muscular pressures are generally involved because the range of lung volumes characteristically used by normal speakers involves relatively low relaxation pressures. Remember that negative muscular pressures are demanded only when the alveolar pressures needed are less than the pressure available through the combined recoil force of the lungs and thorax (including the diaphragm and abdomen). Another feature that distinguishes the muscular pressure problem in conversational speech from that in sustained utterances is that during conversational speech there are frequent demands for rapid changes in muscular pressure. These may be viewed as "pulsatile" variations in muscular pressure that are provided in addition to the usual background level of alveolar pressure for steady utterances. These pulsatile variations are of great linguistic significance as, for example, in stress (emphasis) contrasts. It is sufficient here to point out that these abrupt changes in muscular pressure are of brief duration (about 75 to 150 milliseconds) and involve magnitudes of change in the neighborhood of 1 to 3 cm H_2O during normal-loudness speech in the midvolume range (Netsell, 1969).

The bellows-spring analogy considered earlier for sustained utterances can be extended to apply to conversational speech. Figure 1–25 shows how the problem may be conceptualized as involving the parallel (i.e., simultaneous) solution of two problems. The left side of Figure 1–25 illustrates that component of the solution which provides a relatively constant alveolar pressure in the face of a continuously changing elastic recoil. There, with the wrists of the operator locked, movements of the arms provide the *gradual* changes in muscular pressure needed for utterance. These changes result from forcing the handles of the bellows toward one another to augment the spring-like background force within the range of lung volumes of interest here. This component of the muscular pressure solution may be designated as the "volume solution" because changing lung volume dictates that a changing muscular pressure adjustment be made. The right side of Figure 1–25 combines this volume solution with the second component, which may be designated

Volume solution   Pulsatile solution

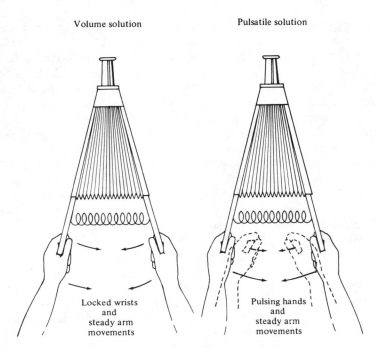

FIGURE 1-25. Spring-bellows analogies portraying the parallel solution of the "volume" and "pulsatile" problems facing the respiratory pump in conversational speech. For explanation see text.

as the "pulsatile solution." There, in addition to the volume solution accomplished by gradual inward movement of the arms, brief and rapid changes in muscular pressure (i.e., pulsatile changes) are accomplished, in analogy, by simultaneous rapid movements of the hands as performed through unlocked wrists. Thus, the problem imposed on the respiratory pump in conversational speech is solved, in analogy, by taking into account the slowly needed muscular pressure adjustments with arm movements and the more rapid variations with sudden and small movements of the hands. Although the nature of muscular pressure changes in running speech is relatively well understood, the muscular events within the respiratory apparatus that govern these changes are not well defined. The following section reviews the essential features of what is known about the specific muscular events.

Electromyographic activity. With positive muscular pressures being required during conversational speech, it follows that expiratory muscles are implicated in the mechanical events of such utterances. Examination of Figures 1–19 and 1–20 reveals that the muscles most important to the maintenance of a relatively steady alveolar pressure within the midvolume range are the internal intercostals. As discussed in the previous section, the "volume solution" for sustained utterances and conversational speech is conceptually identical. Accordingly, the important aspect to be discussed in this section is the manner in which the so-called "pulsatile" pressure changes are accomplished within the midvolume range. A great deal of controversy surrounds the activity of muscles in supplying these "pulsatile" variations (Draper et al., 1959; Hardy, 1967; Hoshiko, 1960; Ladefoged, 1967; Ladefoged, Draper, and Whitteridge, 1958; Stetson, 1951). Although there is general agreement that thoracic muscles are the chief regulators of muscular pressure changes under these circumstances, it is not agreed as to which specific muscles or groups of muscles are involved or what their specific involvements are. Most experimental study has centered on the intercostal muscles. The preponderance of available evidence suggests that the internal intercostal muscles are among the principal generators for pulsatile variations of typical magnitude. These small and fast-acting muscular generators appear to provide bursts of electrical activity in association with their discrete and brief contractions when the conditions of utterance call for rapid and small pressure variations of respiratory origin. Assuming that these bursts cause displacements of the thorax, the available evidence suggests that the muscles of greatest importance to everyday speech are the internal intercostals. They are so positioned and of such a size that they can importantly influence rib cage volume and introduce rapid and small variations in the driving pressure supplied to the larynx and upper airway. There is further evidence (Ladefoged et al., 1958) to suggest that very large pulsatile changes, such as those associated with very emphatic utterances, involve activity of the abdominal muscles. Such information, in conjunction with existing knowledge about respiratory mechanics, makes it seem reasonable to speculate that pulsatile variations of substantial magnitude may involve expiratory muscles in addition to the internal intercostals and abdominals.

It should be noted that the foregoing discussion pertains to the regulation of pulsatile pressure variations within the midrange of the vital capacity. Out of this range, and especially at higher lung volumes, the muscular forces governing alveolar pressure may operate in quite another manner (Hardy, 1970; Ladefoged et al., 1958). At least part of the capability for developing pulsatile variations at high lung volumes seems related to the ability to decrease rapidly and momentarily the counteracting muscular forces that may be used to oppose the recoil of the lungs and thorax. The external intercostal muscles have been implicated in this type of activity (Ladefoged et al., 1958) by the fact that they can decrease their counteracting force briefly and permit the spring-like background force of the respiratory apparatus to exert rapid increases in pressure. Such a mechanism can be considered with reference to the bellows analogy: If the handles of the spring-bellows system were initially spread wide and the arms of the operator used in opposition to the strong recoil provided by the spring at large chamber volumes, very rapid releases of the wrists of the operator would bear functional analogy to rapid and brief decrements in external intercostal activity within the chest. Under these circumstances, the driving forces to the bellows are provided by the spring, with the spring being able to exert these brief increases in pressure only during intermittent relaxation of the hand-wrist component.

NEUROPHYSIOLOGICAL MECHANISMS. Although discussion up to this juncture has been dominated by consideration of consciously controlled muscular events within the torso, there is evidence that load compensating reflexes within the intercostal muscles also are operative during speech (Sears and Newsom Davis, 1968). Such reflexes are in response to mechanical valving (i.e., articulatory gestures) within the larynx and the upper airway, valving which by its action causes very rapid loading and unloading of the respiratory pump. Variations in load cause transient changes in pressure and flow, which, in turn, result in small but rapid changes in lung volume. Such volume changes are in addition to those produced by the conscious driving of the respiratory muscles. When the pump is loaded during conversational speech, such as is the case when the larynx closes abruptly, a transient pressure build-up is reflected back to the torso, and a small volume increase results. Conversely, when the pump is unloaded during conversational speech, such as is the case when the larynx opens abruptly and air escapes rapidly from the lungs, a slight reduction in lung volume occurs. In the face of these rapid volume changes, the gamma-loop system[10] functions at the spinal level as a servomechanism that performs an automatic length stabilization of the intercostal muscles to compensate for the transient loading changes through which the muscles must work. The gamma-loop system is capable of serving this function by virtue of its sensitivities to length and rate of change in length of intercostal muscles (Matthews, 1964). To the extent that intercostal adjustments relate to overall respiratory function, these sensitivities represent displacement equivalents of volume and flow, respectively (Agostoni and Fenn, 1960). As transient length changes occur in the muscles of the torso, intercostal spindle receptors are deformed by these changes and the gamma-loop makes reflexive stabilization adjustments of which the speaker is totally unaware (Matthews, 1964). The responses are such that when loading on contracting inspiratory or expiratory intercostal muscles is made to increase, there is an associated increase in their

---

[10]Following Smith (1969) and Abbs (1971), the gamma-loop system is defined at a segmental level and includes (1) the gamma efferent fibers, (2) the spindle fiber controlled by the efferent fibers, and (3) the synaptic connections made by the spindle afferent fibers with alpha motor neuron. See Campbell (1964), and Ruch, Patton, Woodbury, and Towe (1965) for more detailed discussions. An excellent account of muscle spindle anatomy and physiology is provided in the motion picture film entitled "The Muscle Spindle" by Dr. Ian A. Boyd, Institute of Physiology, University of Glasgow. This film is available through John Wiley and Sons Film Library.

respective electrical activities; conversely, when loading on them is decreased, there is a decrease in their electrical activities (Sears and Newsom Davis, 1968). In addition to positive experimental evidence that reflex responses are elicited by artificially imposed load variations during spontaneous breathing (Newsom Davis, Sears, Staff, and Taylor, 1966) and during utterance (Sears and Newsom Davis, 1968), two other observations about speech breathing seem to accord well with the general nature of the reflex stabilization. Outward displacements of the torso wall, for example, have been shown (Cooker, 1963), to be systematically associated with laryngeal and upper airway valving during speech. These displacements follow transient pressure changes related to loading of the respiratory pump and, as such, they may be viewed as reflections of articulatory events within the head and neck. If outward displacements are assumed to indicate volume increases (Hixon, 1970b), and thus variations in intercostal muscle length, it seems reasonable to suppose that the gamma-loop system responds to these variations by stabilizing the demanded length changes of the muscles. For another example, multiple bursts of electrical activity have been recorded from intercostal muscles during utterance segments when respiratory loading could account for the electrical activity as well, if not better, than could specific voluntary commands to muscle generators (Ladefoged, 1968).

Finally, the operation of the gamma motor system during speech may be far more complex than has been suggested by the foregoing description of function at a gamma-loop reflex level alone. There appears to be good evidence for gamma system activity at supraspinal levels and for involvement of the gamma system in both the initiation and control of voluntary movement (Abbs, 1971; Campbell, 1964, 1968; Sears, 1966). Study of the gamma system has shown it to have specific cortical representation very similar to that for the alpha motor neuron system and for its activity to precede that of alpha motor neurons during spontaneous movements (Mortimer and Akert, 1961). One of the possible functional linkages between the gamma and alpha systems that has been suggested is a parallel driving of the intrafusal and extrafusal muscle systems. Given this arrangement, it may be conceptualized that the alpha system provides the coarse action of the respiratory muscles and the gamma system provides fine adjustments in the muscles (Campbell, 1968; Granit, 1955). For speech, which is a learned motor skill, the rapid variations in respiratory load may become predictable through repeated performance and therefore anticipated and compensated for by appropriately regulated activities of both gamma and alpha motor systems (Sears and Newsom Davis, 1968). In view of what is becoming known about the neurophysiology of respiration, there may soon be valid physiological bases for choosing among possible explanations of speech breathing data and for determining their implications for theoretical models of speech breathing mechanics (Ladefoged, 1968) and the clinical management of clients (Hixon, 1970a).

REFERENCES

Abbs, J. (1971). *The influence of the gamma motor system on jaw movement during speech*. Doctoral Dissertation, University of Wisconsin.

Agostoni, E. (1964). Action of respiratory muscles (pp. 377–386). *In* W. Fenn and H. Rahn (Eds.): *Handbook of physiology. Respiration 1, Sect. 3.* Washington, DC: American Physiological Society.

Agostoni, E., and Fenn, W. (1960). Velocity of muscle shortening as a limiting factor in respiratory air flow. *Journal of Applied Physiology, 15;* 349–353.

Agostoni, E., and Mead, J. (1964). Statics of the respiratory system (pp. 387–409). *In* W. Fenn and H. Rahn (Eds.): *Handbook of physiology. Respiration 1, Sect. 3.* Washington, DC: American Physiological Society.

Bouhuys, A., Proctor, D., and Mead, J. (1966). Kinetic aspects of singing. *Journal of Applied Physiology, 21;* 483–496.

Campbell, E. (1958). *The respiratory muscles and the mechanics of breathing.* Chicago: Year Book Medical Publishers, Inc.

Campbell, E. (1964). Motor pathways (pp. 535–543). *In* W. Fenn and H. Rahn (Eds.): *Handbook of physiology. Respiration 1, Sect. 3.* Washington, DC: American Physiological Society.

Campbell, E. (1968). The respiratory muscles. *Annals of the New York Academy of Science, 155;* 135–140.

Cherniack, R., and Cherniack, L. (1961). *Respiration in health and disease.* Philadelphia: W. B. Saunders Co.

Comroe, J., Jr. (1965). *Physiology of respiration.* Chicago: Year Book Medical Publishers, Inc.

Comroe, J., Jr., Forster, R. II, DuBois, A., Briscoe, W., and Carlsen, E. (1962). *The lung: Clinical physiology and pulmonary function tests* (2nd ed.). Chicago: Year Book Medical Publishers, Inc.

Cooker, H. (1963). *Time relationships of chest wall movements and intraoral pressures during speech.* Doctoral Dissertation. University of Iowa.

Draper, M., Ladefoged, P., and Whitteridge, D. (1959). Respiratory muscles in speech. *Journal of Speech and Hearing Research, 2;* 16–27.

Eblen, R. (1963). Limitations of the use of surface electromyography in studies of speech breathing. *Journal of Speech and Hearing Research, 6;* 3–18.

Granit, R. (1955). *Receptors and sensory perception.* New Haven, CT: Yale University Press.

Hardy, J. (1967). *Electromyographic evidence of syllable pulses in respiratory muscles.* Paper presented at the Annual Convention of the American Speech and Hearing Association, Chicago.

Hardy, J. (1970). *Discrete contractions of respiratory musculatures associated with /CV/ syllable trains.* Paper presented at the Annual Convention of the American Speech and Hearing Association, New York.

Hixon, T. (1970a). *Clinical implications of recent advances in speech breathing mechanics.* Paper presented at the Annual Convention of the American Speech and Hearing Association, New York.

Hixon, T. (1970b). *Respiratory mechanics during speech production.* Paper presented at the meeting of the American Association for the Advancement of Science, Chicago.

Hixon, T., Mead, J., and Goldman, M. (1970). *Separate volume changes of the rib cage and abdomen during speech.* Paper presented at the Annual Convention of the American Speech and Hearing Association, New York.

Hixon, T., Minifie, F., Peyrot, A., and Siebens, A. (1968). *Mechanical behavior of the diaphragm during speech.* Paper presented at the fall meeting of the Acoustical Society of America, Cleveland.

Hixon, T., Siebens, A., and Ewanowski, S. (1968). *Respiratory mechanics during speech production.* Paper presented at the spring meeting of the Acoustical Society of America, Ottawa.

Hoshiko, M. (1960). Sequence of action of breathing muscles during speech. *Journal of Speech and Hearing Research, 3*; 291–296.

Konno, K., and Mead, J. (1967). Measurement of the separate volume changes of rib cage and abdomen during breathing. *Journal of Applied Physiology, 22*; 407–422.

Konno, K., and Mead, J. (1968). Static volume-pressure characteristics of the rib cage and abdomen. *Journal of Applied Physiology, 24*; 544–548.

Ladefoged, P. (1967). *Three areas of experimental phonetics.* London: Oxford University Press.

Ladefoged, P. (1968). Linguistic aspects of respiratory phenomena. *Annals of the New York Academy of Science, 155*; 141–151.

Ladefoged, P., Draper, M., and Whitteridge, D. (1958). Syllables and stress. *Miscellania Phonetica, 3*, 1–15.

Matthews, P. (1964). Muscle spindles and their motor control. *Physiological Review, 44*; 219–288.

Mead, J., Bouhuys, A., and Proctor, D. (1968). Mechanisms generating subglottic pressure. *Annals of the New York Academy of Science, 155*; 177–181.

Mead, J., and Martin, H. (1968). Principles of respiratory mechanics. *Journal of the American Physical Therapy Association, 48*; 478–494.

Mead, J., and Milic-Emili, J. (1964). Theory and methodology in respiratory mechanics with glossary of symbols (pp. 363–376). *In* W. Fenn and H. Rahn (Eds.): *Handbook of Physiology. Respiration 1, Sect. 3.* Washington, DC: American Physiological Society.

Mortimer, E., and Akert, K. (1961). Cortical control and representation of fusimotor neurons. *American Journal of Physical Medicine, 48*; 228–248.

Netsell, R. (1969). A perceptual-acoustic-physiological study of syllable stress. Doctoral Dissertation, University of Iowa.

Newsom Davis, J., Sears, T., Staff, D., and Taylor, A. (1966). The effects of airway obstruction on the electrical activity of intercostal muscles in conscious man. *Journal of Physiology.* (London) *185*; 19P.

Pappenheimer, J., Comroe, J., Jr., Cournand, A., Ferguson, J., Filley, G., Fowler, W., Gray, J., Helmholz, H., Jr., Otis, A., Rahn, H., and Riley, R. (1950). Standardization of definitions and symbols in respiratory physiology. *Federation Proceedings, 9*; 602–615.

Radford, E., Jr. (1964). Static mechanical properties of mammalian lungs (pp. 429–449). *In* W. Fenn and H. Rahn (Eds.): *Handbook of physiology. Respiration 1, Sect. 3.* Washington, DC: American Physiological Society.

Rahn, H., Otis, A., Chadwick, L., and Fenn, W. (1946). The pressure-volume diagram of the thorax and lung. *American Journal of Physiology, 146*; 161–178.

Rouse, H., and Howe, J. (1953). *Basic mechanics of fluids.* New York: John Wiley & Sons.

Ruch, T., Patton, H., Woodbury, J., and Towe, A. (1965). *Neurophysiology* (2nd ed.) Philadelphia: W. B. Saunders Co.

Sears, T. (1966). The respiratory motorneuron: Integration at spinal segmental level (pp. 33–47). *In* J. Howell and E. Campbell (Eds.): *Breathlessness.* Oxford, England: Blackwell Scientific Publications.

Sears, T., and Newsom Davis, J. (1968). The control of respiratory muscles during voluntary breathing. *Annals of the New York Academy of Science, 155*; 183–190.

Siebens, A. (1966). The mechanics of breathing. *In* C. Best and N. Taylor (Eds.): *The physical basis of medical practice* (8th Ed.). Baltimore: Williams & Wilkens Co.

Smith, J. (1969). *Fusimotor neuron block and voluntary arm movement in man.* Doctoral Dissertation, University of Wisconsin.

Stetson, R. (1951). *Motor phonetics.* Amsterdam: North-Holland Publishing Co.

Taylor, A. (1960). The contribution of the intercostal muscles to the effort of respiration in man. *Journal of Physiology, 151*; 390–402.

CHAPTER **2**

Some New Techniques For Measuring the Biomechanical Events of Speech Production: One Laboratory's Experiences

Thomas J. Hixon

T he human speech production apparatus is a remarkably engineered machine. Its function, at least from a mechanical viewpoint, seemingly is unequaled in complexity when compared with other learned motor skills that most of us perform routinely. Attempts to analyze speech function comprehensively in mechanical terms must bring to bear information on the structure of the speech apparatus, the muscular and nonmuscular forces applied to and by its various parts, and the movements of those parts as manifested geometrically and through volume and flow events. The variety of information required for such an analysis, together with the variety of body parts

Reprinted by permission of the publisher from *American Speech and Hearing Association Reports*, Number 7, pp. 68–103, © 1972, American Speech-Language-Hearing Association, Rockville, MD.

constituting the speaking machinery, demand that the investigator have a substantial armamentarium of techniques for evaluating the mechanical events of speech. This chapter focuses on some recent additions to this armamentarium, additions that are of importance to the study of both normal and abnormal speech production. Because space limitations require some selectivity, the decision has been made to emphasize new techniques that, with one exception, currently are being used in a single laboratory (that of the author). Even with this provincial restriction, space dictates that discussion be devoted to only a few of this one laboratory's recent developments, and even those not in much detail. The majority of techniques chosen for discussion reside in custom-designed prototype or first-generation equipment systems whose development has been directed toward the ends of providing (1) precision in measurements, (2) minimal or no encumbrances to the natural speech production process, (3) minimal hazards to those being studied, and (4) real-time data. The primary focus will be on the techniques themselves and the nature of the information that can be obtained from their application. Measurement principles will be emphasized and little attention will be devoted to conventional hardware items in the various systems. Calibration procedures will not be considered.

It is beyond the scope of this chapter to consider specific data; however, many new insights about the speech production process already have been gained through use of some of the techniques to be considered. Many of these techniques are being used routinely in laboratory situations in the evaluation of organically based speech abnormalities. The general approach is to apply the techniques to the study of normal speakers, and, while acquiring data on normal function, to use those data as a reference against which to compare abnormal speakers. This turns out to be an excellent exchange between two major areas of study, because the study of the abnormal often tells one as much about normal function as the study of the normal contributes to the understanding of the abnormal. It will be obvious to the reader that at this time some of the techniques are more applicable clinically than others. Discussion begins with respiratory measurements and then moves on to the larynx and orofacial complex. Roughly equal attention will be devoted to each category. The general areas to be discussed include the following:

I. Volume-Pressure Body Plethysmography
II. Plethysmographic Measurement of Alveolar Pressure
III. Body-Surface Measurements
IV. Partitioning of Mechanical Forces: The Diaphragm as an Example
V. Forced Oscillation Procedures: The Study of Laryngeal Mechanics
VI. Strain-Gauge Measurements of Articulatory Events: Motion and Force

VOLUME-PRESSURE BODY PLETHYSMOGRAPHY

In the respiratory pump, the net displacements of structures become expressed as volume changes. Volumes displaced by pulmonary structures of the pump are reflected in equivalent volume displacements of the body surface because the chest wall is essentially incompressible. It is possible, therefore, to measure changes in lung volume through procedures that provide information on the volumes displaced by the body surface (Mead, 1960). Information of this nature is important in the study of speech physiology, primarily because many of the mechanical events of speech breathing are lung-volume dependent. One method for measuring lung volume changes during speech is illustrated schematically in Figure 2–1. In this figure, a subject is seated inside a multipurpose wooden body chamber,[1] which, in this instance, is configured as a volume-pressure body plethysmograph (Mead, 1968). As shown, the subject is totally encased, except for the head and neck, which protrude through the top of the chamber. The lower part of the neck is encircled by a collar made of rubber dental dam and filled with tiny glass bubbles. This collar is shaped on each subject to provide an airtight seal between the chamber outlet and the neck; it is then hardened by active suction (Mead and Collins, 1954). An adjustable air conditioner recirculates air within the chamber to keep the subject comfortable. As the subject performs breathing activities, chamber pressure increases with net inspiratory volume changes and decreases with net expiratory volume changes. As these volume changes occur, gas is displaced through a fine metal screen built into the front wall of the chamber. This screen acts as a linear flow-resistance so that the flow through it is directly proportional to the pressure differential between the chamber and atmosphere (P chamber). For slow changes in lung volume, essentially all of the volume change is included in the gas displaced through the metal screen. When rapid events are involved, however, part of the lung volume change goes into gas compression or expansion. No matter how rapid

---

[1]This chamber is custom-designed for speech research and incorporates into a single system the functional features of several systems developed as prototypes for research on respiratory mechanics. Jere Mead, Professor of Physiology, Harvard School of Public Health, made many useful suggestions with regard to the design of the overall chamber.

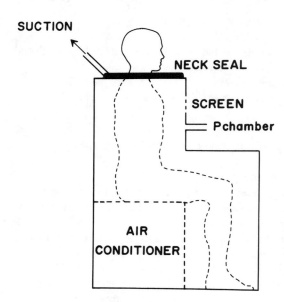

FIGURE 2-1. Body chamber configuration for making plethysmographic measurements of changes in lung volume during speech.

the volume events, all of the volume change can be taken into account at every instant by knowing the volume displaced through the screen and the volume change associated with gas compression or expansion. A measure of the volume displaced into and out of the chamber can be obtained by integrating the flow-proportional pressure signal sensed by a pressure transducer attached to the plethysmograph. Conveniently, the same chamber pressure signal provides a measure of the volume displacement related to gas compression or expansion (Mead, 1968). Because the total volume displacement is the sum of that related to gas compression or expansion and that related to displacement of gas into and out of the chamber, a measurement of the true lung volume change can be achieved by summing these two electronically (Grimby, Takishima, Graham, Macklem, and Mead, 1968). Under the circumstances described, the accuracy with which rapid changes in lung volume can be recorded during speech is limited only by the response of the transducer selected and the speed of sound in air (Mead, 1968).[2] The system discussed here, then, meets the frequently raised criticism against using body plethysmographs in speech research (Lubker, 1970)—namely, that the response of such systems is too poor to permit accurate measurement of the volume events associated with rapid speech movements. Furthermore, the present

---

[2]Although the major concern in this section is lung volume events, similar considerations about measurement accuracy, of course, apply to rates of volume change (flows) and volume accelerations. These latter two can be obtained as the first and second derivatives of lung volume change, respectively.

method is more accurate than techniques that try to measure lung volume changes at the mouth during speech (Hardy and Edmonds, 1968), because volume recordings at the mouth (1) neglect lung volume changes due to gas compression or expansion (Agostoni and Mead, 1964), (2) include volume displacements not only of the lungs but also of the articulators, which themselves displace volumes during speech (Gilbert and Hixon, 1969), and (3) require that corrections be made to account for water vapor temperature changes in the gas (Collins, 1957). Finally, it is important to note that, because the subject's head is unencumbered in the present approach, there are no problems in making accurate acoustic recordings or of interfering with natural speech articulation, as is the case in procedures that require the subject to be coupled to a mouthpiece or facemask of some type (Hardy and Edmonds, 1968; Lubker, 1970).

PLETHYSMOGRAPHIC MEASUREMENT OF ALVEOLAR PRESSURE

The speech apparatus is a three-dimensional (acoustic) system whose net unbalanced forces are manifested in the form of pressures. Nearly continuous pressure fluctuations occur within the apparatus during speech, there being several regions along the airways where pressure measurements are especially telling of physiological mechanisms. Alveolar pressure is of particular interest in mechanical analyses of speech, because it represents the instantaneous net sum of all muscular and nonmuscular forces contributing to the respiratory driving pressure (DuBois, Botelho, and Comroe, 1956). Figure 2–2 schematically illustrates a method for measuring alveolar pressure events during speech (Hixon and Warren, 1971). In this illustration, the multipurpose chamber is configured without a neck seal and with a hinged, lucite dome swung down over the subject's head and latched hermetically to the top of the chamber. Recall, from the foregoing discussion, that during lung volume measurements the subject's airway opening (mouth) was connected to the outside of the chamber (i.e., was free to the room). Volume changes measured under such circumstances are due both to the compression (and decompression) of gas within the subject and to the displacement of gas by the subject, the latter component being of far greater magnitude than the former. In the present configuration, the subject is totally encased and the airway opening is coupled at different times during measurements either to a closed valve or to the inside of the chamber (i.e., is in free communication with the chamber). In both airway-opening conditions only the component of volume change related to gas compression (and decompression) is seen by the chamber. There is no displacement component when the subject is on a closed valve, because volume cannot be exchanged between the subject and the chamber. As for free breathing inside the chamber, the gas displaced into

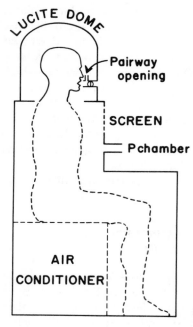

LUCITE DOME

Pairway opening

SCREEN

Pchamber

AIR CONDITIONER

FIGURE 2–2. Chamber configuration for making plethysmographic measurements of alveolar pressure (Palv) during speech.

and out of the subject occupies the space created within the chamber by equivalent displacements of the body surface, and the converse. The essence of alveolar pressure measurement by this approach is to determine alveolar pressure changes from values of compressional (and decompressional) volume changes as measured with the plethysmograph (Arutjunjan, Granstrem, and Kozhevnikov, 1967; Hixon and Warren, 1971). Such an approach capitalizes on the compressible nature of gas contained within the lungs and airways and the potential for quantifying the pressure-volume behavior of that gas through Boyle's law. In practice, measurements are made by first having the subject open the glottis and alternately compress and expand the gas within the subject by attempting to pant slowly through a mouthpiece against a closed valve. During this maneuver, simultaneous measurements are made of compressional volume changes and airway pressure changes. The former are accomplished as in volume-pressure body plethysmography (see earlier description), the latter by a pressure transducer attached to a side tap on the mouthpiece. Because pressure is equal throughout a static fluid system, the pressure measured at the mouthpiece during compressional changes also is a measure of alveolar pressure at every instant. By relating airway pressure changes to volume changes measured at the body surface, a calibration is established that enables volume measurements to be used as measures of alveolar pressure at the absolute lung volume of concern. So calibrated, the subject comes off the mouthpiece-valve assembly, maintains the prevailing lung volume momentarily, and then speaks into the free space of the chamber. When lung volume displacements are relatively small, such as for short utterances, only a single pre-utterance calibration maneuver needs to be performed. Utterances encompassing larger segments of the vital capacity require calibrations both before and after utterance to account for the changing calibration factor with changes in absolute lung volume (Hixon and Warren, 1971). When large absolute lung volume changes are involved, an alternate means of calibration adjustment is on-line correction of the plethysmographic volume signal by adding to it an electrical signal proportional to the subject's instantaneous absolute lung volume (Finucane et al., 1970). Whatever the approach to calibration, once the subject is off the mouthpiece-valve assembly, the volume changes recorded by the plethysmograph represent real-time alveolar pressure measurements. Such measurements also can be taken as excellent approximations of subglottal pressure events during speech. This is possible because the impedance from the alveoli to the subglottal space (i.e., along the lower airway) is sufficiently low to cause only a small pressure loss between the two regions (Bouhuys, Proctor, and Mead, 1966; Hixon and Warren, 1971). If highly accurate subglottal pressure estimates are required, this small impedance loss can be taken into account, although it appears to be an unimportant correction for most speech research purposes. Contrasted with other available techniques for estimating subglottal pressure (Draper, Ladefoged, and Whitteridge, 1959; Kunze, 1964; Perkins and Koike, 1969; Van den Berg, 1956), the technique discussed here appears to hold several distinct advantages, the most important being that it (1) involves no discomfort for the subject, (2) presents no risk to the subject, (3) does not require the placement of measuring devices inside the body, and (4) does not require the assistance of a physician. Such advantages are of obvious interest to both the investigator and the subject, the first three being of heightened significance in the case of neurologically impaired subjects, for whom other procedures are generally impractical and often intolerable.

BODY-SURFACE MEASUREMENTS

From a functional perspective, the chest wall can be viewed as a two-part mechanical system, the parts being the rib cage and diaphragm-abdomen (Konno and Mead, 1967). Each part moves basically as a unit during speech, although there exists a substantial potential for independence of motion between the two. Witness to the latter is the ability to change lung volume mainly with either the rib cage or the diaphragm-abdomen component, and the ability to produce paradoxical movements of one or the other of the subdivisions during breathing maneuvers. As each part moves during speech and displaces volume, points within the part go through motions that are related uniquely to the volumes displaced. More specifically, the volumes displaced by either the rib cage or the abdomen are essentially linearly related to the linear motions of points within the respective parts (Konno and Mead, 1967; Peyrot, Hertel, and Siebens, 1969). The investigator can take advantage of this relationship and estimate the separate volume displacements of the rib cage and abdomen during speech by measuring the anteroposterior diameter changes of the two parts (Hixon, Mead, and Goldman, 1970). As in total lung volume change during speech, measurements of the separate volume displacements of the rib cage and abdomen are important because many of the mechanical events within these subdivisions of the respiratory pump are volume-dependent. Measurements are accomplished along the lines illustrated in Figure 2–3. Changes in the diameter of the rib cage and abdomen generally are measured at the torso midline and at the levels of the nipples and slightly above the umbilicus, respectively. Measurements are made through the use of either of two transducer systems: the magnetometers (Mead, Peterson, Grimby, and Mead, 1967) depicted in panel (A) of Figure 2–3 or the variable inductance linear displacement transducers (French, 1966) portrayed in panel (B). The magnetometer system consists of two pairs of coils, each pair having a coil to generate a magnetic field and an identical mate to sense the field generated. Distance changes between the mates (i.e., diameter changes in the res-

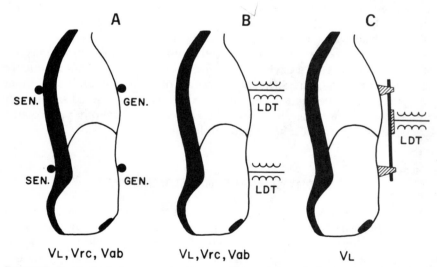

FIGURE 2–3. Methods for measuring changes in lung volume (V_L), rib cage volume (V_{rc}), and abdominal volume (V_{ab}) from body surface movements during speech. (A) Four-coil magnetometer system. (B) Two linear displacement transducers. (C) A single linear displacement transducer and a rigid strut.

piratory part of interest) are indicated by voltages induced in the sensing coil, with the magnitude of the voltage being inversely proportional to the cube of the distance between the two coil mates. Because the range of torso motions encompassed during most speech is small compared with the absolute intercoil distances, the relationship between induced voltage change and diameter change is nearly linear. The linear displacement transducers used are custom-built electromechanical devices. Each of these transducers indicates with a relative DC output voltage the position of a point in reference to a fixed point in line with the axis of the device. A simple way to conceptualize the action of the devices is to consider their two coils as forming voltage dividers. As a ferrite armature is passed through the center of the coils, the relative inductance and, therefore, the impedance of each coil changes. The result is an output voltage that varies directly and linearly with the position of the armature. The armature itself is made of ferrite tubing attached to a spring-loaded fiberglass rod that is placed directly on the surface whose displacement is to be sensed. Although the results obtained with the magnetometer and displacement transducer systems are basically identical, the displacement transducer system is somewhat more difficult to use because the subject must maintain relatively stable posture against a back support. During measurements with the magnetometer system, the subject is permitted much greater freedom of movement. From data on the changes in anteroposterior diameter of the rib cage and abdomen, not only are the separate volume contributions of the two functional parts of the chest wall known, but it also is possible to determine the change in total lung volume during speech by summing the two diameter signals graphically or electronically (Hixon, 1970). Electrical summation results in a signal that over a wide range of lung volumes is a practical equivalent of the volume events measured by more conventional techniques (Mead et al., 1967). A variation on the theme of measuring lung volume changes from body surface movements is illustrated in panel (C) of Figure 2–3, where a simple mechanical device and a single linear displacement transducer are used to obtain data on lung volume changes during speech. Because the chest wall is functionally a two-degree-of-freedom system, the displacements of the rib cage and abdomen can be resolved into a single displacement that is proportional to lung volume change (Peyrot et al., 1969). This is accomplished easily by running a post between the rib cage and abdomen and finding the point on this post that does not move during voluntary shifting of volume between the two parts of the system (the rib cage and abdomen) under iso-volume conditions (i.e., with the glottis closed). Once the location of this point is determined empirically, measurement of the displacement of the point during breathing or speech activities provides another means of recording total lung volume changes. Thus, without interference to acoustic recording or encumbrance to the natural speech articulation process, the techniques discussed in this section permit the measurement of changes in the separate volumes of the rib cage and abdomen, and in the total lung volume during speech. The advantages discussed earlier for plethysmographic recording of volume events during speech over volume recordings at the airway opening also apply as advantages of these techniques.

PARTITIONING OF MECHANICAL FORCES: THE DIAPHRAGM AS AN EXAMPLE

Like many other complex machines, the behavior of the speech production apparatus is governed by the actions of a number of different mechanical parts. Because the actions of these parts are influenced by both muscular and nonmuscular forces, it is important to the understanding of speech mechanics to be able to partition these forces during measurements. One approach used to obtain information on the forces regulating the behavior of one of these parts—namely, the diaphragm—is illustrated schematically in Figure 2–4A. The strategy in this approach is to combine two measurement techniques, one to provide information on the electrical activity of the muscular portion of the diaphragm (Hixon, Minifie, Peyrot, and Siebens, 1968) and the other to provide information on the structure's transmural pressure (Agostoni and Rahn, 1960; Bouhuys et al., 1966). The electrical activity of the diaphragm is sensed by a custom-designed EMG electrode (Hixon, Siebens, and Minifie, 1969). This electrode, shown in Figure 2–4B, is a bipolar surface unit that is passed pernasally into the esophagus and positioned at the level of the esophageal hiatus. The distance between the poles of the electrode (i.e., the two silver spheres) is adjusted to obtain optimal recordings and then the electrode is anchored in the hiatus through inflation of a gastric balloon attached to the unit. In the hiatus, the electrical activity of the crurae (pillars) of the diaphragm is sensed, activity that is comparable to that of the more major muscular portions of the structure (the costal fibers) (Hixon et al., 1969). With the electrode in position, the nearest skeletal muscles, other than the diaphragm, are the psoas and quadratus lumborum. Because hip flexion maneuvers do not modify the electromyogram, it seems highly unlikely that recordings could be contaminated by electrical activity from these or other, more distant muscles. In addition to being recorded in its raw form, the EMG signal from the crurae is conditioned electronically through custom-built equipment which accomplishes a real-time elimination of the electrocardiogram interference and provides a voltage equivalent of the first integral of the raw signal (French and Siebens, 1969). To measure transmural pressure, simultaneous recordings of esophageal and gastric pressures are made using recently improved conventional latex balloon techniques (Milic-Emili, Mead, Turner, and Glauser, 1964) or using the miniature pressure transducers shown in Figure 2–4B (Hixon, Minifie, Peyrot, and Siebens, 1968). The latter are

A

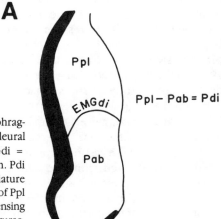

$$Ppl - Pab = Pdi$$

FIGURE 2-4. (A) Factors influencing diaphragmatic behavior during speech. Ppl = pleural pressure. Pab = abdominal pressure. EMGdi = electromyographic activity of the diaphragm. Pdi = transdiaphragmatic pressure. (B) Miniature pressure transducers for obtaining estimates of Ppl and Pab, and a bipolar surface electrode for sensing the electrical signal from the diaphragmatic crurae.

B

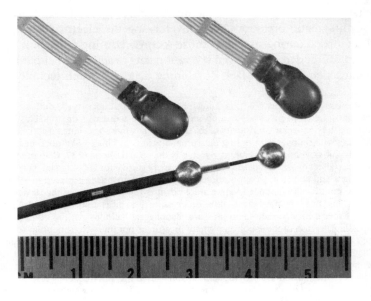

commercially available sensors with excellent frequency response, although in some ways they are less desirable to work with and less accurate than balloon procedures.[3] Whichever sensing system is used, the devices are passed pernasally, one to the level of the middle third of the esophagus and the other into the stomach. The pressure recorded from the esophageal unit is taken as a measure of pleural pressure (Mead and Milic-Emili, 1964), and the gastric pressure signal is used to estimate abdominal pressure (Agostoni and Rahn, 1960). Gastric and abdominal pressures actually differ by an amount depending on the muscle tone of the stomach and the hydrostatic pressure gradient between the pleural surface and the stomach (Duomarco and Rimini, 1947). To a close approximation, the magnitude of this difference is indicated by the minimum difference between gastric and pleural pressures during relaxation above the resting expiratory level (Bouhuys et al., 1966). This difference is subtracted from the gastric pressure to correct it to abdominal pressure. As portrayed in Figure 2–4A, because the pressure acting on the pulmonary side of the diaphragm (pleural pressure) as well as that acting on the abdominal side of the partition (abdominal pressure) can be specified, the transmural or transdiaphragmatic pressure acting on the structure at every instant can be designated (Bouhuys et al., 1966). When the pressure differential across the diaphragm together with its own electrical activity is known, the net forces regulating the structure into components of both muscular and nonmuscular origin can be analyzed (Hixon, Minifie, Peyrot, and Siebens, 1968). A typical approach to such an analysis would be first to have the subject relax the respiratory pump against an infinite resistance at different lung volumes throughout the vital capacity while simultaneously recording electrical activity and transdiaphragmatic pressure. Then, by relating the electrical and pressure signals recorded during speech to those recorded during relaxation, it is possible to interpret departures from relaxation data as activity of either muscular or nonmuscular origin. In fact, combining data from such techniques with

---

[3]One inconvenient aspect of using miniature pressure transducers is the difficulty in zeroing them to atmosphere once they are in a position within the esophagus or stomach. Other problems relate to the temperature sensitivity of the devices. They must be calibrated at the temperature at which they will be operating during measurements in situ. This can be done in a water bath heated to the subject's body temperature, which is in the neighborhood of 37°C. In situ temperature variations also affect measurements; however, these are negligible for measurement purposes within the esophagus and stomach. In applications in which the transducer is placed in a flow stream (e.g., in the mouth), flow-induced temperature changes render the use of the devices difficult. Finally, it should be recognized that esophageal pressure (Pes) measurements made with miniature transducers reveal local variations in pressure. Esophageal balloons, on the other hand, when encompassing a region of the esophagus where pressure is not uniform from point to point, will provide a measurement of pressure that approximates the most negative value in the region (Mead and Milic-Emili, 1964). Because it is the most negative value of pressure that is usually most significant from a mechanical perspective, the esophageal balloon would be preferred. Indeed, although miniature pressure transducers provide some advantages in size and frequency response, and perhaps even durability, the nature of the measurements to be made dictates whether they are reasonable substitutes for standard esophageal balloon techniques.

data on the separate volume changes of the rib cage and abdomen (Hixon, Minifie, Peyrot, and Siebens, 1968) allows reasonable inferences to be made concerning the nature of muscular activity—namely, whether it is isotonic, isometric, or pliometric. Aside from the unique mechanical information that the procedures described here provide, techniques of this type have the obvious advantage over x-ray procedures of permitting extensive study of the part in question without hazard to the subject. The discussion here has considered the study of diaphragmatic behavior only. The principles involved, however, have general applicability to the study of many other parts of the speech production apparatus (Hixon, Siebens, and Ewanowski, 1968).

FORCED OSCILLATION PROCEDURES: THE STUDY OF LARYNGEAL MECHANICS

Forced oscillation techniques are a new and powerful approach to the study of the mechanics of speech and voice production. These techniques involve a wide variety of forced applications of either known pressure or volume changes to various parts of the speech apparatus. The results of such applications can be interpreted in terms of changes in the behavior of these parts, or in terms of changes in various aspects of the acoustic signal. For purposes of discussion here, consideration will be given to only one of the many possibilities for applying forced oscillations in speech research, the application of forced transglottal pressure changes in the study of the mechanics of voice production. One of the approaches used involves the application of forced sinusoidal pressure oscillation to the body surface (Hixon, Klatt, and Mead, 1970). Figure 2–5 illustrates this approach schematically. A subject is seated in the multipurpose chamber, which is configured in this instance as a pressure-oscillation device. The subject's head and neck protrude unencumbered through the top of the chamber and a loose-fitting but hardened collar encircles the subject's neck at the chamber outlet. Four loudspeakers, two series sets in parallel, are coupled to the back of the chamber and are controlled through a power amplifier by an oscillator. This chamber configuration permits sinusoidal pressure changes to be provided within the chamber (at the body surface) over a wide range of frequencies and at amplitudes of up to 6 cmH$_2$O peak to peak. The lower part of Figure 2–5 depicts an electrical analogue of the mechanical situation of the chamber containing a subject. The loudspeakers (1) see in parallel the following: the gas in the chamber as a compliance (2), the leak across the loose-fitting neck seal as a resistance (3), and the subject as a complex, lumped component (4). The pressure applied to the subject during oscillation is spent in a complex fashion among opposing pressures of resistances, compliances, and inertances. At one particular frequency of oscillation—namely, the resonant frequency of the respiratory pump—opposing pressures related to inertance and compliance

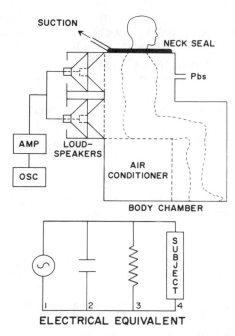

FIGURE 2-5. Upper: Body chamber configuration for applying forced oscillatory changes in pressure at the body surface (Pbs). Lower: Electrical equivalent of the mechanical situation illustrated in the upper part of the figure. See discussion in text.

are equal and of opposite sign and thus cancel (DuBois, Brody, Louis, and Burgess, 1956; Grimby et al., 1968; Peslin, Hixon, and Mead, 1971). At this frequency, the impedance of the respiratory apparatus is represented entirely by a flow-resistive term (Goldman et al., 1970). This frequency can be determined empirically in each subject by varying the frequency of applied pressure until flow, as measured by a flowmeter at the subject's airway opening, is exactly in phase with transrespiratory pressure (i.e., the pressure differential between the body surface and the airway opening). Under the conditions described, pressure changes generated at the body surface are realized as slightly smaller pressure changes at both the pleural surface and the subglottal space, because there is a small resistive pressure loss across the chest wall (Hixon, Klatt, and Mead, 1970). Thus, it is possible to impart known forced subglottal pressure changes to the larynx through the application of known forced body surface pressure changes corrected for this loss (Hixon, 1971b). In addition, it is possible to depart from the resonant frequency of the subject under certain circumstances and still have a good estimate of subglottal pressure changes from body surface pressure changes, because the high magnitude of the series resistance offered by the larynx during voice production renders the reactive components of the mechanical system relatively unimportant (Hixon, Klatt, and Mead, 1970).

Before considering the nature of the information that can be obtained about laryngeal function through the use of forced oscillation, a second mode for applying forced pressure changes transglottally warrants discussion. This mode, shown schematically in Figure 2–6, involves the generation of sinusoidal pressure changes at the subject's airway opening (Grimby et al., 1968; Hixon, Klatt, and Mead, 1970; Lieberman, Knudson, and Mead, 1969). The configuration shown has the subject coupled at the mouth to the multipurpose chamber through a low resistance and low inertance tubing arrangement. A bias flow of constant magnitude is used to circulate air through the system and, thereby, reduce dead space. A long tube within the chamber and with one end to atmosphere accommodates the needed vent for the bias flow and for breathing and, at the same time, offers high inertial impedance at the frequencies of oscillation used for experimental manipulation. This latter feature makes it possible to develop the desired pressure levels within the chamber, despite the substantial vent leak (Grimby et al., 1968). The entire setup is so arranged that changes in the mechanical impedance of the subject (e.g.,

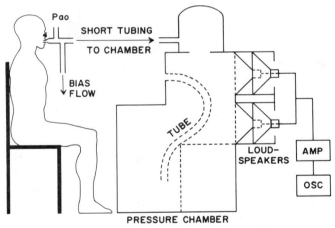

FIGURE 2–6. Upper: Chamber configuration for applying forced oscillatory changes in pressure at the airway opening (Pao). Lower: Electrical equivalent of the mechanical situation illustrated in the upper part of the figure. See discussion in text.

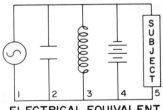

ELECTRICAL EQUIVALENT

increases in laryngeal impedance) have little influence on the pressure delivered at the airway opening. The bottom part of Figure 2–6 shows the electrical equivalent of the mechanical situation depicted in the top of the figure. In this case, the loudspeakers (1) see in parallel the following: the gas in the chamber as a compliance (2), the gas in the long tube as an inertance (3), the DC bias flow as a battery (4), and the subject as a complex, lumped component incorporating compliances, resistances, and inertances (5). As with the body surface configuration, control of the four loudspeakers through an oscillator and power amplifier permits regulation of chamber pressure and, thereby, permits variation of the pressure seen on the downstream (supraglottal) side of the larynx. Thus, with either of the two techniques discussed, it is possible to impose forced transglottal pressure changes, with these changes being applied to the pulmonary side of the larynx in the one case and to the upper airway side in the other.

With the capability for providing controlled changes in pressures acting on the larynx, investigators are in a position to study the influence of transglottal pressure events on various acoustical aspects of voice production and on the mechanical behavior of the laryngeal valve. Most of the information gathered to date has been obtained through application of forced oscillations while speakers phonate sustained vowels (Hixon, Klatt, and Mead, 1970; Lieberman et al., 1969). It is assumed that during such utterances, vocal fold adjustment remains constant so that changes in vocal output are attributable solely to variations in transglottal pressure. Although laryngeal electromyography eventually must be consulted in this regard, the observation that DC pressure and flow do not change when going from normal phonation to phonation under oscillation conditions suggests that contributory laryngeal adjustments are not made during oscillatory applications. Forced oscillation procedures, therefore, provide a means for parceling out the contribution of the respiratory pump under conditions in which both the respiratory and laryngeal systems can influence various acoustical parameters of the voice (e.g., vocal fundamental frequency and vocal intensity). These techniques, in addition, provide a means for studying the mechanical behavior of the larynx in response to pressure changes, that behavior being revealed in part through pressure-flow measurements during phonation. In this regard, it should be noted that oscillatory resistance measurements (Peslin et al., 1971) can be made during phonation without inserting various devices inside the body to estimate subglottal pressure. Comparing the two modes of applying pressure, the body surface configuration has a distinct advantage over the airway opening application in that the subject's speech apparatus is unencumbered and, therefore, interference with natural utterance or acoustic recording is not a problem.

STRAIN-GAUGE MEASUREMENTS OF ARTICULATORY EVENTS: MOTION AND FORCE

Some parts of machines move and exert forces, and so it is with the articulatory machinery. To describe articulatory function at a mechanical level comprehensively, it must be possible to quantify the relation of motion to force in accordance with physical laws. Such quantification permits an understanding of the underlying mechanisms and properties of the speech production apparatus. The mechanical actions of the articulators are difficult to measure because of both the complexity of speech behavior and the difficulties involved in tracking rapidly moving and, in some cases, relatively inaccessible structures. Recent advances in recording technology now make it possible to obtain real-time data on the motions and forces associated with various articulator activities. Some of these advances are in the form of strain-gauge systems. As examples of these, four recently developed systems and their applications to studies of the mandible, lips, and velum are considered.

An example of strain-gauge application to the monitoring of jaw displacement is illustrated in Figure 2–7. The unit depicted (Abbs, 1971) was constructed after a prototype by Sussman and Smith (1970). The subject wears an adjustable headband and support system, to which one end of a phosphor-bronze strip is clamped. The other end of the strip presents an attached rubber knob that rests on the skin over the mental protuberance of the mandible such that some degree of initial strain is placed on the strip. Strain gauges are bonded to both sides of this metal strip and wired to form two arms of a four-arm Wheatstone bridge circuit. In the position shown, vertical movements of the jaw exert bending forces on the metal strip that are realized as resistance changes in the strain gauges. The result is an output voltage signal that is directly proportional to the component of mandibular motion that is resolved into the vertical dimension. Because the transducing system is fixed relative to the head, the subject is allowed reasonably free movement without risk

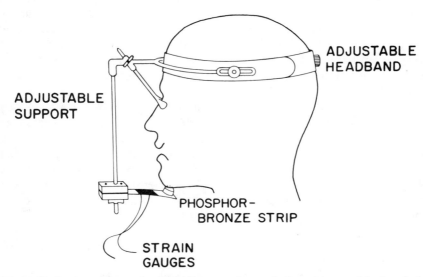

FIGURE 2–7. Strain-gauge transducer for measuring vertical movements of the jaw during speech.

of recording artifact. It has been shown that jaw movement transducing in this configuration is subject to negligible artifact from anteroposterior jaw movements in the range of movements characteristic of speech. More specifically, maximum jaw openings in the vertical dimension are about 5% smaller than those along the true movement path of the jaw as influenced by the temporomandibular joint articulation (Abbs, 1971). In addition to using the voltage output from the transducer as an analogue of jaw displacement, measurements can incorporate differentiation of the voltage signal to obtain information on both the velocity and acceleration components of jaw motion (Abbs and Netsell, 1970). The latter component appears to provide information not discernible from visual analyses of displacement tracings alone and, in fact, may well provide a means of examining the net muscular forcing function of the mandibular articulator (Abbs and Netsell, 1971).

Lip displacement during speech can be measured in a way similar to that just described for the jaw. As with the prototype of the jaw displacement transducer just discussed, the system for making lip measurements was developed by Sussman and Smith (1970). As shown in Figure 2–8A, this system is composed of two separate transducers, one for each lip. Each unit consists of a T-shaped phosphor-bronze strip with the bar portion of the T in contact with the lip. These strips are extremely flexible and present no significant interference with lip movement (Sussman and Smith, 1970). The transducers are positioned so that in a mouth-open position there is some initial strain on each strip. The resultant recoil of the metal strips and surface forces from the moist lip mucosa are sufficient in combination to keep the bars of the Ts in contact with the lips. As with the jaw transducer, pairs of strain gauges form two arms of a four-arm Wheatstone bridge for each unit, so that, when lip displacements place bending forces on the metal strips, resistance changes occur in the strain-gauge elements. The result is a changing output voltage that varies in direct proportion to the vertical displacement component of the lip being monitored. Again, as with the jaw-transducing unit, the analogue signals are in real-time and can be differentiated to determine the velocity and acceleration components of movement.

Figure 2–8B illustrates schematically a strain-gauge transducer developed to measure the force of lip activity (Kim, 1971). This unit provides a voltage output directly proportional to the net force generated by the activity of the two lips combined. As shown, a rigid strut supports a circular-shaped flat metal deflection beam whose ends come into contact with the upper and lower lips. The net displacement of the two lips induces a net strain on the metal beam that is reflected in the changing resistances of two strain gauges bonded to opposite sides of the circular beam. These gauges act as two arms of a four-arm Wheatstone bridge. Because the circular deflection beam functionally is similar to a spring, the net force generated by the lips in deflecting the ends of the beam is equal to the product of the spring constant and the net displacement of the beam's ends. Within the range of displacements involved in speech, the system behaves in a manner predictable by Hooke's law. Thus,

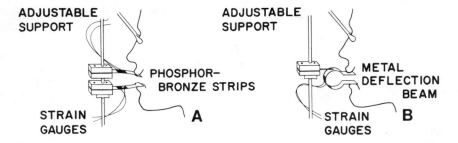

FIGURE 2-8. (A) Strain-gauge transducer for measuring vertical movements of the lips during speech. (B) Strain-gauge transducer for measuring the net force of lip activity during speech.

it is possible to estimate the net force of lip activity during speech in terms of the net displacement of the two ends of the deflection beam. Although this transducer system presents some interference to labial activity, it appears to represent as good a system as is available for measuring this aspect of speech mechanics.

As a last example of strain-gauge systems of recent origin, Figure 2-9 depicts a velar displacement transducer. This unit was fabricated directly after the prototype transducer built by Christiansen and colleagues (Christiansen and Moller, 1971; Moller and Christiansen, 1969; Moller, Martin, and Christiansen, 1971). The sensing unit consists of two strain gauges mounted on a cantilever beam that attaches by an orthodontic band or a tooth clip to a maxillary molar. A wire guard fixed to the assembly protects the cantilever beam inferiorly so that tongue movements will not create measurement artifacts by exerting forces on the beam. A finger spring extends from the cantilever beam to contact the velum at the midline and at about its middle third longitudinally. Vertical movements of the velum during speech result in displacements of the finger spring that in turn are resolved into bending of the cantilever beam. Strain gauges bonded to the beam respond to the bending forces, and, thereby, change the resistance in two arms of the Wheatstone circuit. The result, as with the other displacement devices just discussed, is an output voltage that represents velar displacement in an analogue form. Finally, as with the other techniques discussed, derivatives of this signal can be taken to determine other components of motion.

ELECTROMAGNETIC MEASUREMENTS OF ARTICULATORY MOTIONS

In addition to measuring articulatory motions with strain-gauge transducers, electromagnetic transducers called magnetometers may also be used (Hixon, 1971a; Mead et al., 1967). The general principles underlying magnetometer measurements were discussed earlier under "Body-Surface

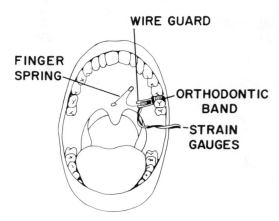

FIGURE 2-9. Strain-gauge transducer for measuring velar movements during speech.

Measurements.'' Unlike body-surface measurements, for which four coils are used, only one generating coil and either one or two sensing coils are used for measurements of articulatory motion. As an example of how electromagnetic techniques can be applied to measure articulatory motions, Figure 2–10A illustrates a method for measuring the vertical displacements of the mandible during speech (Hixon, 1971a). A generating coil (encased in polyethylene) is fixed to the undersurface of the jaw with the long axis of the coil oriented perpendicular to the sagittal plane. An identically oriented sensing coil is positioned atop the head so that it cannot be moved by facial gestures. Recall from earlier discussion (see ''Body-Surface Measurements'') that with the long axes of the generating and sensing coils oriented parallel, the voltage induced in the sensor is inversely proportional to the cube of the distance between the coils. Therefore, with the upper coil serving as a stable reference, vertical movements of the generating coil on the jaw induce voltage changes in the sensor and, thereby, provide a continuous real-time electrical equivalent of what may be conceptualized as the unidimensional movement of a point on the jaw. For practical purposes, this equivalent is related linearly to coil displacement, because the range of jaw motion encompassed in speech is small compared with the absolute intercoil distance. The sensing coil can be stabilized in other locations above or below the generating coil, but placement atop the head has the advantage of allowing the subject relatively free movement. Movement of the skin over the mandible results in some measurement artifact; however, the use of the generating coil on a special device attached to the lower incisors (Ohala, Hiki, Hubler, and Harshman, 1968) shows nearly comparable results to those obtained with the generator on the undersurface of the jaw. Additional information bearing on this point has been provided by Dr. Ronald W. Netsell (personal communication, March, 1970), who found displacement of a point on the undersurface of the jaw to

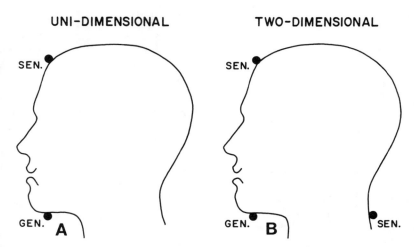

FIGURE 2-10. (A) Magnetometer coil arrangement for measuring vertical movements of the jaw during speech. (B) Coil arrangement for measuring simultaneous vertical and anteroposterior movements of the jaw.

agree, within a few percentage points, with vertical measurements obtained from tracings of cinefluorographic films showing displacement of the bony mandible.

Figure 2–10B shows a method for recording manidibular motions in two dimensions. In this method another sensing coil is added, this one positioned on the back of the subject's neck. Like its equivalent atop the head, the neck coil affords continuous measurement of the distance the generator is moved toward or away from it. With the two sensing coils stabilized and the generating coil riding with the mandible, simultaneous recordings of the two-dimensional movements of the generator are obtained. By displaying these two movements relative to each other, the two-dimensional movement of a point on the jaw within the sagittal plane can be visualized (Hixon, 1971a).

Attempts to measure the movements of other articulators have been encouraging; however, existing coils are too large (2 cm in length and 0.5 cm in diameter) for use within the vocal tract without significantly interfering with natural speech. This particular problem might be solved by constructing miniature coils that are mounted on tiny suction cups that will fix the coils to intraoral structures. Figure 2–11 shows some of the strategic points that may possibly be tracked in various dimensions during speech. Circles show locations on the lips, mandible, tongue (three points), velum, and posterior pharyngeal wall. The rectangle illustrates the long axis coil positioning that might be employed to study lateral pharyngeal wall movement. Of course, with the electromagnetic procedures considered in this section the investigator

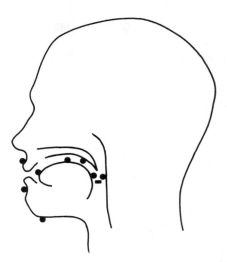

FIGURE 2-11. Strategic generating coil placements on the articulators where measurements with miniature magnetometers should be profitable.

has the option of examining both the velocity and acceleration of movements of the various articulatory structures, as was seen to be the case for strain-gauge displacement monitors.

Finally, those wishing to pursue techniques based on electromagnetic principles also might consider the use of recently developed magnistors,[4] which are tiny magnetic-sensing transistor chips. These devices show promise of further miniaturization than may be possible with magnetometer coil systems.

UPPER AIRWAY AND TRANSGLOTTAL
FLOW MEASUREMENTS

An important manifestation of motion in the speech production apparatus is flow. Flow measurements are of interest in a number of locations, two of the most important of which are at the airway opening (at the mouth, the nose, or both) and transglottally (across the larynx). One of the procedures used to measure flow from the upper airway during speech is illustrated in Figure 2–12. The system is a slightly improved version of a prototype system designed by Mead (Mead, 1960; Klatt, Stevens, and Mead, 1968). A large mask is placed over the subject's face and secured by a head harness. This mask contains a rubber diaphragm with a center opening into which the subject's face is fitted and which facilitates formation of an airtight seal between the subject and the mask. The perimeter of the mask is firm but sufficiently compliant to permit

---

[4]Manufactured by the Hudson Corporation, Box 867, Manchester, NH 03105.

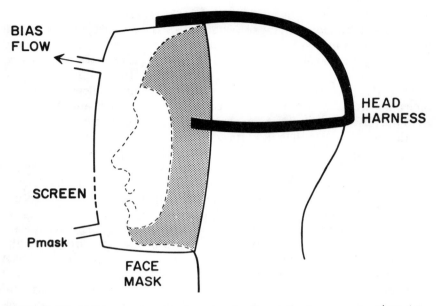

FIGURE 2-12. Full-face mask system for measuring flow at the airway opening (V̇ao) during speech.

the subject's articulators (including the jaw) relatively free motion without significant encumbrance to natural articulation. The front wall of the mask is formed by a lucite face plate and contains a relatively large opening covered by a metal screen. This screen serves as a linear resistance to flow into and out of the mask during speech or breathing activities. A bias flow moves air at a constant rate through the mask and thereby has several useful purposes: it prevents condensation of moisture on the metal screen (otherwise screen resistance would change), it helps to reduce dead space within the mask, and it helps to keep the subject relatively cool and comfortable. Pressure within the mask is sensed by a transducer and taken as a measure of flow through the metal screen at every instant. The mask is built so that a metal screen area of various sizes is available for different studies. Selection of screen size depends on the range of flows to be encountered in a given study and is made to ensure that the mask pressure signal will be related linearly to flow through the screen. The part of the mask pressure signal related to the bias flow can be taken into account as baseline offset or it can be zero suppressed electronically (Klatt et al., 1968). As the subject speaks into the mask system, flow from the airway opening is sensed along with flow related to changes in mask volume caused by displacements of various articulatory structures and the walls of the mask itself. The latter component of flow is an artifact for most measurement purposes; however, it is relatively small for most speakers and dependent on the speech sampled. The overall system described here surmounts many of the measurement system objections that are raised routinely against the use of other types of masks for speech research (Hardy, 1965; Hixon, 1966; Lubker, 1970; Lubker and Moll, 1965; Subtelny, Worth, and Sakuda, 1966). First, the present system places insignificant restriction on natural articulatory movements. Second, the bias flow feature surmounts all of the physiological objections that have been raised to the use of masks, such as problems with their dead space and discomfort for the subject. These are objections that can be met in any mask system simply by incorporating a bias flow feature.

Techniques previously have not been available for measuring flow across the larynx during speech, except to the extent that such measurements can be made at the airway opening during utterances when the articulators are relatively stationary (e.g., sustained vowels) and, therefore, are not themselves creating flows (Gilbert and Hixon, 1969). A procedure to circumvent the articulatory displacement problem and, thus, obtain a measure of transglottal flow, is illustrated schematically in Figure 2–13. The subject is seated in the multipurpose chamber, the door of the chamber being open in this configuration. A collar is used to form an airtight seal between the subject's neck and the top of the chamber through which the subject's head and neck are protruding. A lucite dome is positioned over the subject's head and latched

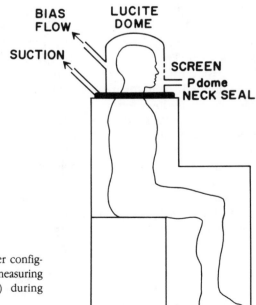

FIGURE 2–13. Chamber configuration (door open) for measuring transglottal flow (Vtg) during speech.

airtight to the top of the chamber. Together, the collar and dome form a small chamber that completely encases the speech apparatus from the larynx outward. A metal screen is built into the wall of the dome and serves as a linear resistance to flow into or out of the chamber. Dome pressure is taken as a measure of flow through this screen at every instant during speech. As in the flow system discussed previously, a bias flow is used to handle the problems of subject comfort, dead space, and moisture collection on the screen. The subject's articulatory apparatus is entirely free of the types of encumbrances offered by other flow-measuring devices used routinely. In addition, because the walls of the head chamber are rigid, unlike those of the face mask system discussed previously, articulatory motions cannot distort the shape of the chamber so that it will itself displace volume. During moments of articulation when the vocal tract is open to the dome, displacements of articulatory structures (e.g., lips, cheeks, neck) are not registered as flow events, because the net volumes of the articulators themselves are not changing. During articulatory events when the vocal tract is closed to the dome (e.g., as during a voiced stop) an estimate of transglottal flow is still obtained, because flow through the larynx is reflected in displacements of the cheeks and neck, which, in turn, cause volumes to be displaced inside the dome, these displacements being realized as flow through the dome screen. A small, but potential, source of error in such measurement is the compression or expansion of gas within the vocal tract. This can be taken into account through simultaneous measurements of oral pressure, although corrections for this factor represent very small adjustments. As discussed here, then, measurements of transglottal flow can be obtained during states when the vocal tract is either open or closed, the latter being a case in which internal flow from the respiratory pump to the upper airway can be measured.[5] This measurement would be recognized by the experimental phonetician as an important bit of mechanical information during the stop phase of voiced plosives when voicing continues momentarily after closure of the vocal tract and flow continues transglottally. Such measurements are impossible with conventional flow-measuring devices (Gilbert and Hixon, 1969; Isshiki and Ringel, 1964) because closure at different valving points along the vocal tract precludes flow from the airway opening.

---

[5]Another approach for measuring transglottal flow during speech uses the plethysmographic principles discussed under "Volume-Pressure Body Plethysmography." After correcting the volume signal from the chamber to make possible the measurement of rapid volume events, the volume analogue can be differentiated to obtain a measure of flow at the chest wall. Such flow differs from transglottal flow only to the extent that part of the motion of the chest wall is related to gas compression (and decompression). This is a small component compared to the volume displacement component, so that flow of the chest wall reflects transglottal flow to a good approximation. The advantage of this approach over the dome approach discussed in text is that the head is unencumbered and accurate acoustic recordings can be made, if desired. The dome technique is emphasized here because it can be combined easily with the technique discussed for measuring alveolar pressure.

SIMULTANEOUS MEASUREMENTS OF ALVEOLAR PRESSURE AND TRANSGLOTTAL FLOW: VARIATIONS ON TWO THEMES

In preceding sections techniques have been considered for measuring transglottal flow and alveolar pressure. Each of these measurements gives information about the mechanical behavior of the speech apparatus. In combination, they become more than additive instructively, revealing much about the status of the laryngeal valve and how the respiratory pump acts on and interacts with the larynx during speech. Figure 2–14 illustrates how these aerodynamic aspects of speech can be measured simultaneously by combining the essential features of the techniques discussed previously under "Plethysmographic Measurement of Alveolar Pressure" and "Upper Airway and Transglottal Flow Measurements" (Hixon and Warren, 1971). The subject is seated inside the chamber and is wearing a neck seal. The door of the chamber is closed, the lucite dome is over the subject's head and secured to the top of the chamber, and the air conditioner is turned on. A fine metal screen built into the body of the neck seal takes the place, in principle, of the screen within the wall of the dome, as described previously. Transglottal flow is measured as the pressure differential between the two sides of this screen (i.e., P dome – P chamber) with flow from the dome being directed back into the body

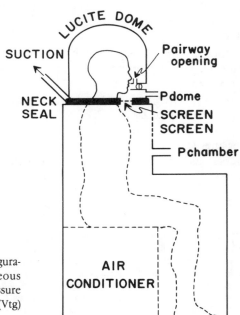

FIGURE 2–14. Chamber configuration for making simultaneous measurements of alveolar pressure (Palv) and transglottal flow (Vtg) during speech.

chamber rather than being permitted to escape to the atmosphere. To ensure accuracy of measurement of rapid events of interest, the mechanical time constants of the dome and body chambers are adjusted empirically to be equal. The feature of not permitting air to escape from the total system dictates that the only volume change sensed by the plethysmograph is that related to compression (and decompression) of gas within the subject. This means that measurements of alveolar pressure can be made along the lines discussed in the section on "Plethysmographic Measurement of Alveolar Pressure." When both transglottal flow and alveolar pressure are in analogue forms, the investigator is able not only to record them continuously but also to make use of on-line electronic computations to provide real-time readouts of aerodynamic power and impedance. Of final concern with reference to the configuration shown in Figure 2–14 is the fact that estimates of changes in lung volume also can be obtained along with measurements of transglottal flow and alveolar pressure. These estimates reside in the first time integral of the transglottal flow analogue, which, as has been seen, is provided via continuous measurement of the pressure differential across the screen of the neck seal (Chistovich and Kozhevnikov, 1969; Hixon and Warren, 1971).

ULTRASONIC SCANS OF THE TONGUE

In speech, the mechanical significance of the upper airway depends in part on the changing geometry of its boundaries. An obvious major determiner of this geometry is the dorsal surface of the tongue, a boundary that can assume a variety of configurations and that runs nearly the entire length coordinate of the vocal tract. A new methodological development which allows the visualization of the tongue's dorsal surface when the tongue is stationary, is ultrasonic scanning. This technique (Minifie, Kelsey, Zagzebski, and King, 1971) provides data in the form of echograms of the dorsal surface of the tongue in different planes. As examples of the types of visualization that are possible, longitudinal and transverse echograms will be considered. In x-ray parlance, these represent the equivalent of lateral and coronal-oblique views, respectively. In the present method, pulsed ultrasound (Kelsey, Minifie, and Hixon, 1968) is generated by a 2.25 MHz transducer and transmitted through the tongue mass to the tissue-air interface along the dorsal surface of the tongue. The impedance change at this interface causes much of the transmitted energy to be reflected back to the generating site, where it is sensed by the same transducer acting as a receiver. The echoes received are processed as a series of dots in a B-scan mode (Kelsey et al., 1968), the resulting composite of echoes providing a two-dimensional view of the tongue that is displayed on the screen of an ultrasonoscope.

Figure 2–15A shows the transducer movement pathway followed to obtain longitudinal echograms of the dorsal surface of the tongue in the midsaggital plane. Such scans are obtained by moving the ultrasonic probe in compound sector motions from a midline position on the anterior neck wall at the level of the larynx upward to the mandibular symphysis. For a complete scan this procedure takes approximately 3 seconds, during which the subject must maintain a constant tongue position. A sample echogram obtained with the procedure described is shown in Figure 2–16. In this figure, the tongue is shown in a resting configuration, with the facial contour also being shown to aid in appreciating the relative position of the tongue within the head. The facial outline was obtained by passing the transducer probe over the subject's face with the ultrasonoscope set at minimum gain. This procedure shows only the changing position of the ultrasonic probe itself. The diverging straight lines in Figure 2–16 are scan lines made by brightening the ultrasonoscope at various points to provide identification of locations for transverse scans that were made in the experiment from which this echogram is taken. Longitudinal echograms of the type shown in Figure 2–16 can be obtained during various speech utterances, the only provision being that the utterances must be of a sustainable nature to allow time for the scan to be completed.

Figure 2–15B depicts the transducer movement pathway for obtaining transverse echograms of the tongue as well as coronal facial contours. There the scanning direction has been rotated 90 degrees relative to the scanning direction for longitudinal echograms of the tongue. Again, scans are obtained by moving the transducer probe in compound sector motions in a given plane. Some sample transverse echograms are shown in Figure 2–17. Each of these was obtained by scanning in the coronal-oblique plane through the inferior surface of the chin and the tongue blade. Figure 2–17A shows a slightly convex curvature of the tongue blade during a sustained /u/ production. Figure 2–17B

FIGURE 2–15. Transducer movement pathways for obtaining ultrasonic echograms of the dorsal surface of the tongue. (A) Longitudinal scan in the midsagittal plane. (B) Transverse scan in a coronal-oblique plane.

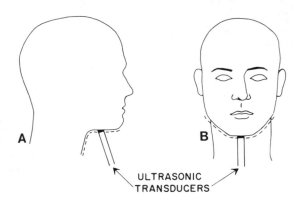

ULTRASONIC TRANSDUCERS

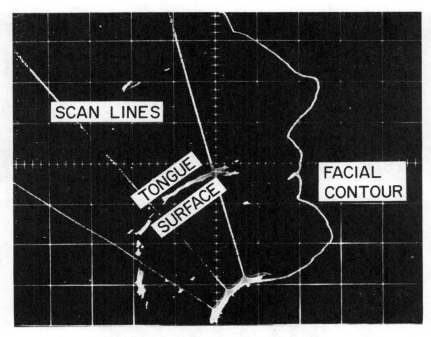

FIGURE 2–16. Longitudinal echogram of the dorsal surface of the tongue at rest. The facial contour is shown, as are three scan lines along which transverse scans usually are made. (From Minifie, F., et al: Ultrasonic scans of the dorsal surface of the tongue. *Journal of the Acoustical Society of America, 49,* 1857–1860, 1971. Used by permission.)

shows the markedly convex tongue blade configuration when the tongue is at rest, whereas Figure 2–17C depicts the concave surface of the tongue blade observed during a production of /ʃ/. Facial contours in the three echograms show the inferior and lateral outline of the jaw.

Taken together the two scan views discussed provide an effective means for mapping tongue contours during sustained utterances. Unfortunately, dynamic articulatory movements cannot be monitored with the techniques described, although such monitoring may be possible in the future. As pointed out by Minifie and colleagues (1971), commercial ultrasonic scanners are now available that make it possible to visualize linear scans at rates of 16 per sec. They suggest that, if such scanners can be modified to provide rapid compound sector scans, it may be possible to monitor dynamic articulatory movements of the tongue during utterance. Such an advancement would be welcomed by speech physiologists concerned with comprehensive studies of tongue dynamics without the hazards of x-ray procedures.

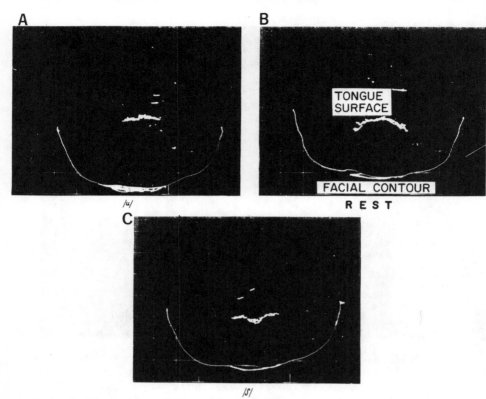

FIGURE 2–17. Transverse (coronal-oblique) echograms of the dorsal surface of the tongue, under three conditions. The jaw contour is shown. (A) Sustained /u/ production. (B) The tongue at rest. (C) Sustained /ʃ/ production. (From Minifie, F., et al: Ultrasonic scans of the dorsal surface of the tongue. *Journal of the Acoustical Society of America, 49,* 1857–1860, 1971. Used by permission.)

LASER HOLOGRAPHIC INTERFEROGRAMS: THE STUDY OF SPEECH MOVEMENTS

Some parts of the speech apparatus are arranged such that portions of their boundaries are visible on the exterior surface of the torso, head, or neck regions (e.g., the abdominal wall and cheeks). Other parts lie deep to these visible surfaces but nevertheless have part of their boundaries revealed through external geometric landmarks that are more or less obvious in different speakers (e.g., the costal margin and the thyroid prominence). Because the activities of both of these types of parts are to some extent reflected by the surface motions they create, it is instructive to be able to visualize the patterns of motion distributed over the exterior of the speech apparatus. A technique that shows rather provocative potential for being able to provide such a visualization is laser holographic interferometry. Although the present laboratory is only beginning to use such methods, the successful use of laser holographic interferograms by Zivi and Humberstone (1970) in the study of respiratory physiology leads to the belief that interferograms will be a useful new tool for speech research. Figure 2–18 illustrates schematically the experimental arrangement used to obtain interferograms of the surface of a subject (Zivi and Humberstone, 1970). Double-pulsed ruby laser holography is used to produce an image of the patterns of motion of a target, which in this instance is the anterior torso, neck, and head regions of a human. The data provided are in the form of a complex diffraction gradient on photographic film, a gradient caused by the interference of two coherent light beams from the same laser source. The target structures are located in one of the beams whereas a reference beam provides wavelength and phase information about the laser output. The reference beam and the light reflected by the target are combined at the photographic film, with the interference between the two beams providing the needed diffraction gradient. Subsequent illumination of the diffraction gradient by a laser simulating the reference beam results in diffracted rays that duplicate those that originally came from the target structure, the result being that a three-dimensional image of the target appears in the position occupied previously by the target. In the use of double-pulsed interferometry (Zivi and Humberstone, 1970) a double-exposure hologram is made of the target. Target movement between the two exposures results in a photographic image that shows the target in the two positions at the instants of the double pulsing of the laser. When the two images reconstructed by the hologram are superimposed, they show interference fringes on the imaged target, fringes that provide quantitative information on the movement of the target between the two exposures. Therefore, without touching the subject, it is possible to both visualize and measure the motions of body surfaces during physiological processes. This capability is illustrated

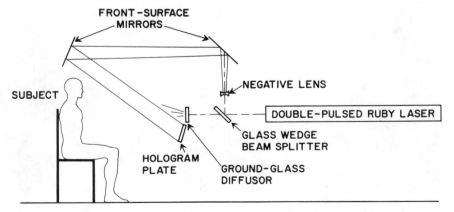

FIGURE 2–18. Experimental arrangement for obtaining laser holographic interferograms of the surface of a speaker. Modified from Zivi and Humberstone (1970).

in Figure 2–19, which shows a photograph of a reconstructed holographic image of a subject performing a maximally forced vital capacity maneuver into a mouthpiece. This somewhat psychedelic image was made by causing a ruby laser to double-pulse with an interval between pulses of 150 μsec. Because the target moved only slightly between pulses, the subject himself does not appear to have moved; however, the interference fringes in the picture indicate

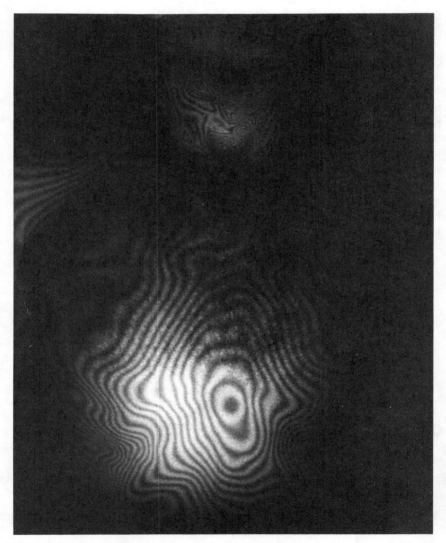

FIGURE 2–19. Photograph of a reconstructed holographic image of a subject during the performance of a maximally forced vital capacity maneuver. Provided by courtesy of S. M. Zivi, Laser Products Manager, Physical Research Center, TRW Instruments, El Segundo, CA 90245.

the nature of the movement pattern which actually occurred between laser exposures. Dark fringes in the image show points on the subject that moved between exposures by an amount such that the light reflected from the second laser pulse was shifted one-half wavelength with respect to the corresponding ray from the first pulse (Zivi and Humberstone, 1970). Although quantitative interpretation of Figure 2–19 is possible, it will suffice here to interpret the interferogram qualitatively. Except for areas where motion of the target is not approximately toward the hologram, all points on a given dark fringe are traveling at the same velocity. Closed loops made by dark fringes indicate that the surface outlined by the loop is becoming more or less curved. The large number of fringes show that considerable movement occurred on the chest-abdomen surface during the vital capacity maneuver. From knowing the direction of body surface displacement, the investigator can infer that the series of closed loops in this area shows the surface to be flattening during the expiration. The maximum displacement appears to be at the torso midline. Much less motion during the maneuver seems to have occurred in the lateral pectoral regions of the chest, because few fringes are noted there. The cheek area shows several closed loop fringes that seem to fit the reasonable interpretation that the cheek is moving outward like a drum membrane because of the large transmural pressure during the forced expiration. Areas of the neck also appear to move somewhat like a drum membrane, as can be noted below the mandible and above the suprasternal notch area.

It only can be conjectured what the potential applications of interferograms in speech research might be. Any application involving the study of the nature of motion patterns is an obvious potential use of the holographic technique. The technique may be useful, for example, in estimating the volumes displaced by various parts of the speech apparatus. When combined with pressure measurements, such estimates may permit estimates of regional resistances and compliances. It already has been demonstrated that the technique can be used to study the influence of vocally induced vibrations as their effect is realized in surface motions of a speaker (Zivi and Humberstone, 1970). Because interferograms provide information about some structures near the external surface of the body, they seem a likely candidate for a method of tracking changes in laryngeal height during speech. Finally, Zivi and Humberstone (1970) have suggested that quantitative measurements could be made of the mechanical response of selected muscles as they are electrically stimulated. Such information would be of obvious value to those who are interested in the speech of subjects with neurologically based disorders.

CONCLUSIONS

This chapter has been an attempt to bring to the reader's awareness some new "ways of knowing" about the biomechanical behavior of the speech apparatus. Some specific applications of these ways of knowing have been considered. The hope is that the chapter at the same time provided a broad enough general treatment of the topics discussed herein that with a minimum of creativity they can be extended to the research and clinical problems of others. On reviewing what is said in this chapter, two things in particular appear striking: The first is how much more probably would be understood about speech mechanisms if, in talking about them, more people considered the speech apparatus in totality rather than as a collection of parts functioning somewhat independently of one another. The second is how many different disciplines have made contributions to the ideas outlined in this chapter (e.g., physiology, speech-language pathology, dentistry, biology, engineering, electronics, acoustics, physics). This second point strikes particularly hard because it seems obvious that humankind would be much further advanced on topics such as those considered here were each worker a little less provincial in his or her approach to problems. This, of course, is what chapters such as this one are all about—broadening interdisciplinary perspective.

ACKNOWLEDGMENT

The preparation of this manuscript was supported by Research Grant No. NS 09656 and Research Career Development Award No. 1 K4 NS 41350 from the National Institute of Neurological Diseases and Stroke.

REFERENCES

Abbs, J. (1971). The influence of the gamma motor system on jaw movement during speech. Doctoral Dissertation, University of Wisconsin.

Abbs, J., and Netsell, R. (1970). *The inferential role of the gamma loop in speech production: A new application of an old technique.* Paper presented at the Annual Convention of the American Speech and Hearing Association, New York.

Abbs, J., and Netsell, R. (1971). *An interpretation of continuous articulator acceleration as a muscle forcing function.* Paper presented at the spring meeting of the Acoustical Society of America, Washington, DC.

Agostoni, E., and Mead, J. (1964). Statics of the respiratory system (pp. 387–409). *In* W. Fenn and H. Rahn (Eds.): *Handbook of physiology. Respiration 1, Sect. 3.* Washington, DC: American Physiological Society.

Agostoni, E., and Rahn, H. (1960). Abdominal and thoracic pressures at different lung volumes. *Journal of Applied Physiology, 15,* 1087–1092.

Arutjunjan, E., Granstrem, M., and Kozhevnikov, V. (1967). *Some characteristics of the respiratory system acting in speech.* Paper presented at the Seventh International Conference on Medical and Biological Engineering, Stockholm.

Bouhuys, A., Proctor, D., and Mead, J. (1966). Kinetic aspects of singing. *Journal of Applied Physiology, 21,* 483–496.

Chistovich, L., and Kozhevnikov, V. (1969). Some aspects of the physiological study of speech (pp. 305–321). *In* L. Proctor (Ed.): *Biocybernetics of the central nervous system.* Boston: Little, Brown.

Christiansen, R., and Moller, K. (1971). Instrumentation for recording velar movement. *American Journal of*

Orthodontics, 59, 448–455.

Collins, W. E., Inc. (1957). *Clinical spirometry: Instructions for use of the Collins respirometer and for calculation and interpretation of data in pulmonary function and basal metabolism testing.* Boston: Warren E. Collins, Inc.

Draper, M., Ladefoged, P., and Whitteridge, D. (1959). Respiratory muscles in speech. *Journal of Speech and Hearing Research, 2,* 16–27.

DuBois, A., Botelho, S., and Comroe, J., Jr. (1956). A new method for measuring airway resistance in man using a body plethysmograph: Values in normal subjects and in patients with respiratory disease. *Journal of Clinical Investigation, 35,* 327–335.

DuBois, A., Brody, A., Louis, D., and Burgess, B., Jr. (1956). Oscillation mechanics of lungs and chest in man. *Journal of Applied Physiology, 8,* 587–594.

Duomarco, J., and Rimini, R. (1947). *La presion intra-abdominal en el hombre.* Buenos Aires: El Aterneo.

Finucane, K., Dawson, S., Phelan, P., Green, I., Wohl, M., and Mead, J. (1970). *Frequency dependence of lower airway resistance in man.* Paper presented at the 54th annual meeting of the Federation of American Societies for Experimental Biology, Atlantic City.

French, J. (1966). A variable inductance linear displacement transducer. *Journal of Medical and Biological Engineering, 4,* 495–497.

French, J., and Siebens, A. (1969). *Real-time elimination of the electrocardiogram from the integrated electromyogram of the diaphragm.* Paper presented at the Eighth International Conference on Medical and Biological Engineering, Chicago.

Gilbert, H., and Hixon, T. (1969). *Oral airflow during stop consonant production.* Paper presented at the Annual Convention of the American Speech and Hearing Association, Chicago.

Goldman, M., Knudson, R., Mead, J., Peterson, N., Schwaber, J., and Wohl, M.

(1970). A simplified measurement of respiratory resistance by forced oscillation. *Journal of Applied Physiology, 28,* 113–116.

Grimby, G., Takishima, T., Graham, W., Macklem, P., and Mead, J. (1968). Frequency dependence of flow resistance in patients with obstructive lung disease. *Journal of Clinical Investigation, 47,* 1455–1465.

Hardy, J. (1965). Air flow and air pressure studies. *Proceedings of the Conference Communicative Problems in Cleft Palate. ASHA Reports Number 1,* 141–152.

Hardy, J., and Edmonds, T. (1968). Electronic integrator for measurement of partitions of the lung volume. *Journal of Speech and Hearing Research, 11,* 777–786.

Hixon, T. (1966). Turbulent noise sources for speech. *Folia Phoniatrica, 18,* 168–182.

Hixon, T. (1970). *Respiratory mechanics during speech production.* Paper presented at the meeting of the American Association for the Advancement of Science, Chicago.

Hixon, T. (1971a). An electromagnetic method for transducing jaw movements during speech. *Journal of the Acoustical Society of America, 49,* 603–606.

Hixon, T. (1971b). *Mechanical aspects of speech production, 1: The respiratory pump.* Paper presented at the Annual Convention of the American Speech and Hearing Association, Chicago.

Hixon, T., Klatt, D., and Mead, J. (1970). *Influence of forced transglottal pressure changes on vocal fundamental frequency.* Paper presented at the fall meeting of the Acoustical Society of America, Houston.

Hixon, T., Mead, J., and Goldman, M. (1970). *Separate volume changes of the rib cage and abdomen during speech.* Paper presented at the Annual Convention of the American Speech and Hearing Association, New York.

Hixon, T., Minifie, F., Peyrot, A., and Siebens, A. (1968). *Mechanical behavior of the diaphragm during speech production.* Paper presented at the fall meeting of the Acoustical Society of America, Cleveland.

Hixon, T., Siebens, A., and Ewanowski, S. (1968). *Respiratory mechanics during speech production.* Paper presented at the spring meeting of the Acoustical Society of America, Ottawa.

Hixon, T., Siebens, A., and Minifie, F. (1969). An EMG electrode for the diaphragm. *Journal of the Acoustical Society of America*, 46, 1588–1590.

Hixon, T., and Warren, D. (1971). *Use of plethysmographic techniques in speech research: Two laboratories' experiences.* Paper presented at the Annual Convention of the American Speech and Hearing Association, Chicago.

Isshiki, N., and Ringel, R. (1964). Air flow during the production of selected consonants. *Journal of Speech and Hearing Research*, 7, 233–244.

Kelsey, C., Minifie, F., and Hixon, T. (1968). Applications of ultrasound in speech research. *Journal of Speech and Hearing Research*, 12, 564–575.

Kim, B. (1971). *A physiological study of the production mechanisms of Korean stop consonants.* Doctoral Dissertation, University of Wisconsin.

Klatt, D., Stevens, K., and Mead, J. (1968). Studies of articulatory activity and airflow during speech. *Annals of the New York Academy of Science*, 155, 42–55.

Konno, K., and Mead, J. (1967). Measurement of the separate volume changes of rib cage and abdomen during breathing. *Journal of Applied Physiology*, 22, 407–422.

Kunze, L. (1964). Evaluation of methods of estimating sub-glottal air pressure. *Journal of Speech and Hearing Research*, 7, 151–164.

Lieberman, P., Knudson, R., and Mead, J. (1969). Determination of the rate of change of fundamental frequency with respect to subglottal air pressure during sustained phonation. *Journal of the Acoustical Society of America*, 45, 1537–1543.

Lubker, J. (1970). Aerodynamic and ultrasonic assessment techniques in speech-dentofacial research. *Proceedings of the Workshop Speech and the Dentofacial Complex: The State of the Art. ASHA Reports Number 5*, 207–223.

Lubker, J., and Moll, K. (1965). Simultaneous oral-nasal air flow measurements and cinefluorographic observations during speech production. *Cleft Palate Journal*, 2, 257–272.

Mead, J. (1960). Volume displacement body plethysmograph for respiratory measurements in human subjects. *Journal of Applied Physiology*, 15, 736–740.

Mead, J. (1968). A summary of one laboratory's experience with body plethysmography. *In* H. Herzog (Ed.): *Respiration*. Basel: S. Karger.

Mead, J., and Milic-Emili, J. (1964). Theory and methodology in respiratory mechanics with glossary of symbols (pp. 363–376). *In* W. Fenn and H. Rahn (Eds.): *Handbook of physiology. Respiration 1, Sect. 3*. Washington, DC: American Physiological Society.

Mead, J., Peterson, N., Grimby, G., and Mead, J. (1967). Pulmonary ventilation measured from body surface movements. *Science*, 156, 1383–1384.

Mead, W., and Collins, V. (1954). The principles of dilatancy applied to techniques of radiotherapy. *American Journal of Roentgenology, Radium Therapy, and Nuclear Medicine*, 71 864–866.

Milic-Emili, J., Mead, J., Turner, J., and Glauser, E. (1964). Improved technique for estimating pleural pressure from esophageal balloons. *Journal of Applied Physiology*, 19, 207–211.

Minifie, F., Kelsey, C., Zagzebski, J., and King, T. (1971). Ultrasonic scans of the dorsal surface of the tongue. *Journal of the Acoustical Society of America*, 49, 1857–1860.

Moller, K., and Christiansen, R. (1969). *Instrumentation for recording velar movement.* Paper presented at the Annual Convention of the American Speech and Hearing Association, Chicago.

Moller, K., Martin, R., and Christiansen, R. (1971). A technique for recording velar movement. *Cleft Palate Journal*, 8, 263–276.

Ohala, J., Hiki, S., Hubler, S., and Harshman, R. (1968). Photoelectric methods of transducing lip and jaw movements in speech. *UCLA Working Papers in Phonetics*, 10, 135–144.

Perkins, W., and Koike, Y. (1969). Patterns of subglottal pressure variation during phonation. *Folia Phoniatrica*, 21, 1–8.

Peslin, R., Hixon, T., and Mead, J. (1971). Variation des resistances thoracopulmonaires au cours du cycle ventilatoire etudiees par methode d'oscillation (Variations of thoraco-pulmonary resistance during the respiratory cycle, studied by forced oscillations). *Bulletin of Physio-Pathological Research*, 7, 173–186.

Peyrot, A., Hertel, G., and Siebens, A. (1969). Pulmonary ventilation measured by a single linear displacement transducer. *Journal of Medical and Biological Engineering*, 7, 1–2.

Subtelny, J., Worth, J., and Sakuda, M. (1966). Intraoral pressure and rate of flow during speech. *Journal of Speech and Hearing Research*, 9, 498–518.

Sussman, H., and Smith, K. (1970). Transducer for measuring mandibular movements. *Journal of Acoustical Society of America*, 48, 857–858.

Van den Berg, J. (1956). Direct and indirect determination of the mean subglottic pressure. *Folia Phoniatrica*, 8, 1–24.

Zivi, S., and Humberstone, G. (1970). Chest motion visualized by holographic interferometry. *Medical Research in Engineering*, 9, 5–7.

CHAPTER 3

Kinematics of the Chest Wall During Speech Production: Volume Displacements of the Rib Cage, Abdomen, and Lung

Thomas J. Hixon
Michael D. Goldman
Jere Mead

I nvestigations of the volume events of speech production have been concerned primarily with lung volume changes, as measured at the airway opening (mouth) with spirometers (Hoshiko, 1965) or flowmeters (volume obtained by integration) (Hardy and Edmonds, 1968), or at the body surface via volume displacement body plethysmographs (Bouhuys, Proctor, and Mead, 1966; Draper, Ladefoged, and Whitteridge, 1959). How such volume changes are partitioned among various parts of the respiratory apparatus (e.g., the rib cage, diaphragm, and abdomen) is unknown, although it is a matter of

Reprinted by permission of the publisher from the *Journal of Speech and Hearing Research,* *16*, pp. 78–115, © 1973, American Speech-Language-Hearing Association, Rockville, MD.

fundamental importance to understanding the physiological bases of both normal and abnormal speech production. This chapter presents data on lung volume changes during speech and how those changes can be ascribed to the separate volume displacements of two respiratory parts, namely the rib cage and the abdomen. The measurement approach used incorporates the essential features of two developments in the field of respiratory physiology: first, a method for estimating separately the volume displacements of the surfaces of the rib cage and abdomen by measuring changes in their respective anteroposterior diameters (Konno and Mead, 1967); and second, an improved transducer system for making such diameter measurements (Mead, Peterson, Grimby, and Mead, 1967). Although the theoretical basis for the measurement approach is discussed in detail elsewhere (Konno and Mead, 1967), it is likely to be unfamiliar to many speech researchers. Therefore, for present purposes and the reader's convenience, the following section offers a brief account of the measurement principles involved.

THEORY

The term *chest wall* is used by speech researchers and respiratory physiologists to mean different things. Speech workers typically use *chest wall* when referring to the visible outer surface of the thorax, whereas physiologists use the term to designate collectively all extrapulmonary parts of the body that share changes in the volume of the lungs. It is in this latter sense that the term *chest wall* is used here; so defined, it includes, except for the lungs and airways, all parts of the respiratory apparatus: the rib cage, the diaphragm, and the abdomen and its contents. From the viewpoint of anatomy, the rib cage, diaphragm, and abdomen constitute three different but interconnected structures, each of which forms a wall, and as a group are arranged to form the two major cavities of the torso. The rib cage and diaphragm form the thoracic cavity, and they delimit most of the surface boundary of the lungs to which they are linked through pleural forces. The abdominal cavity is defined by the diaphragm and abdominal wall. The contents of this cavity are the hydraulic equivalent of so much liquid, and as such they represent an incompressible mass lying between the diaphragm and abdominal wall. (The volume of gas in the intestinal tract is small—about 100 milliliters [ml] on the average—and may be neglected.) Given this property of the abdominal contents, it becomes profitable to think of the diaphragm, abdominal contents, and abdominal wall as a single structure, albeit a thick one, of which the diaphragm and abdominal wall represent the inner and outer surfaces of the structure and the abdominal contents represent the major bulk. From this viewpoint, the three-structure anatomical model of the chest wall (i.e., the rib cage, diaphragm, and abdomen and its contents) is reduced conceptually to a two-structure model involving the rib cage and the "diaphragm-abdomen."

To a useful approximation, the rib cage and diaphragm-abdomen may be regarded as individual parts of the chest wall, a part being defined in kinematic terms as a mechanism that displaces volume as it moves. In the case of the chest wall, one surface of each of these parts is visible externally, whereas together they encompass an area on the body that is coextensive with that of the torso. Because volumes displaced by the body surface are equal to those displaced by pulmonary structures, the combined displacements of the rib cage wall and the abdominal wall reflect the total lung volume change. Each of the two parts seems to move as a unit during breathing and, despite their sharing a common boundary at the costal margin, there is considerable functional separation between them. Witness to the latter is the ability to change lung volume mainly through displacement of either the rib cage wall or the abdominal wall, and the ability to produce paradoxical movements in which the volume displacement of one or the other of the parts is contradictory in sign to lung volume change. An example of the latter is an expiration in which the rib cage is decreasing in size and the abdomen is simultaneously displacing outward.

Two investigations have shown empirically (Konno and Mead, 1967; Peyrot, Hertel, and Siebens, 1969) that under most circumstances each of the two parts of the chest wall has volume change as the only independent variable with respect to its motion. Stated otherwise, each part has a single degree of freedom or way in which to move, so that it exhibits a fixed shape at any particular volume of the part. The chest wall itself, because it is an arrangement of moving parts that displace volume, constitutes a "system." The number of degrees of freedom in this system depends on whether it is open or closed. With the respiratory airways open to atmosphere, the system can exchange volume with its surroundings and has two degrees of freedom (i.e., two different ways in which to move), one for each of the two moving parts, the rib cage wall and the abdominal wall. This is the condition that prevails in ordinary breathing in which volume exchange is permitted with the surroundings through the open larynx and upper airway. Under such circumstances, changes in lung volume can be accomplished with either part of the chest wall, or through any combination of relative displacements of the two parts, there being two parallel pathways (the rib cage wall and the diaphragm-abdomen) capable of sharing volume changes with the lungs. By contrast, when the system is closed, it cannot exchange volume with its surroundings (i.e., its volume is constant), and any changes in volume must take place between the two parts of the system (the rib cage and the abdominal wall). When either the larynx or upper airway is closed, therefore, the system's parts are serially arranged and the chest wall has only one way in which to move or one degree of freedom. Unlike the open-system condition, in which the two parts can displace volume relatively independently, the closed-system condition represents a circumstance in which the volumes displaced by the two parts of the system are highly interdependent. Because, when the system is closed, volume can only be exchanged between the two parts, once the volume displaced by either the rib cage or the abdomen is determined, that of the other part must be equal and opposite. Figure 3-1 illustrates schematically these closed-system relationships with reference to changes in the configuration of the chest wall. The system is shown in three different conditions, all having in common the same lung volume. Panel (A) shows the chest wall relaxed at the functional residual capacity (FRC), whereas in panels (B) and (C), also at FRC, as much volume as possible has been shifted into and out of the rib cage, respectively. The displacement of volume in this manner and the accompanying change in chest wall configuration are accomplished through the use of respiratory muscles. The displacement of volume back and forth between the two parts of the system at constant lung volume is called an "isovolume maneuver." Although a complete isovolume maneuver involves the maximal shifting of volume back and forth between the surfaces of the rib cage and abdomen, a general appreciation for the maneuver can be gained by alternately contracting and relaxing one's abdominal muscles with the larynx closed.

To the extent that each of the two parts of the chest wall exhibits a fixed shape at a given volume of the part, all motions of points within a part must bear fixed relationships to the volumes that part displaces. It follows that volume displacements can be estimated from measurements of motions of a single point within the part in question, after, of course, the relationship

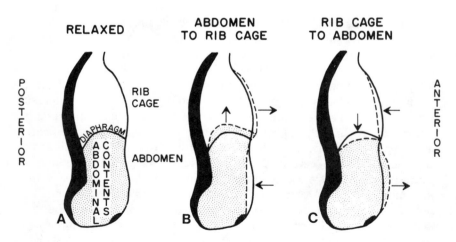

FIGURE 3-1. Schematic illustration of chest wall configuration in which the system is closed at FRC and relaxed (A), or distorted by muscle activity (B) and (C) to maximally displace volume into the rib cage and abdomen, respectively.

between volume displacement and linear motion of that point is determined. The simplest means of establishing such a relationship is to displace volumes into and out of a part while simultaneously measuring changes in its anteroposterior diameter when the degree of vertebral extension is constant. Isovolume maneuvers provide a convenient way to accomplish these displacements, because subjects can use their own respiratory muscles to displace volumes without the need for externally produced volume displacements. As discussed previously, isovolume maneuvers involve equal and opposite volume displacements by the surfaces of the rib cage and abdomen. By performing a series of isovolume maneuvers at different known lung volumes, a family of data can be generated to reveal the functional relationships between the relative motion of the two parts. From these data, it is possible to derive the volume-motion relationships for each part through procedures that are the graphical equivalents of removing one part (i.e., reducing the number of degrees of freedom to one) (Konno and Mead, 1967), or as is described in a subsequent section, through a more convenient procedure of modifying the gains of the magnetometer outputs so that the two signals correspond to identical volume displacements in the data display. In principle, this latter procedure consists of adjusting the magnetometer signals to be equal and opposite for the two parts (rib cage and abdomen) during isovolume maneuvers in which the volumes displaced by the surfaces of the rib cage and abdomen are equal and opposite. By graphically displaying the relative motion relationships determined with lung volume constant (i.e., during the isovolume maneuvers) together with relative motion data obtained when lung volume is unconstrained (e.g., during speech), it is then possible to estimate the separate volume contributions of the rib cage and abdomen to changes in lung volume for the latter. The reader will better appreciate the concepts outlined in this paragraph after reading the discussion under "Data Displays: Orientation and Interpretation" in the *Results* section.

METHOD

Subjects

Six healthy adult men served as subjects in this investigation. Each met the selection criteria of normal articulation, voice, and hearing, and no known anatomical or physiological abnormalities of the speech apparatus. A further criterion for inclusion in the investigation was that each subject was a "good relaxer," in the sense that he could voluntarily relax his respiratory apparatus against a closed upper airway at different lung volumes throughout his vital capacity. The ability of subjects to relax their respiratory muscles was tested by the standard method of relaxation pressures (Rahn, Otis, Chadwick, and

Fenn, 1946). The subject used his respiratory muscles to establish different lung volume levels; at each of these he then relaxed as completely as possible against a closed airway. Pressures measured at the subject's airway opening (mouth) were plotted against measures of the prevailing lung volumes, thus allowing the static relaxation volume-pressure relationship to be described. As used by respiratory physiologists (see Agostoni and Mead, 1964), the term good relaxer designates those subjects whose relaxation volume-pressure data are highly consistent in repeated performances of relaxation maneuvers. Five subjects met this criterion in both the upright and supine positions. Relaxation pressure data for the sixth subject (TH) were equivocal for the supine position, so he was included only in studies of the upright position.

Five subjects spoke General American English; the remaining subject (AG) spoke Spanish and an intelligible English containing linguistic remnants of his native tongue. Only one subject (TH) had training in phonetics, and all subjects had participated in respiratory experiments many times. The more pertinent physical characteristics of each subject are given in Table 3–1.

Equipment

Figure 3–2 is a schematic diagram of the electronic equipment used. Changes in anteroposterior diameters of the rib cage and abdomen were sensed with electromagnetic transducers (i.e., magnetometers). The devices used were somewhat smaller (coils 2 cm in length and about 0.5 cm in diameter), but basically of the same design as prototype units whose specifications are reported in detail elsewhere (Mead et al., 1967). Only the important functional features of the system will be discussed here. The basic principle of diameter measurements with magnetometers is that of sensing with one coil, the strength of a magnetic field generated by a coil mate. Two generator-sensor pairs were used, one pair to sense rib cage diameter changes and the other pair to sense abdominal diameter changes. (For coil placements, see the following section.) Each generating coil was driven sinusoidally at its resonant frequency, and its respective coil mate sensed the magnetic field produced. At the driving frequencies used (1.53 kHz for the rib cage and 0.69 kHz for the abdomen),

Table 3–1. *Pertinent Physical Characteristics of Each Subject*

Subject	Age (yr)	Height (cm)	Weight (kg)	Vital Capacity (L)
MG	33	172.7	87.7	5.1
AG	31	187.3	93.2	6.4
JB	29	177.8	70.5	6.2
DL	37	186.7	79.5	5.7
JM	49	188.0	86.4	6.3
TH	28	177.8	88.2	5.2

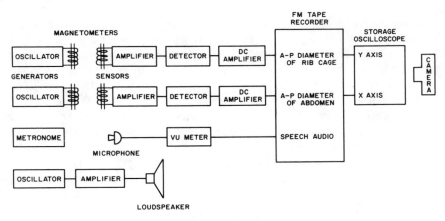

FIGURE 3-2. Block diagram of electronic equipment used.

body tissues and air have negligible effects on the strengths of the magnetic fields produced, a fact of crucial importance to biological applications of the devices. With the long axes of a generator-sensor coil pair oriented parallel, the voltage induced in the sensor is inversely proportional to the cube of the distance between the two mates. As the devices were used in this investigation, distance changes between the generating and sensing coils were small relative to the absolute distance between the coils, so that the relationship between voltage change and distance change was essentially linear over nearly the entire range of motion of both the rib cage and the abdomen.

Processing of each magnetometer signal involved amplification of the amplitude-modulated output from the sensor, half-wave rectification, filtering (to prevent cross-talk between the two pairs of coils), and passage of the signal through a DC amplifier. The voltage related to the absolute distance between coil mates was zero suppressed at the DC amplifier, and only the voltage equivalent of intercoil distance change was amplified. With both the generating and sensing coils movable, the output of the sensing coil indicates changes in distance between it and the generator, whether there is movement of one or both coils. If one coil in a pair is relatively stable, as was the case for the back coils in the measurements made here, the output of a sensor may be thought of as providing a continuous measurement of the unidimensional change in the position of a point in reference to a fixed point (i.e., the coil on the back).

The processed signals from the magnetometers were fed to two channels of an FM tape-recording system where they were stored for subsequent playback into a storage oscilloscsope. During playback, the diameter signals for the rib cage and abdomen were displayed against one another on the oscilloscope, the rib cage on the Y axis and abdomen on the X axis (for details, see *Results* section on "Data Displays: Orientation and Interpretation"). Data displays on the screen of the oscilloscope were stored and then recorded permanently by photographing the screen with a Polaroid camera.

Three portions of the electronic equipment arrangement provided information to the subjects to guide them in certain of their utterances. Acoustic signals were sensed by a unidirectional microphone and fed through a VU meter to a direct record channel of the FM tape recorder. The VU meter served as an index of speech intensity. A loudspeaker, driven by a power amplifier and controlled by an oscillator, provided pure tone frequency standards against which the subjects could match their vocal fundamental frequency. Finally, an electronic metronome was used for certain conditions to pace each subject in his rate of speech utterance.

General Procedure

After removal of local body hair, the magnetometer coils (encased in polyethylene) were attached to the body surface with an adhesive spray. Two generating coils were positioned at the midline on the anterior surface of the chest wall, one for the rib cage at the level of the nipples and one for the abdomen immediately above the umbilicus. Sensing coil mates were positioned on the posterior surface of the body, also at the midline, and at the same axial levels as their respective generator mates (see Fig. 3–3). All four coils were oriented with their long axes perpendicular to the sagittal plane.

Experimental tasks were performed in two body positions: upright and supine. For recordings in the upright position, subjects stood on a footplate attached to a tilt table oriented approximately 15 degrees off vertical toward supine (Fig. 3–3). With his head and neck supported by a pillow, each subject leaned backward against the table, which was covered with a thick polyurethane pad. The segment of the pad supporting the torso had a rectangular indentation running vertically at the midline to provide a space within which the coils on the subject's back were free to move. The off-vertical position was selected for study of the upright position because it was more comfortable than free standing for long periods and because it proved an easier task than free standing for maintaining a consistent body posture (i.e., a constant degree of extension of the vertebral column) throughout the investigation. Preliminary measurements on three subjects (JM, MG, and TH) showed no differences between data obtained in the free standing position and those obtained in the off-vertical position. For recordings in the supine position, the tilt table was adjusted to horizontal. Investigation of both the upright and supine positions was done in a single experimental session, with the upright position studied first. To preclude measurement artifacts, subjects were cautioned to avoid raising their arms and shifting their torso position (i.e., extending or flexing their vertebral column) during recordings. Metal

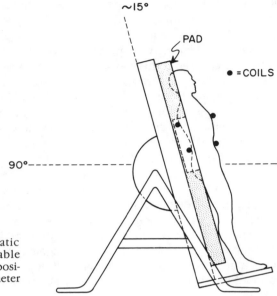

FIGURE 3-3. Schematic illustration of tilt table configuration, subject positioning, and magnetometer coil placements.

objects were removed to prevent interference with the magnetometer signals. Magnetometer calibration signals were placed on tape both before and after the recordings were made for each position.

Two types of activities were performed—respiratory maneuvers and utterances—which are discussed in the next two sections. The entire group of activities was repeated on separate occasions (several months apart) at least once by each subject and three times by two subjects (TH and MG) over a period of 2 years. Because data from repeated experiments were highly consistent, only the results of the first session are reported in this paper.

RESPIRATORY MANEUVERS. Recordings were made during the performance of four nonspeech respiratory activities. These included vital capacity maneuvers, resting breathing, relaxation of the respiratory apparatus against a closed airway at various lung volumes, and isovolume maneuvers at predetermined lung volumes. Each of the four activities was done several times, both before and after the utterance tasks (see next section) in each position. Except for resting breathing, which was done nasally, each subject performed these activities while wearing a noseclip.

Vital capacity maneuvers were done by having each subject inspire to the total lung capacity (TLC) and expire completely to the residual volume (RV) through a mouthpiece coupled to a spirometer.

Recordings of resting breathing were made while subjects breathed quietly for a minute after inspiring to TLC and then relaxing to the functional residual capacity (FRC) without equipment at the airway opening.

Relaxation maneuvers were performed following inspiration to TLC, after which the subject relaxed his respiratory apparatus as completely as possible (usually for 3 to 5 secs) against a closed glottis at successive descending volume steps, encompassing the entire vital capacity range. As it was desired to have data at many levels within the vital capacity (at least within each 5% VC), a number of repetitions of the descending volume steps procedure were elicited. Each performance of a series of relaxations was done following the consistent volume history of inspiring to TLC and then descending in steps through the vital capacity. To provide intermittent experimental checks on data consistency, subjects were asked to relax at TLC, FRC, and RV periodically during the utterance tasks described in the next section. Data for the upper part of the vital capacity range also were checked on occasion for consistency by a procedure that provided information comparable to that generated by the descending step activity. In this procedure, the subject relaxed his respiratory apparatus from TLC to FRC during a single continuous slow expiration through a very high resistance leak provided by a tight pursing of his lips.

Isovolume maneuvers were performed at 80, 60, 40, and 20% levels of the vital capacity. Each subject inspired to TLC and slowly expired to the 80% VC level through a mouthpiece coupled to a spirometer. At that level, the subject closed his glottis, relaxed, and then slowly performed a number of isovolume maneuvers (usually taking about 5 secs each) by displacing volume back and forth between the rib cage and abdomen (see earlier section on *Theory*). Shifting from relaxation toward the inspiratory direction of the abdomen (i.e., forcing the abdominal wall outward from its relaxation position) was done in the supine position only, because preliminary measurements in the upright position showed no speech to occur at abdominal diameters exceeding those during relaxation at corresponding lung volumes. After the performance of several isovolume maneuvers at the 80% VC level, the subject opened his glottis, expired slowly to the 60% VC level, and repeated the isovolume tasks done at 80% VC. Similarly, the subject repeated the procedures by descending to the 40% and 20% VC levels. As with the relaxation maneuvers, a single pass through the VC was insufficient to complete the investigative tasks because of the need to breathe. Therefore, the isovolume activities were done a number of times—each, however, with the volume history of inspiring to TLC and then descending to a predetermined lung volume level. As an intermittent verification of data consistency, isovolume maneuvers were done at FRC periodically during the utterance tasks described next.

UTTERANCES. A core of utterances was produced by each subject, and additional special activities were performed by randomly selected subjects. The core activities each were performed a minimum of two times consecutively in each position studied and in the same order for each position.

The first group of activities consisted of four speech tasks and one singing task. Each of these activities was performed subsequent to standardization of the recent lung volume history, which consisted of having each utterance activity preceded by a near maximal inspiration, a relaxed expiration to FRC, and several resting breathing cycles during which the subject was instructed in the utterance task. The speech and singing tasks were:

1. Two minutes of spontaneous conversation with an investigator
2. Normal reading of a standard declarative paragraph (the first paragraph of "The Rainbow Passage" by Fairbanks [1960])
3. Soft reading of the same paragraph in 2 above
4. Loud reading of the same paragraph in 2 above
5. Normal singing of the first verse of the American National Anthem.

The one bilingual subject (AG) in the study performed Task 1 in both English and Spanish and Tasks 2 through 4 in Spanish from his own written translation of the paragraph. For Task 5 he sang the national anthem of Argentina.

The second group of utterances performed by each subject consisted of a sustained vowel activity and four syllable repetition activities, each performed at either three loudnesses or three utterance rates, and throughout nearly the entire vital capacity range. After performing the same volume history as in the first group of activities, subjects were instructed to make their final pre-utterance inspiration to near TLC and then to do the activities on a single expiration until they could no longer perform the task (i.e., to near RV). Subjects were guided in their performances by one or more of the three monitoring systems discussed earlier (see "Equipment" section): speech intensity, vocal fundamental frequency, and rate of syllable utterance. The vowel and syllable repetition tasks were as follows:

1. Sustained production of the vowel /ɑ/ at a vocal fundamental frequency of 130 Hz, and at each of three loudness levels—normal, soft, and loud
2. Repetition of the syllable /pʌ/ at an utterance rate of 3 per sec, at normal pitch, and at each of three loudness levels—normal, soft, and loud
3. Repetition of the syllable /pʌ/ at normal loudness, normal pitch, and at each of three utterance rates—3 per sec, 5 per sec, and maximum
4. Repetition of the syllable /hʌ/ at an utterance rate of 3 per sec, at normal pitch, and at each of three loudness levels—normal, soft and loud
5. Repetition of the syllable /hʌ/ at normal loudness, normal pitch, and at each of three utterance rates—3 per sec, 5 per sec, and maximum.

Finally, selected subjects performed one or more special speech activities, described later during the illustration of various points of discussion.

RESULTS

Data Displays: Orientation and Interpretation

Figure 3–4 is a schematic drawing, illustrative of data displays used in this section to present the results. The display shown is for the upright position, although the principles involved in its construction are equally applicable to data for the supine position. Anteroposterior diameter of the rib cage is shown on the *Y* axis, increasing upward. Abdominal anteroposterior diameter is displayed on the *X* axis, increasing to the right. *X-Y* displays of this type, because they reveal the motions of both the rib cage and abdomen simultaneously, are termed motion-motion or relative motion charts.

The curved, dashed line in Figure 3–4 depicts the relative motion relaxation line. This line is described by the series of data points generated during relaxation against a closed glottis at different lung volumes (see earlier discussion on "Respiratory Maneuvers" in *Method* section). Open circles on the relaxation line represent points corresponding to each 20% of the vital capacity, the upper and lower extremes being the total lung capacity (TLC) and the residual volume (RV), respectively. The pathway defined by the relaxation line reveals the nature of changes in the shape of the two-part chest wall system during voluntary relaxation at different lung volumes. The

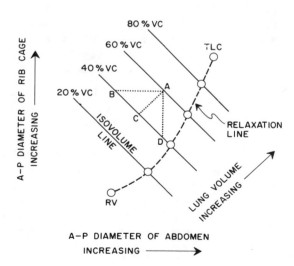

FIGURE   3–4. Schematic drawing of a relative motion chart (rib cage versus abdomen) like those constructed for data display.

relaxation line likewise represents the relative motion pathway that presumably would be followed were the respiratory muscles paralyzed and the system driven passively through different volumes by a mechanical respirator.

The four solid diagonal lines intersecting the relaxation line at 20% VC increments are isovolume lines. These depict the pathways followed on the chart during the shifting of volume back and forth between the surfaces of the rib cage and abdomen with lung volume constant (see earlier discussion on "Respiratory Maneuvers" in *Method* section). Segments of the isovolume lines to the left of the relaxation line involve rib cage diameters in excess of and abdominal diameters less than their relaxation diameters at the prevailing lung volume. The converse holds for isovolume-line segments to the right of the relaxation line. Moving up and down any isovolume line involves the shifting of volume from the surface of the abdomen to the surface of the rib cage and vice versa, respectively. All isovolume lines in Figure 3–4 have slopes of – 1, indicating that for any shift in volume between the rib cage and abdomen there are equal signals from the two magnetometer sets. Unlike this situation, charts calibrated for absolute diameters of the rib cage and abdomen have isovolume slopes of less than – 1 (i.e., change in abdominal diameter exceeds that of the rib cage). Such charts can be interpreted for the separate volume changes of the two parts by solving graphically the relationship between diameter change and volume change for each part (Konno and Mead, 1967). A more direct and convenient procedure is to adjust the slopes of the isovolume lines empirically to – 1 values, as in the schematic chart of Figure 3–4. This has been done for all relative motion charts to be presented here through adjustment of the relative gains of the rib cage and abdominal diameter signals for the isovolume line nearest FRC (at 40% VC upright and 20% VC supine). With equal displacements on the charts then representing equal volume displacements by the surfaces of the rib cage and abdomen, the relative motion chart takes the form of a relative volume chart. Thus modified, such charts provide an easily read and direct graphic display of changes in lung volume, of the relative volume contributions of the rib cage and abdomen to changes in total volume, and of the separate volume displacements of the rib cage and abdomen (i.e., of the configuration of the chest wall).

Change in lung volume between any two points on the chart is given by the distance between them perpendicular to the isovolume lines. Upward and to the right on the chart indicates an increasing lung volume. Decreasing lung volume is downward and to the left. The pathways labeled AB, AC, and AD in Figure 3–4 each show 20% VC decreases in lung volume. Conversely, their reversals show 20% VC increases in lung volume. Were the vital capacity 5 L, each of the pathways would encompass a 1 L change in lung volume. Movement in either direction along the pathway BCD in Figure 3–4 does not involve a change in lung volume, because all points on the pathway represent the same lung volume (i.e., they describe the 40% VC isovolume line). As an aid to the reader's conceptualization of reading volume change directly from charts, the entire chart can be rotated 45 degrees counterclockwise so that the isovolume lines in Figure 3–4 are horizontal. This makes them analogous to a series of X axes where vertical displacements are proportional to lung volume changes.

The relative volume contributions of the rib cage and abdomen to the total volume change are given by the slope of the line between any two points on the chart. Again, considering the three dotted pathways in Figure 3–4, the total volume change is identical for each, whereas the relative volumes displaced by the surfaces of the rib cage and abdomen are markedly different. For the horizontal pathway (AB), the total volume change is accomplished by displacement of the abdomen, rib cage volume remaining constant. The vertical pathway (AD) shows the converse, with rib cage displacement alone accounting for the total volume change. Slopes between these two extremes (AB and AD) result from different relative contributions on the part of the rib cage and abdomen, the magnitude of the slope being proportional to the percentage contribution of each part to the total volume change. The pathway showing a + 1 slope (dotted line AC), for example, shows the adjusted surface displacements of the rib cage and abdomen as contributing equally to the total volume change.

The separate volumes of the rib cage and abdomen (those specifying the configuration of the chest wall) are given by position along the vertical and horizontal axes of the relative volume chart, respectively. Upward on the chart indicates an increasing rib cage volume. Toward the right constitutes an increasing abdominal volume (i.e., an outward displacement of the abdominal surface). Because location on the relative volume chart specifies the separate volumes of the rib cage and abdomen, every point on the chart defines a different chest wall configuration. A pathway on the chart, because it is a series of points, constitutes a record of the changing shape of the moving chest wall. Pathways AB, AC, and AD in Figure 3–4 all start at a rib cage volume equivalent to that obtained during relaxation at 75% of the vital capacity and show, respectively, no change in rib cage volume, a decrease to a size equivalent to that obtained upon relaxation at the 60% VC level, and a decrease to a size equal to that obtained upon relaxation at the 45% VC level. For the same three pathways (AB, AC, and AD), the volume of the abdomen at the beginning of each is equivalent to that for relaxation at 35% of the vital capacity. The pathways AB and AC show reductions in abdominal volume to levels equivalent to those obtained during relaxation at the 5% and 15% VC levels, respectively. The pathway AD shows no abdominal volume change.

Respiratory Maneuvers

Figure 3–5 presents relative motion displays for data obtained during respiratory maneuvers in both positions. As discussed earlier, only segments of the isovolume lines to the left of the relaxation line are shown for the upright

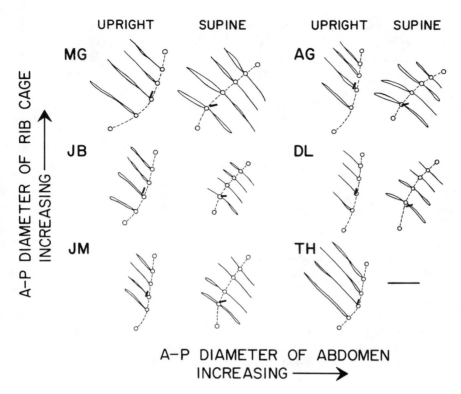

FIGURE 3-5. Relative volume charts for all subjects in the upright and supine positions showing data obtained during respiratory maneuvers. Dashed lines depict relaxation characteristics; thin solid lines, configurations assumed during isovolume maneuvers; and short thick lines, resting breathing patterns.

position. The relative volume data for respiratory maneuvers in each position are qualitatively similar across subjects. Relaxation lines show both the rib cage and abdomen to decrease in diameter with decreases in lung volume, whereas over the entire vital capacity range the volume change of the rib cage exceeds that of the abdomen. For the upright position, relaxation lines are slightly concave toward the Y axis with the major part of the abdominal volume change occurring below FRC. By contrast, the supine position shows relaxation lines to be convex toward the Y axis. For each subject, the isovolume line nearest FRC (i.e., the 40% VC isopleth upright and the 20% VC isopleth supine) is set to approximate a -1 slope following the rationale discussed in the previous section. The roughly 20% VC difference in FRC level between the two positions is as would be predicted on mechanical grounds (Agostoni and Mead, 1964). In the upright position, gravity acts in an expiratory direction on the rib cage and in an inspiratory direction on the abdomen. A shift to supine finds the gravitational effect to be expiratory on both the rib cage and abdomen. An expiratory influence on the latter causes the abdominal mass and diaphragm to be driven headward and a reduction in lung volume to result. For the most part, the isovolume lines are essentially single-valued, flat loops or single lines, each being linearly or approximately so. The single-valued character of the isopleths supports the assumption that the chest wall has basically two moving parts and demonstrates further that the relative diameter relationships of the two parts are not influenced significantly by the direction of volume shift between them (i.e., there is little or no hysteresis in the isopleths). The fact that the isopleths are roughly linear suggests that the ratio of linear diameter change to volume displacement is similar for the diameters studied in the two parts. That the isopleths are approximately parallel across the different lung volumes indicates that the diameter-volume relationships between the rib cage and abdomen are essentially independent of the configuration of the opposite part. In the charts, the isopleths for each subject are approximately equidistant for equal volume increments. This means that the relationship between diameter change and volume change is approximately linear for each part. Although they are not displayed, intermediate isopleths generated at each odd 20% VC were parallel to those shown and spaced uniformly midway between the even 20% isovolume lines.

Of final interest with respect to the respiratory activites are the short solid lines showing resting breathing patterns. These show that subjects covered about 10% of their vital capacity during quiet breaths. For the upright position, slopes of the lines reveal that changes in lung volume were the result of both rib cage and abdominal displacements, the rib cage contribution far exceeding that of the abdomen for all subjects. Conversely, lines for the supine position show that the abdomen contributed much more to total volume change than did the rib cage. In the upright position, subjects breathed essentially along the relaxation line, whereas for the supine position they breathed toward the right of it. Subjects were instructed to breathe in as relaxed a manner as possible. As long as they attended consciously to the task, they breathed in the manner shown in Figure 3–5. It should be noted, however, that at other informal moments during the investigation of the upright position, subjects continued to breathe parallel to the relaxation line, but often their tracings were displaced somewhat to the left on the chart. Such departures from the relaxation line are consistent with some expected abdominal muscle tone in the upright position and may reflect more accurately the manner in which subjects typically breathe.

Conversation, Reading, and Singing

Figures 3–6 through 3–9 show utterance data for conversation, reading, and singing in the upright and supine positions. Data tracings are superimposed on a series of relative volume charts, each repeating from Figure 3–5 the

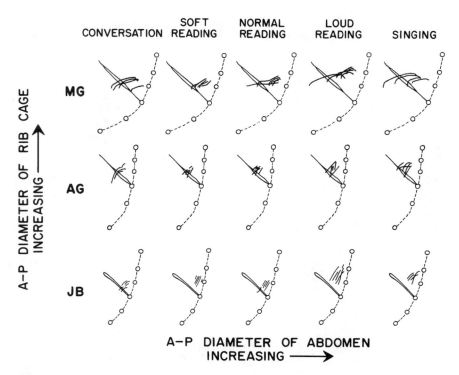

FIGURE 3-6. Relative volume charts for subjects MG, AG, and JB in the upright position, showing data obtained during conversation, reading, and singing. Relaxation characteristics and 40% VC isopleths are repeated from Figure 3–5.

appropriate relaxation line and isopleth nearest FRC for reference. Tracings included in Figures 3–6 and 3–8 are representative of the variety of tracings obtained for repeated performances of the various tasks. Only the expiratory limbs of the recorded relative volume loops are shown, and then only a few loops for each task so as to avoid cluttering the charts. The discussion that follows, however, is based on the entire data pool from which these tracings have been selected for display. No significant differences were found between the Spanish and English data sets generated by the one bilingual subject (AG) in this study. The tracings shown in Figures 3–6 to 3–9 are for his Spanish utterances, the data set in which he also performed a singing task.

LUNG VOLUME. Lung volume was restricted to the midrange of the vital capacity (the middle 60% VC) for the vast majority of utterances involving conversation, reading, and singing. Without exception, expiratory limbs (speech breathing phrases) were initiated from above FRC. Nearly all phrases,

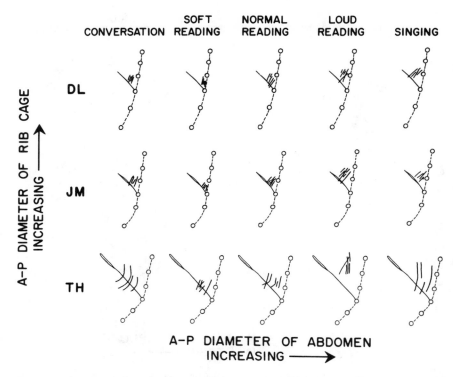

FIGURE 3-7. Relative volume charts for subjects DL, JM, and TH in the upright position, showing data obtained during conversation, reading, and singing (details same as for Figure 3–6).

in fact, were initiated from above the end-inspiratory level for resting breathing (i.e., outside the tidal volume range) in each position. For conversation and normal reading, most expiratory limbs started from within a relatively narrow range of lung volumes, encompassing approximately 60%–50% VC in the upright position and 50%–30% VC in the supine position. Soft reading also was initiated from within these approximate volume limits, but in contrast to normal reading, usually from slightly lower volumes. For the loud reading passage, breathing phrases characteristically were started from substantially higher lung volumes than for the other reading tasks, typically between 10%–20% VC higher. Thus, in the three readings, the subject group demonstrated a trend of initiating utterances from successively higher lung volumes with successive increases in loudness, the increase between normal and loud reading being especially prominent in this regard. Findings were mixed with respect to the initiation levels for singing. One subject (MG) began his singing phrases in both positions from volume levels comparable to those he used for normal reading. Others (AG and TH) initiated expiratory limbs

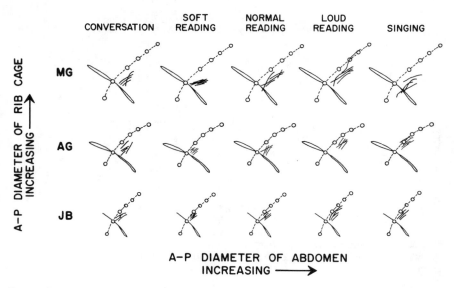

FIGURE 3-8. Relative volume charts for subjects MG, AG, and JB in the supine position, showing data obtained during conversation, reading, and singing. Relaxation characteristics and 20% VC isopleths are repeated from Figure 3-5.

from levels similar to those characteristic of their loud reading, and still others (JB, DL, and JM) sang from starting levels comparable to normal reading in one position and loud reading in the other.

For the most part, expiratory limbs during conversation, reading, and singing were terminated above or approximately at the FRC level. Exceptions were confined primarily to two subjects (MG and TH) in the upright position and usually involved only moderate encroachment upon the expiratory reserve volume. For conversation and normal reading, subjects typically expired 10%-20% VC during breathing phrases, with occasional expiratory limbs covering up to 30% of the vital capacity (e.g., see MG and TH upright for conversation and singing). The majority of breathing phrases for conversation and normal reading were terminated between approximately 50%-30% VC in the upright position and 35%-20% VC in the supine position. Soft reading was terminated within the same relative limits; however, the volumes expired when reading softly often were less than those expired for normal reading (see DL in both positions). Expired volumes for loud reading were equal to or frequently in excess of those for the normal reading task, with some subjects (see TH upright and AG supine) terminating their loud phrases at higher volumes than for the first three tasks. Thus, over the three readings of the standard passage, the volume expired per phrase tended to increase with loudness for some subjects (AG and JM upright and MG and DL supine), the

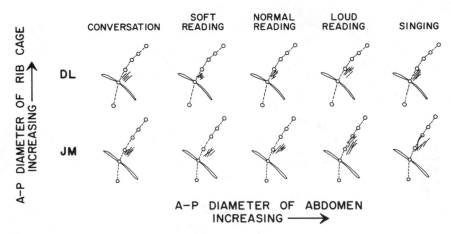

FIGURE 3-9.   Relative volume charts for subjects DL and JM in the supine position, showing data obtained during conversation, reading, and singing (details same as for Figure 3–8).

most marked differences in expired volume being between the loud task and the other two readings. Volumes expired during singing were comparable to those for normal reading by some subjects (JB upright) and those for loud reading by others (AG and TH upright). Termination levels for singing were generally similar to those for the first three tasks, with certain subjects (JB upright and AG supine) showing a tendency to end some limbs at slightly higher VC levels.

RELATIVE VOLUME DISPLACEMENTS OF THE RIB CAGE AND ABDOMEN. The observed changes in total volume during the utterances resulted from a wide range of relative displacements by the rib cage and abdomen. Not only did the relative contribution of the two parts differ among subjects, tasks, and within tasks, it also often changed within single expiratory limbs. The extremes of relative contribution occurred for subjects MG and TH. MG typically showed a predominance of abdominal displacement during his utterances, there being times when he used little or no motion of his rib cage (see normal reading, upright). Conversely, TH demonstrated a predominance of rib cage displacement, his total volume change being accounted for at times entirely by motion of the rib cage, as in loud reading (see exception at lower volumes during conversation). For the upright position, the remaining four subjects demonstrated contributions ranging from various degrees of rib cage predominance (DL and JM on the first two tasks) to roughly equal contributions by the two parts (DL and JM on singing), abdominal predominance being rare. In the supine position, the subject group (except MG) tended toward less rib cage displacement on the same tasks than upright, there being more limbs in which rib cage and abdominal displacements were equal or in which the abdomen was predominant. Individual subjects differed in their response to the positional shift. One (AG) showed little change; others (JB, DL, and JM) contributed less with their rib cages in the supine than in the upright position on most tasks; and one (MG) typically contributed more with his rib cage in the supine than in the upright position. The only positional effect shared by all subjects was the trend toward less rib cage contribution in the supine than in the upright position during soft reading.

Aside from the positional influence, there were relative contribution differences among tasks within each position. In general, pathway slopes for conversational speech indicated as much, or slightly more, rib cage contribution than those for normal reading. Across reading passages, changes in relative contribution were idiosyncratic for different subjects and positions. For readings in the upright position, two subjects (AG and JB) showed no change across loudness; one (TH) showed an increased rib cage contribution with increases in loudness; and three (JM, DL, and MG) showed decreases in rib cage contribution with increases in loudness, especially in soft versus normal and loud reading. The supine position, on the other hand, found two subjects (MG and AG) demonstrating substantially less rib cage contribution for soft versus normal and loud readings. The remaining subjects (JB, DL, and JM) demonstrated their smallest rib cage contribution during normal reading as compared to soft and loud. Relative displacements during singing were similar to those for loud reading by some subjects (MG and JM upright) and involved a somewhat less rib cage contribution for loud reading by others (see DL upright and AG supine).

As noted previously, the relative contributions of the rib cage and abdomen often changed within single expiratory limbs. Four subjects, in particular, showed various degrees of slope change for some of their utterances (e.g., see conversational speech upright), three (AG, JB, and MG) demonstrating tracings that tended concave toward the Y axis, showing an increasing rib cage contribution with decreasing lung volume, and one (TH) showing just the opposite. Maximum slope changes for single limbs were found for MG and TH. During conversation TH showed instances of all rib cage displacement above FRC to predominantly abdominal displacement at lower volumes. MG, by contrast, often went from predominantly abdominal motion at higher volumes to mainly rib cage motion at lower volumes (see singing upright). In addition to showing the maximum slope changes for single limbs, MG and TH also frequently demonstrated paradoxical displacements of the rib cage and abdomen. These are revealed in tracings in which the sign of volume displacement of one or the other of the parts is opposite to that of lung volume change (i.e., one part is displacing volume in an inspiratory direction, whereas the net total volume change is expiratory). Paradoxical motions of this nature were demonstrated by TH, for example, during conversation, loud reading, and singing, when at times his abdominal wall moved outward while his lung volume and rib cage volume were decreasing. The volume displaced by the rib cage, therefore, exceeded the total volume change by an amount equal to the inspiratory displacement of the abdomen. Paradoxical movement in the opposite sense was demonstrated by subject MG during the early stages of many of his utterances for loud reading and singing. At such times, MG decreased both his lung volume and the volume of his abdomen while simultaneously increasing the volume of his rib cage. For these circumstances, then, the abdomen displaced more volume than did the lungs by an amount equal to the inspiratory displacement of the rib cage.

SEPARATE VOLUMES OF THE RIB CAGE AND ABDOMEN: CHEST WALL CONFIGURATION. In both positions, nearly all conversation, reading, and singing took place within the range of rib cage and abdominal diameters (volumes) associated with relaxation at TLC and RV. With rare exception, expiratory limbs were initiated at rib cage volumes in excess of those for relaxation at FRC, and usually for those at the end-inspiratory level for resting breathing. In the first three tasks, most limbs were initiated within a small range of rib cage volumes, encompassed by rib cage sizes during relaxation at 70% and 50% of the vital capacity for the upright position and at 40% and 30% VC for the supine postion. Within these ranges, soft reading often was initiated at lower rib cage volumes than conversation or normal reading, whereas loud reading typically was initiated at much higher rib cage volumes than for the first three tasks. Consistent with the earlier noted increase in starting lung volume with increases in loudness, expiratory limbs were initiated from successively higher rib cage levels with successive loudness increases during reading. For singing, one subject (MG) performed in both positions from starting rib cage sizes comparable to those for his normal reading; others (AG, JM, and TH) started limbs at levels similar to those for loud reading; and two subjects (JB and DL) matched their loud reading starting levels in the upright position and their normal reading levels for supine.

Conversation, reading, and singing generally were terminated at rib cage volumes above or approximately at those at relaxed FRC levels (for an exception, see MG singing supine) and, excepting subjects MG and AG supine, typically above the end-inspiratory volume levels for resting breathing. For the first three tasks, limbs were terminated at rib cage volumes equal to those attained upon relaxation between 60% and 50% VC upright and 30% and 20% VC supine. During loud reading and singing, however, limbs were sometimes terminated at somewhat higher or lower rib cage volumes (e.g., see TH reading loud upright and MG singing supine). Typical rib cage excursions encompassed changes on the order of those for 10% to 20% VC changes in relaxed rib cage volume through the vital capacity midrange. On loud reading, subjects frequently expired through a greater rib cage range than for the first three tasks (see JB upright and JM supine). This completed a trend across readings for rib cage excursions to increase with loudness, especially for soft and normal versus loud speech (JM upright and DL supine). Singing appeared similar to loud reading with regard to rib cage excursion in the upright position, the findings for supine being mixed between performances similar to normal reading (MG, JB, and DL) and those similar to loud reading (AG and JM).

Generally speaking, the abdomen was confined to smaller volumes than those for relaxation at FRC upright and to larger volumes than those for relaxation at FRC supine. Upright, the size of the abdomen at the initiation of utterances usually ranged between the sizes obtained during relaxation at the 40% and 20% VC levels. Only AG departed substantially from this range by using volumes smaller than those for relaxation at 20% VC. Unlike pre-utterance rib cage volume, which was higher for successively louder readings and singing, abdominal volume at the initiation of limbs was similar for all tasks (see MG and JM). In league with rib cage data, this means that speech from higher lung volumes for certain tasks was produced with pre-utterance increases in rib cage volume and without similar changes in abdominal volume. The abdominal volumes on termination of limbs in the upright position encompassed a range that included, for the most part, volumes equal to those between 30% VC and RV during relaxation. Typical utterances for conversation, reading, and singing involved abdominal excursions equal to those associated with 10% to 20% VC changes upon relaxation.

Unlike the case with the upright position, the volume of the abdomen at the initiation of utterances differed with various tasks performed supine. For the first three tasks, limbs were started from abdominal volumes equal to those attained between 60% and 40% VC relaxed, with soft reading generally showing the lowest initiation volumes (JM was an exception). By contrast, loud reading started at much larger abdominal volumes than the preceding tasks, with a trend existing for abdominal volume to be greater at the start of limbs for successively louder readings. Note that unlike the upright position, in which only the rib cage assumed higher pre-utterance volumes with increases in loudness, both the rib cage and abdomen were at larger volumes to begin utterances in the supine position. Results for singing were subject dependent, some similar to normal reading (MG) and others similar to loud reading (AG). Abdominal excursions for supine speaking approximated those for 10% to 20% VC changes in the relaxed abdomen. Most phrases ended at volumes equal to those assumed by the abdomen between 40% and 20% VC relaxed (JM was somewhat higher), with some phrases ending at larger volumes for loud reading (AG and DL) and singing (AG).

Considering the separate volume data for the rib cage and abdomen during speech relative to those for relaxation, it is found that upright speech took place well to the left of the relaxation configuration of the chest wall. Thus, the rib cage was relatively more and the abdomen correspondingly less expanded than they were in the relaxed state at the same lung volume. By contrast, supine speech occurred to the right of the relaxation configuration

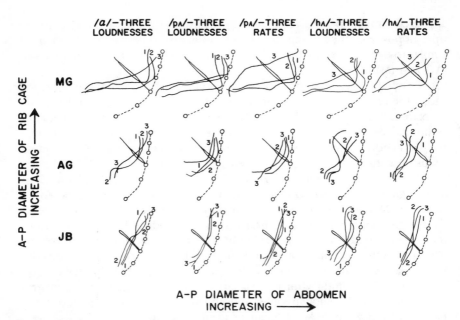

FIGURE 3-10. Relative volume charts for subjects MG, AG, and JB in the upright position, showing data obtained during a sustained vowel and four syllable repetition activities, each performed at either three loudnesses or three utterance rates, and throughout most of the vital capacity. Numbers 1, 2, and 3 denote pathways for successive increases in either loudness (soft, normal, loud) or syllable utterance rate (3 per sec, 5 per sec, maximum). Relaxation characteristics and 40% VC isopleths are repeated from Figure 3-5.

on the charts, meaning that the rib cage was relatively less and the abdomen correspondingly more expanded than they were during relaxation at the prevailing lung volumes.

Sustained Vowel and Syllable Repetition Utterances

Figures 3-10 through 3-13 contain data for the sustained vowels and syllable repetitions performed in the upright and supine positions. Relaxation lines and isopleths nearest FRC are repeated from Figure 3-5. Only utterance tracings for the first performance of each activity are shown, differences among repeated tasks having been subtle. The numbers 1, 2, and 3 on the different charts denote, respectively, successive increases in either loudness or rate, as defined previously.

RELATIVE VOLUME DISPLACEMENTS OF THE RIB CAGE AND ABDOMEN. A wide variety of rib cage and abdominal displacements were used during the vowel and syllable utterances. Pathway slopes were relatively constant for some utterances (see JM upright), whereas for others they differed

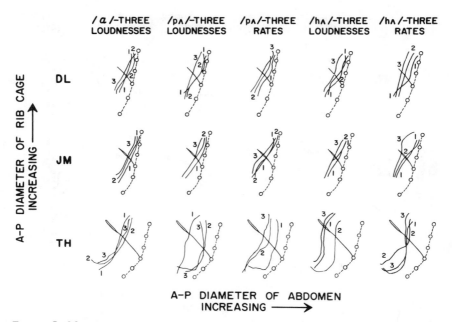

FIGURE 3-11. Relative volume charts for subjects DL, JM, and TH in the upright position, showing data obtained during a sustained vowel and four syllable repetition activities, each performed at either three loudnesses or three utterance rates, and throughout most of the vital capacity range (details same as for Figure 3–10).

markedly with lung volume (MG upright and supine). The range of relative contributions was as great as that observed for conversation, reading, and singing and was reflected within single tracings for MG in the upright position (see soft utterance of /hʌ/ in Figure 3–10).

Results differed between positions. Most tracings for the upright position tended to be concave toward the Y axis and involved a predominance of rib cage displacement at higher lung volumes (see MG on maximum rate /pʌ/ for an exception). This predominant rib cage contribution continued in varying degrees through the lower volumes on four subjects (JB, DL, JM, and TH), with TH at times showing either equal relative contributions or abdominal predominance near the end of utterances (i.e., below 10% VC). The remaining two subjects (AG and MG) performed differently than the other four subjects after reaching the midvolume range. AG frequently showed equal or mainly abdominal displacement from the vicinity of FRC downward, whereas MG typically demonstrated marked abdominal predominance over the same range. (Maximum rate utterances were notable exceptions.) Pathways for the supine position usually were convex toward the Y axis. At high lung volumes, initial motions ranged from marked rib cage predominance (see many of JB's tracings) to marked abdominal predominance (see many of AG's tracings), the majority

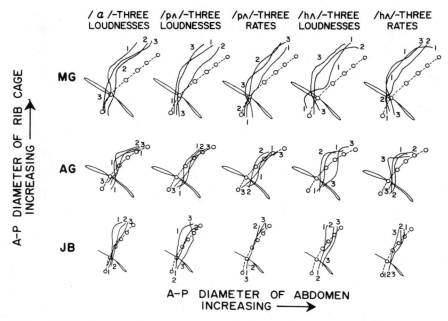

FIGURE 3-12. Relative volume charts for subjects MG, AG, and JB in the supine position, showing data obtained during a sustained vowel and four syllable repetition activities, each performed at either three loudness or three utterance rates, and throughout most of the vital capacity. Numbers 1, 2, and 3 denote pathways for successive increases in either loudness (soft, normal, loud) or syllable utterance rate (3 per sec, 5 per sec, maximum). Relaxation characteristics and 20% VC isopleths are repeated from Figure 3-5.

of pathways revealing approximately equal two-part contributions or a slight predominance by the rib cage. For most utterances, reductions in lung volume were accompanied by increases in the relative contribution of the rib cage, with pronounced rib cage displacement exhibited from the midvolume range downward.

Loudness and utterance rate did not systematically influence the relative displacements of the rib cage and abdomen across the subject group. The only between-subject trend occurred in the upright position in the form of relatively more abdominal contribution at higher lung volumes during the loudest and fastest utterances of a number of subjects (see MG and DL). When individual subjects demonstrated effects, these also were confined mainly to the upright position. Subject MG in particular showed strikingly different relative contributions at similar lung volumes for his utterances at different loudnesses and rates. In contrast to the influence of these factors on MG's performance upright was DL's highly similar pathways for different loudnesses and utterance rates in the supine position.

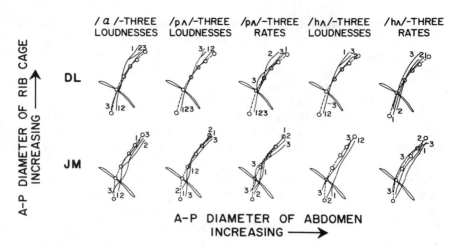

FIGURE 3–13.   Relative volume charts for subjects DL and JM in the supine position, showing data obtained during a sustained vowel and four syllable repetition activities, each performed at either three loudnesses or three utterance rates, and throughout most of the vital capacity (details same as for Figure 3–12).

As with conversation, reading, and singing, paradoxical displacements occurred during the vowel and syllable utterances. Abdominal paradoxing frequently was exhibited in the upright position at the higher lung volumes, especially during soft and normal utterances and at the lower utterance rates (e.g., see MG on many of his utterances). Paradoxing of the rib cage was observed at very low volumes in the upright position (e.g., see TH especially). For supine, only MG demonstrated frequent paradoxing, occurring at very low volumes when his abdomen moved outward in contradiction to the expiratory change in lung volume.

SEPARATE VOLUME DISPLACEMENTS OF THE RIB CAGE AND ABDOMEN: CHEST WALL CONFIGURATION. During vowel and syllable utterances, rib cage volume usually was restricted to the range of volumes covered during relaxation. Notable exceptions occurred at very high lung volumes for TH upright and MG supine. Generally speaking, utterances were initiated at rib cage volumes in excess of those attained on relaxation at 90% VC in both positions for the subject group. From there, a major segment of the relaxed rib cage volume range was covered for utterances, sometimes essentially the entire range (see TH and JB upright and MG, DL, and JM supine). The only significant departure from the group trend was MG upright, who went through substantially less rib cage excursion than other subjects, his rib cage never becoming appreciably smaller than its size at the relaxed FRC position (i.e., at 40% VC).

Abdominal excursions during vowels and syllable repetitions stayed within the relaxed VC abdominal range in the supine position for all subjects and generally within that range in the upright position for JB, DL, and JM. For the remaining subjects upright (MG, AG, and TH), the abdomen often decreased to a size smaller than that attained at relaxed RV. Utterances were initiated over a wide range of abdominal volumes by the subject group, as exemplified by subject TH upright and subjects DL and JM supine. TH often initiated utterances from smaller abdominal volumes than for relaxed RV (see the /hʌ/ utterances). By contrast, DL and JM supine invariably initiated their utterances from very large abdominal volumes, typically in the range equal to that for relaxation between TLC and 80% VC. Abdominal excursions varied for different utterances, subjects, and positions. Upright, the abdomen often decreased to a size substantially smaller than that attained upon relaxation at RV (see MG, AG, and TH). In addition, some utterances involved more change in abdominal volume than that which occurred during relaxation throughout the vital capacity range (see MG upright). For supine, the large majority of utterances (MG notably excepted) did not involve abdominal sizes less than those for relaxation at FRC (i.e., not smaller than the size of the abdomen when relaxed at 20% VC).

It was noted previously that for some subjects the relative contribution of the rib cage and abdomen differed with loudness and utterance rate. The configuration of the chest wall also differed for some subjects across loudnesses and rates. These differences are manifested by position of the tracings on the relative motion chart. For supine, trends were few, one being that for the fastest utterance of /hʌ/, pathways were displaced more leftward than for slower repetitions by four subjects (AG, JB, DL, and JM). In the upright position, some subjects (e.g., see especially MG, DL, and JM) showed both louder and faster utterances to be displaced more leftward on the chart than softer and slower utterances. These findings for the two positions indicate that the abdomen was smaller and the rib cage correspondingly larger for certain louder and faster utterances than they were for softer and slower utterances at the same lung volumes.

In accord with findings for conversation, reading, and singing, all vowel and syllable utterances took place to the left of the relative volume relaxation line in the upright position. In the supine position, however, tracings usually began to the left of the relaxation line and proceeded to cross it to the right in going to lower volumes. This cross-over point, where the speech configuration of the chest wall was identical to that during relaxation, typically occurred in the midvolume range (see AG, JB, and DL) or lower (see MG), and at higher lung volumes with increases in loudness for some subjects (see AG and JB). Only JM proved to be an exception to this trend, in that he generally remained on the relaxation line or to the right of it for his supine utterances. As noted earlier, conversation, reading, and singing took place to the right of the relaxation line in the supine position. Except for MG on the vowel and syllable utterances, tracings generally crossed the relaxation line to the right above FRC where conversation, reading, and singing were found to occur. Slopes for the pathways generally were not similar for the two sets of data (see Figs. 3–8 and 3–9 versus Figs. 3–14 and 3–13), however, so that tracings for utterances throughout the vital capacity in the supine position cannot be viewed as extrapolations of those for conversation, reading, and singing. When the two sets of data for the upright position are contrasted, however (see Figs. 3–6 and 3–7 versus Figs. 3–10 and 3–11), it is tempting to view many of the vowel and syllable utterances as extrapolations of those that occurred during conversation, reading, and singing.

DISCUSSION

As reflected by the present measurements of lung volume change, humans nearly continuously change their body size during the acts of speaking and singing. They alternate between getting larger and smaller, the latter occurring during all utterances in the English language. Changes in lung volume for the present subjects generally were restricted to the midrange of the vital capacity and showed no systematic differences in expired volumes during identical utterances in the two positions. Identical utterances occurred at lower volumes in the supine than upright position, with differences observed between positions following both the direction and approximate magnitude of the shift

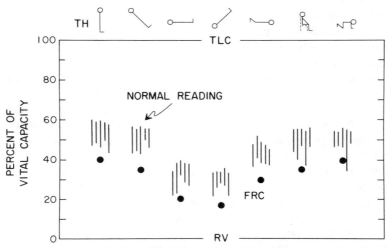

FIGURE 3-14. Lung volumes encompassed for successive expiratory limbs (left to right) during normal readings of a standard passage in various body positions by a single subject. Filled circles depict FRC levels in the different positions.

in FRC level between them. More specifically, the resting expiratory level was about 20% VC lower in the supine than in the upright position, and speech was produced at a similarly lower level. Additional observations on two subjects during resting breathing and speech events in a wide variety of body positions revealed that the volume levels through which speech occurs are highly dependent on the resting level of the system. This is illustrated for subject TH in Figure 3–14, where the FRC levels for different body positions are shown, together with the volumes expired during readings of a standard passage. It can be concluded from these observations that speech events are tied closely to the equilibrium level of the respiratory apparatus and that they shift within the vital capacity in accordance with shifts in FRC level. Factors governing the shift in FRC with body position are discussed in detail elsewhere (Agostoni and Mead, 1964). The principal factor is that of axial displacement of the diaphragm brought about by the influence of gravity on the abdominal contents.

It was observed that the expired volume varied from limb to limb during the speech events. Typically, it encompassed 10% to 20% of the vital capacity. Differences in average flow, as for example across loudness, undoubtedly accounted to some extent for these limb to limb variations. Another major factor, however, was the linguistic content of the utterances. For the most part, expiratory limbs were terminated at either sentence or phrase boundaries, especially during the reading activities. Only in the case of loud reading did subjects cross sentence boundaries without pausing to inspire. A typical example was the utterance of two short sentences on a single expiration. Thus, with subjects pausing to inspire at sentence and phrase boundaries, the volume expired for a given limb was governed by the length of the phrase and sentence units and the average flow from the respiratory apparatus (i.e., through the larynx) over those units.

Speech and singing were initiated from above the resting end-inspiratory level (i.e., outside the tidal breathing range) in both positions for the subjects, a finding consistent with those of Hoshiko and Blockcolsky (1967) and Bouhuys and colleagues (1966) for the upright position. The observation that relatively few utterances extended below the FRC level is inconsistent with that of the latter authors; however, different reading passages for the two studies may account for the different findings. It should be noted that in generally restricting utterances to the midvolume range, humans depart minimally from the volume levels used to fulfill their usual ventilatory needs. In addition, they operate within the least demanding portion of their vital capacity range with respect to the muscular cost required against the spring-like background force (i.e., relaxation pressure) of the respiratory apparatus. Speech produced outside the midvolume range requires greater expenditures of muscular energy because the respiratory apparatus becomes less and less compliant or stiffer as the extremes of the vital capacity are approached.

Compared to soft and normal speech, subjects went to higher lung volumes for loud speech and, in some cases, expired greater amounts of air on single expiratory limbs. Both of these observations are consistent with the data of Bouhuys and colleagues (1966). Greater expired volumes related in part to higher average flows for loud speech by some subjects and also in part to longer utterance times for single limbs. With loud speech demanding a higher driving pressure, the shift to higher volumes for such speech apparently takes advantage of the higher respiratory recoil forces available there. Although the present subjects easily could initiate loud speech at lower volumes by providing a higher muscular pressure, they chose to accomplish the task by expending part of the additionally required muscular pressure on the inspiratory side of the respiratory cycle through stretching the lungs–chest wall unit to a larger size initially. This suggests that the mechanism involved may be one of maintaining a roughly similar patterning of muscular pressure events during speech, but superimposing this patterning on a successively higher background force with successive increases in loudness. The virtue of such a strategy is that by using the greater recoil forces at higher volumes to raise the average driving pressure for louder speech, the system can continue to function around a fairly relaxed state where large variations in muscular pressure are not required for the speech events.

Both mechanical and linguistic factors influenced lung volume events during utterance; however, these factors have been treated somewhat independently thus far. Some insight into their interaction is provided in Figure 3–15, in which data are presented for two subjects instructed to read a standard passage normally, first starting at a high lung volume and then starting at a low volume. For the high volume start, the subjects spoke from near TLC to the 80% VC level, inspired shallowly, spoke to lower volumes, and inspired, until after several breaths they were speaking within the usual midvolume range. For the low volume start, subjects spoke well into the expiratory reserve, inspired, spoke again, and inspired, and again within several breaths were operating within their usual volume range. The observation that subjects moved toward the midvolume range when the system intentionally was set into activity at points well removed from it, attests to the strong mechanical influence involved. The volume history for the utterances shows, however, that subjects continued to impose their usual inspiratory interruptions at sentence boundaries. Were the influence considered here purely mechanical, it would be anticipated that the return to the midvolume range from the high starting volume condition would proceed without interruption for breaths. Rather, the situation exists in which the respiratory apparatus is moving toward an operating range consistent with its optimal performance for speech, while simultaneously the superimposition of a linguistic problem is solved as usual through highly ingrained regulatory patterns. Beyond the examples of Figure 3–15, numerous tasks can be designed to demonstrate either primarily linguistic or mechanical effects on lung volume events during utterance. Linguistic aspects can be shown, for example, through sentences of sufficient length that when a subject is instructed to begin reading from near TLC, he or she will read naturally to FRC on a single breath (Bless and Miller, 1972) without the inspiratory interruptions shown in Figure 3–15. This can be contrasted with the reading of long sentences starting at low lung volumes. In this case, mechanical considerations prevail, because the speaker is forced to inspire at unconventional locations in the reading passage to accommodate the system's demands to resupply for continued utterance.

Although total volume changes were similar for different subjects, they were achieved through a wide range of relative volume contributions by the rib cage and abdomen. For conversation, reading, and singing, the most consistent group trend was a relative decrease in rib cage contribution with the shift from the upright to supine. Within the range of volumes used for utterances, this change was in the same direction as that for relative compliance of the two parts, with the shift in position. Subsequently, it will be shown that for the same utterances, different muscular forces probably operate in the two body positions so that solely relative compliance differences between them cannot account for the observed relative contribution differences.

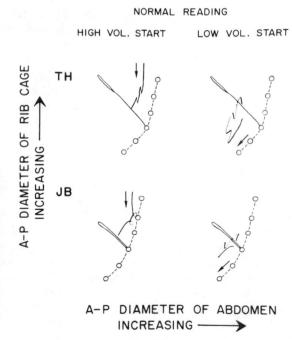

FIGURE 3–15. Relative volume charts for two subjects in the upright position, showing data obtained during normal reading of a standard passage intitiated from high and low lung volumes. Expiratory and inspiratory activities are represented by solid and dotted line segments, respectively. Relaxation characteristics and 40% VC isopleths are repeated from Figure 3–5.

Certainly, the changes in relative compliance cannot account for the differences observed for the vowel and syllable utterances, because they differed substantially in relative contributions at corresponding lung volumes in the two positions.

It is unclear why individual subjects performed so differently on the same utterance tasks when it came to relative contributions. For the respiratory maneuvers studied, including resting breathing, data were similar among subjects. Consequently, the different patterns exhibited for speech cannot be attributed to an overlay on different ingrained patterns of normal ventilation. In addition, no structural features of the subjects appeared to be correlated in any way with the relative contributions used for speech. Quite to the contrary, the two subjects (MG and TH) who set the extremes for relative contributions were judged to be the most physically similar of the subjects (see Table 3–1). Even though there seems to be no immediate mechanical explanation for the different performances by subjects, the results are not surprising when other data on respiratory function and speech articulation are considered. For example, although subjects as a group perform very similarly in relative contributions for resting breathing, they may perform very differently in relative contributions as individuals when they are compared during ventilation in exercise (Drs. Michael D. Goldman, Gunnar Grimby, and Jere Mead, personal communication, June, 1972). Concerning an articulation example, observations of the jaw-tongue system are relevant. If the jaw-tongue is viewed as a unit that can change vocal tract configuration, there are innumerable relative motions of the two structures that can achieve similar effects in changing the dimensions of the upper airway. That different speakers may use one or the other of the structures relatively more to change vocal tract configuration is evidenced by substantial differences in jaw motion for structurally similar subjects during the same speech tasks (Abbs, Netsell, and Hixon, 1971). Important with respect to these examples and the present data is the notion that there are a number of ways to achieve acceptable motions for utterances (i.e., there are a number of degrees of freedom in performance), whether the motion be in the chest wall or vocal tract. The motion strategy chosen by a subject and the manner in which its patterning becomes neurologically ingrained probably depend largely on how the subject has learned to use the muscular system most effectively against the passive mechanical properties of the respiratory apparatus.

Being aware of the highly repeatable relative contributions for individual speakers, it is equally important to note that subjects were able to depart from their usual patterns easily and at will. Evidence of this ability is contained in Figure 3–16, which shows the relative volume pathways followed by two subjects upright during special productions of a sustained vowel at constant normal loudness and pitch and through most of the vital capacity range. For

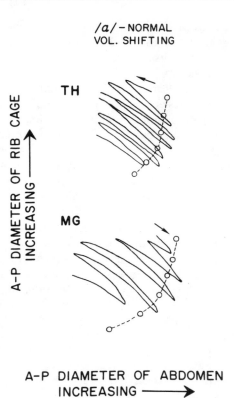

/a/ – NORMAL
VOL. SHIFTING

FIGURE 3–16. Relative volume charts for two subjects in the upright position, showing data obtained during a normal sustained vowel production from near TLC to near RV while displacing volume back and forth alternately between the rib cage and abdomen (i.e., in a manner akin to the isovolume maneuver). Relaxation characteristics are repeated from Figure 3–5.

these phonations, speakers were instructed to displace volume back and forth alternately between the rib cage and abdomen in a manner akin to the isovolume maneuver. As with a usual isovolume maneuver (see section on *Theory*), the reader can gain a general appreciation for this task by alternately contracting and relaxing the abdominal muscles during vowel production or normal speech. Nearly continuous paradoxical displacments of the rib cage and abdomen occurred in one form or another during the phonated isovolume maneuver. As with the paradoxing noted earlier, expiratory utterance dictates that one part of the chest wall must be reducing in size faster than the other part is increasing, the implication being that the volume displaced by one of the parts actually exceeds the total expiratory displacement of the lungs. Beyond the observations of Figure 3–16, subjects given biofeedback in the form of a storage oscilloscope display of a relative volume chart could voluntarily trace out a wide variety of prescribed relative volume pathways while speaking, including those in which they used either all rib cage or all abdomen when instructed to do so. Subject TH became particularly adept at controlling the configuration of his chest wall, as can be seen in the tracings of Figure 3–17. The upper chart shows a pattern of prescribed limbs generated during successive sustained vowel utterances over a large portion of the vital capacity. The lower chart shows the remarkable respiratory gymnastics TH could perform when his glottis was open and he attempted to trace out a complex pattern (his name in writing) by changing his chest wall configuration. This pattern was traced left to right with a combination of inspiratory and expiratory excursions by the two parts of the chest wall. The main point to be made from the data in Figures 3–16 and 3–17 is that an innumerable variety of relative displacement patterns can be generated by the two-degree-of-freedom chest wall system, the only limitation placed on the system for speech being that the combination of displacements is consistent with net expiration. The wide range of acceptable displacements of the chest wall is similar in some respects conceptually to the potential motions acceptable by the jaw-tongue unit discussed earlier. Speakers can change patterns of jaw and tongue motion voluntarily in a trading relationship to maintain normal speech. Case in point is the re-organization of motions that must occur when the pipe smoker

SAMPLE CONTROL UNDER BIOFEEDBACK

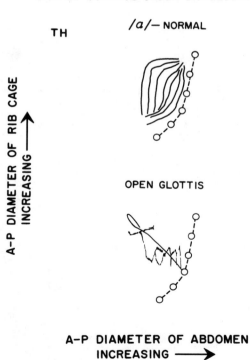

FIGURE 3–17. Relative volume charts showing data obtained for one subject in the upright position under conditions of visual feedback of chest wall configuration from a storage oscilloscope display. Tracings in the upper chart are for repeated sustained utterances of a vowel. The tracing in the lower chart was generated with the larynx open. Relaxation characteristics and the 40% VC isopleth are repeated from Figure 3–5.

maintains normal articulation after clenching his teeth and using compensatory articulatory motions of the tongue and other oral structures.

To this juncture, displacements of the rib cage and abdomen have been considered in themselves and apart from their causes. The relative motion chart also can be used to infer underlying muscular mechanisms associated with the various utterances. Such inferences are based on the possible muscular actions that could account for chest wall configuration (i.e., shape) at every instant. Interpretations of this nature depend, for the most part, on comparisons of chest wall shape during speech and relaxation, departures from the relaxed shape at corresponding lung volumes implying some form of muscular activity; some, because, given relative volume data alone, the combination of muscular forces involved cannot be specified unequivocally, there being more than a single way to maintain any specified shape, as is discussed here.

During utterance, the chest wall was nearly continuously distorted from its relaxed configuration, meaning that muscular forces were acting on it. In the upright position, all utterances occurred to the left of the relaxation line on the chart. Consequently, forces were operating to make the rib cage larger and the abdomen correspondingly smaller than they were during relaxation at the prevailing lung volume. Muscular activities that could bring about distortion of this nature include: (1) net[1] inspiratory forces operating on the rib cage, (2) expiratory forces operating on the abdomen, (3) a combination of net inspiratory forces operating on the rib cage and expiratory forces operating on the abdomen, and (4) a combination of expiratory forces operating on both the rib cage (net) and abdomen, but with the abdomen in predominance. Note that for the alternatives listed, only actions of the rib cage wall and abdominal wall are considered. The diaphragm is not included, in view of observations that its action alone does not cause departure from the relaxation configuration of the chest wall, but rather drives the rib cage and abdomen along their own passive characteristics (up and down the relaxation line on the chart) (Goldman and Mead, 1970). On the basis of relative motion data it is not, therefore, possible to specify whether or not the diaphragm was active to any degree during the utterance tasks.

---

[1]As used in this chapter, the term *net* encompasses situations in which either inspiratory or expiratory muscles of the rib cage are active alone, or in which both are active simultaneously either equally or with one or the other in predominance. When active equally, the result is a net zero that is the functional equivalent of relaxation as far as departure from the relaxation line is concerned. It cannot be said with certainty on the basis of the relative volume chart whether or not opposing muscular forces are operating. In cases of departure from the relaxation line, it can simply be stated that the net force is such that the system is distorted in one manner or another. For the four alternatives listed, net is specified for the rib cage only and not for the abdomen. This is because the muscles of the rib cage wall are so arranged that the structure is capable of generating pressures of two signs, inspiratory and expiratory. The abdominal wall, on the other hand, can actively generate pressure in the expiratory sign only. Hereinafter, the term *net* also is used in reference to activity between the two parts of the chest wall. For example, the net force generated by the rib cage and abdomen can be considered in the same terms as discussed here.

It can be reasoned as to which of the various alternatives is more likely than others on the basis of the sign and magnitude of the muscular pressure required for the different utterances. Estimates of such muscular pressure demands are based on knowledge of the approximate alveolar pressures required for the different utterances and the typical recoil pressures available at the prevailing lung volumes for normal subjects such as these (Bouhuys et al., 1966). Generally speaking, positive muscular pressure probably was required for the utterances studied in the upright position. That is, muscular forces had to be provided to supplement the spring-like background force generated by the respiratory apparatus. These positive muscular pressures also had to increase with decreasing lung volume during the utterances. Exceptions to the application of positive muscular pressure most likely would occur during very soft utterances requiring alveolar pressure that might be less than that provided by passive forces, and at very high lung volumes when the recoil forces might be in excess of those needed. In these two instances, the muscular pressure demands would be negative. For these reasons, it is believed that alternatives 2 or 4 probably account for the leftward departure from the relaxation line during most conversation, reading, and singing. It seems relatively certain that one of these alternatives would be operating below FRC. Thus, it would appear that the abdomen was active for these utterance tasks in the upright position. Whether this is with or without concomitant activity on the part of the rib cage, cannot be determined from the present data alone. The only instances in which it seems possible that one of the other two alternatives may explain the data is during the initial portions of soft reading phrases when some inspiratory checking might be called for. For utterances occurring throughout high lung volumes (especially soft utterances) it seems likely that alternatives 1 or 3 might be operating. Because both of these involve some form of inspiratory force, they are likely candidates for providing the negative muscular pressure required to check excessive recoil forces of the respiratory apparatus at high volumes. Thus, utterances performed throughout nearly the entire vital capacity range in the upright position probably require more than a single alternative to maintain departure to the left of the relaxation line on the chart, the alternative in operation being determined by lung volume and alveolar pressure requirements.

In addition to just position on the chart (i.e., being to the left of the relaxation line), the specific pathways followed (the history of position) are supportive of the various alternatives selected previously. From the mid-volume range downward, at which a positive muscular pressure is assumed to be operating, nearly all utterance tracings typically involve decreases in the diameter of both the rib cage and abdomen. This observation is consistent with alternatives 2 and 4. It likewise is consistent with alternative 3; however, it seems a rather improbable option, because it includes inspiratory forces in a range of volumes at which positive muscular pressures are required. In cases for which it was reasoned that negative forces would be involved at higher lung volumes, it was noted that for many of the sustained utterances—

particularly the soft and normal ones—there often is a sloping of the tracings back toward the relaxation line (i.e., the rib cage is getting smaller and the abdomen larger). Such observations are consistent with either alternatives 1 or 3, 1 being supportive of the interpretation of Bouhuys and colleagues (1966) that inspiratory muscles of the rib cage operate to control its descent when negative muscular pressures are called for. The outward movement of the abdominal wall in this case may reflect a passive displacement of the relaxed structure.

Observations for sustained vowels and syllable repetitions in the upright position revealed that for some subjects pathways often were displaced leftward on the chart with increases in loudness and utterance rate. This means that as louder speech and faster speech were produced, the abdomen was smaller and the rib cage correspondingly larger at the same lung volumes. It also was observed that with some subjects upright, there was relatively greater abdominal contribution at higher volumes for louder and faster speech. It seems likely that both of these observations reflect greater activity on the part of the abdomen for louder and faster utterances. For loudness, at least, such an interpretation is consistent with the greater muscular pressure required for increases in loudness (Bouhuys et al., 1966).

Distortions of the chest wall from it relaxed configuration in the supine body position were quite different from those observed for upright. For conversation, reading, and singing, tracings were to the right of the relaxation line on the chart. Thus, forces were operating on the chest wall to make the rib cage smaller and the abdomen correspondingly larger than they were when relaxed at the prevailing lung volume. Muscular activities that could cause distortion of this nature are (1) net expiratory forces operating on the rib cage, and (2) a combination of expiratory forces operating on both the rib cage (net) and abdomen, but with the rib cage in predominance.

The shift from upright to supine results in an increased relaxation pressure at all lung volumes, due principally to the influence of gravity on the abdomen (Agostoni and Mead, 1964). Because speech in the supine position occurs at lower lung volumes, at which the relaxation pressure is approximately equal to that for upright speech, however, the muscular pressure demands for conversation, reading, and singing are similar supine to those just described for upright. Given the need for positive muscular pressures for these utterances, either alternative 1 or 2 could explain the data. In either case the rib cage must be active in the expiratory direction, whether or not the abdomen is relaxed or less active than the rib cage. The slopes of the tracings for supine speech are consistent with either of the potential alternatives offered so that slope information is not of use in differentiating between the two alternatives.

Sustained vowels and syllable repetitions were not restricted to the right side of the relative volume relaxation line for the supine position, but were at times to either side of the line or on it. Various alternatives for being to the left or right of the line were just considered. To be on the line during speech requires a net muscular activity of zero, wherein the inspiratory and expiratory forces of the system are in balance. The only possible exception to this is during moments when the relaxation pressure is equal to that demanded for utterance and the system is relaxed. Although there were exceptions, high-to-mid lung volumes generally involved leftward departures from the relaxation line. This is consistent with the negative muscular pressure required in this range, there being a need for such pressure at lower volumes supine than upright because of the higher recoil forces generated by the supine system at identical lung volumes. The general trend for rightward departure from the relaxation line at lower volumes probably is the result of expiratory forces working to provide positive muscular pressures in that range. For several cases, the levels of intersection between the pathways and relaxation line occurred at higher lung volumes with increases in loudness, a trend consistent with the possibility that at these intersections the apparatus might be relaxed and driven entirely by passive forces. In many other cases, however, intersection levels did not bear a systematic relationship to loudness. It seems likely, therefore, that in many instances in which the apparatus is identical in configuration to that achieved upon relaxation, it is being maintained in that configuration by muscular forces. Furthermore, in those instances in which substantial segments of utterance tracings lie essentially on the relaxation line, changing muscular forces clearly are required to stay on the line if alveolar pressure is to be maintained relatively constant. As noted earlier, the sustained vowel and syllable repetition tracings were not extrapolations of those for supine conversation, reading, and singing. Thus, it seems reasonable that different mechanisms may account for the two types of activities within the common range of lung volumes involved.

Considering the distortion of the chest wall from its relaxed configuration, it is of interest that changes in the configuration at which speech took place did not have to do with changes in the pressure required for utterance. Earlier it was noted that the configuration of the chest wall could be changed dramatically during a "phonation isovolume maneuver" (see Fig. 3–16), an instance in which the alveolar pressure was presumed constant. During running speech, changes in alveolar pressure can be relatively large, yet substantial displacements are not seen on the charts corresponding to these pressure changes (i.e., the tracings were relatively smooth and did not show major "jogs" for the pressure changes). Only in the case of speech involving very great stress (emphasis) or high flows did corresponding motion jogs occur. Such an example is presented in Figure 3–18 for MG upright from his production of a series of discrete emphatic /hʌ/ syllables starting from a high lung volume. Leftward jogs accompanied the actual syllable productions, whereas downward motions occurred between utterances. Given that major jogs did not occur in charts for what might be considered typical utterances

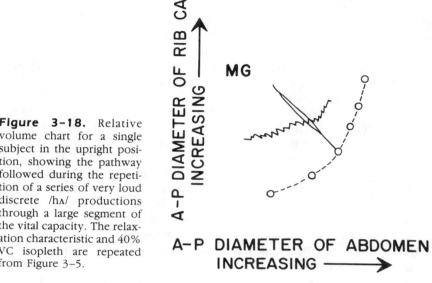

DISCRETE /hʌ/
VERY LOUD

Figure 3-18. Relative volume chart for a single subject in the upright position, showing the pathway followed during the repetition of a series of very loud discrete /hʌ/ productions through a large segment of the vital capacity. The relaxation characteristic and 40% VC isopleth are repeated from Figure 3-5.

(conversation or reading), it would appear that humans distort the chest wall from its relaxed configuration but do not further substantially distort it in developing variations in pressure (i.e., in providing the compressional volume changes required for utterance). This is interpreted to mean that the general distortion of the chest wall from its relaxed configuration constitutes a form of posturing of the system, off which the speaker then minimally distorts the chest wall to provide the rapid compressional volume changes (pressure fluctuations) needed to drive the larynx and upper airway. With respect to this situation, it is useful to conceptualize the workings of the chest wall in speech as involving the simultaneous or parallel solution of two problems. One is a rather gross kinematic problem, wherein a volume solution is provided and, in effect, used as a "platform" from which to solve the second problem of developing the required alveolar pressure. It is tempting to speculate that speakers set the chest wall in this platform configuration so that certain of its muscles are placed at their optimal mechanical advantage for generating rapid pressure changes without further major changes in the shape of the system. In any event, it is apparent that speakers can solve the problem of chest wall configuration quite separately from that of alveolar pressure.

Finally, there remains the problem of describing precisely the forces responsible for setting the configuration of the chest wall and for developing the pressure changes needed to drive the larynx and upper airway for speech. This problem has been addressed in studies of the separate volume-pressure behaviors of the rib cage and abdomen. The results of this work are presented in Chapter 4, which deals with various dynamic aspects of chest wall function for speech.

ACKNOWLEDGMENT

The preparation of this manuscript was supported by Special Research Fellowship NS-02038, Research Grant NS-09656, and Research Career Development Award NS-1 K4 41,350 from the National Institute of Neurological Diseases and Stroke, by Research Grant GM-12564 from the National Institute of General Medical Sciences, and by Research Grant AP-00229 from the National Air Pollution Control Administration.

REFERENCES

Abbs, J., Netsell, R., and Hixon, T. (1971). *Variations in mandibular displacement, velocity, and acceleration as a function of phonetic context.* Paper presented at the fall meeting of the Acoustical Society of America, Denver.

Agostoni, E., and Mead, J. (1964). Statics of the respiratory system (pp. 387-409). *In* W. Fenn and H. Rahn (Eds.): *Handbook of physiology. Respiration 1*, Sect. 3. Washington, DC: American Physiological Society.

Bless, D., and Miller, J. (1972). *Influence of mechanical and linguistic factors on lung volume events during speech.* Paper presented at the Annual Convention of the American Speech and Hearing Association, San Francisco.

Bouhuys, A., Proctor, D., and Mead, J. (1966). Kinetic aspects of singing. *Journal of Applied Physiology, 21*, 483-496.

Draper, M., Ladefoged, P., and Whitteridge, D. (1959). Respiratory muscles in speech. *Journal of Speech and Hearing Research, 2*, 16-27.

Fairbanks, G., (1960). *Voice and articulation drillbook (2nd ed.).* New York: Harper and Row.

Goldman, M., and Mead, J. (1970). The passive volume-pressure characteristics of the rib cage. *Physiologist, 13*, 208.

Hardy, J., and Edmonds, T. (1968). Electronic integrator for measurement of partitions of the lung volume. *Journal of Speech and Hearing Research, 11*, 777-786.

Hoshiko, M. (1965). Lung volume for initiation of phonation. *Journal of Applied Physiology, 20*, 480-482.

Hoshiko, M., and Blockcolsky, V. (1967). A respirometric study of lung function during utterance of varying speech material. *Speech Monographs, 34*, 74-79.

Konno, K., and Mead, J. (1967). Measurement of the separate volume changes of rib cage and abdomen during breathing. *Journal of Applied Physiology, 22*, 407-422.

Mead, J., Peterson, N., Grimby, G., and Mead, J. (1967). Pulmonary ventilation measured from body surface movements. *Science, 156*, 1383-1384.

Peyrot, A., Hertel, G., and Siebens, A. (1969). Pulmonary ventilation measured by a single linear displacement transducer. *Journal of Medical and Biological Engineering, 7*, 1-2.

Rahn, H., Otis, A., Chadwick, L., and Fenn, W. (1946). The pressure-volume diagram of the lung and thorax. *American Journal of Physiology, 146*, 161-178.

CHAPTER 4

Dynamics of the Chest Wall During Speech Production: Function of the Thorax, Rib Cage, Diaphragm, and Abdomen

Thomas J. Hixon
Jere Mead
Michael D. Goldman

I n the preceding chapter, data were presented on various kinematic aspects of chest wall function during speech production. As is denoted by the term *kinematic*, these data dealt solely with motions of the chest wall, apart from their causes. Here attention is devoted to various *dynamic* aspects of chest wall function during speech via observations of both the motions of the chest wall and the various forces applied to and by its different parts in creating those motions. The approach uses two types of respiratory measurements:

Reprinted by permission of the publisher from the *Journal of Speech and Hearing Research,* 19, pp. 297–356, © 1976, American Speech-Language-Hearing Association, Rockville, MD.

one, the method described previously for estimating the volume displacements of the surfaces of the rib cage and abdomen by measuring changes in their respective anteroposterior diameters (see Chapter 3), and the other, the use of catheter-balloon techniques for estimating pleural and abdominal pressures from measurements of esophageal and gastric pressures, respectively (Bouhuys, Proctor, and Mead, 1966; Milic-Emili, Mead, Turner, and Glauser, 1964). Using data obtained from these two types of measurements, relative motion charts and various forms of motion-pressure charts are constructed, from which mechanical behaviors of the chest wall, thorax, rib cage, diaphragm, and abdomen can be determined. To provide a framework within which to appreciate such measurements, the next section presents a theoretical basis for chest wall function in general and for the measurement approach in particular.

MEASUREMENT FRAMEWORK

The human chest wall is a complicated biomachine consisting of all extrapulmonary parts of the respiratory apparatus that share volume changes with the lungs. So defined, it includes the rib cage, the diaphragm, and the abdomen and its contents. The functional importance of the chest wall to breathing lies in its potential for action as a reciprocating bellows. Motions of this bellows provide for adjustments in alveolar pressure (compression and decompression) and for adjustments in the size of the chest wall (displacements). Each of the parts of the chest wall—rib cage, diaphragm, and abdomen—may exhibit motion during breathing. These motions sum up to be the same as those of the lungs. The chest wall and lungs are concentric parts of the respiratory apparatus operating in mechanical series. The chest wall itself presents two mechanically parallel pathways through which motion may occur. Parallel arrangement allows that the motion in each pathway may be different or even independent of that in the other. One surface of each pathway is visible externally on the torso—the rib cage wall and the abdominal wall—and manifests the motion in that particular pathway.

Motions of the chest wall and its parts are caused by forces that deform them. These forces come from two sources, one inherent and the other volitional. Inherent force arises from the elasticlike properties of different parts of the chest wall, properties that cause these parts to behave in ways analogous to coil springs. The sign (either inspiratory or expiratory) and the magnitude of the inherent force provided by each part depends on the prevailing volume (position) of the particular part and on the position of the body. Contributors to inherent force are the natural recoil of muscles, cartilages, and ligaments in the different parts and the influence of gravity on the parts. Volitional force capability is vested in the more than two dozen muscles that are a part of the substance of the different parts of the chest wall and that can power them variously. Volitional force can be supplied in different combinations of signs in the different parts and in magnitudes that depend on the will of the individual and are limited only by the strength of the respiratory muscles in a given sign within the part in question.

The task of any comprehensive attempt to analyze chest wall behavior during breathing is to specify both the motions of the chest wall's different parts and the forces, both inherent and volitional, that bring about those motions. The motions and forces of concern are distributed within the different parts in an extremely complicated fashion so that their specification is a major technical problem. Fortunately, however, motions of the parts sum up to volume displacements that are accessible to measurement at certain locations, and forces are fairly uniformly distributed at certain points where they result in measurable pressures. Thus, the comprehensive analysis task is approachable from a volume-pressure perspective, or in the lexicon of the bioengineer, a strain-stress perspective.

Relevant volume displacements for such an analysis include those of the chest wall (the same as for the lung), rib cage wall, abdominal wall, and diaphragm (Fig. 4–1A). Measurements of the first three of these are rather straightforward. This is due to the fact that motions of the visible outer surfaces of the two parallel pathways of the chest wall, namely the rib cage wall and the abdominal wall, have volume displacement as the only independent variable with respect to their individual motion. Accordingly, measurements of anteroposterior diameter changes of the rib cage and abdomen can be used to determine the individual volume displacements of these separate parts, and the combined diameter changes of the parts can be used to determine the volume displacement of the chest wall and the lungs. By shifting volume back and forth alternately between the surfaces of the rib cage wall and the abdominal wall with the upper airway closed, data can be generated to reveal the functional relationship between the relative motions of the rib cage wall and the abdominal wall at the prevailing lung volume. When done at a number of different fixed lung volumes distributed throughout the vital capacity, this volume shifting—termed an "isovolume maneuver" (see Chapter 3)—provides a family of data from which it is possible to derive the volume-motion relationships for each of the two chest wall pathways and for the entire chest wall through procedures that are the graphical equivalents of removing one of the pathways. By graphically displaying this family of data from isovolume maneuvers together with data obtained when lung volume is unconstrained, as for example during normal breathing or speech breathing, it is then possible to estimate the separate volume contributions of the rib cage wall and the abdominal wall to total chest wall volume (lung volume) for the unconstrained conditions. The reader will better appreciate the concepts mentioned here after reviewing pages 94 to 97 in Chapter 3 and after reading the section of this chapter dealing with "Data Displays: Orientation and Interpretation." There is no totally satisfactory means for determining precisely the volume

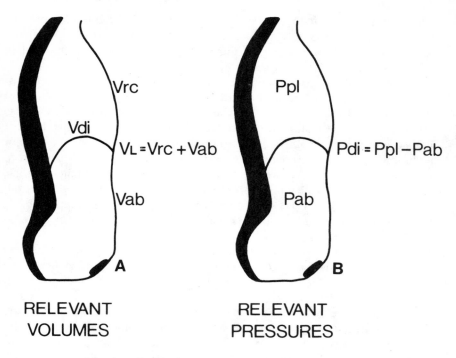

RELEVANT
VOLUMES

RELEVANT
PRESSURES

FIGURE 4-1. The relevant volume displacements (A) and pressures (B) of concern for any comprehensive analysis of chest wall function. Capital letters V and P represent volume displacement and pressure. Subscripts in panel (A) indicate the following: L = lung; rc = rib cage wall; ab = abdominal wall; di = diaphragm. Those in panel (B) indicate the following: pl = pleural; ab = abdominal; di = transdiaphragmatic.

displacement of the diaphragm. Under certain restricted conditions the diaphragm's volume displacement is reflected accurately in abdominal wall volume displacement. Previous work has used total lung volume change as an index of diaphragmatic volume displacement (Bouhuys et al., 1966; Hixon, Siebens, and Ewanowski, 1968), a convention followed here for lack of a better substitute given the current state of the art.

Relevant pressures, for purposes of a comprehensive analysis of chest wall behavior, include pleural, abdominal, and transdiaphragmatic (Fig. 4–1B). Two measurements lead to determinations of these three pressures: the measurement of esophageal pressure and the measurement of gastric pressure. Esophageal pressure is used as a measure of the relevant pleural-surface pressure. Pleural pressure cannot be sensed directly in humans without risk or measurement artifact and so it is commonly measured indirectly from the esophagus, where it is manifested accurately through the esophageal wall.

Actually, esophageal pressure represents pleural pressure accurately somewhere near axial midlung because pleural pressure systematically differs slightly in magnitude from the top to the bottom of the thorax. The differences are small, however, and can be neglected for practical purposes. Thus, esophageal and pleural pressures are functionally synonymous. Gastric pressure is measured directly from the stomach as a means of estimating abdominal pressure. As with pleural pressure, abdominal pressure cannot be measured directly without risk and so it is commonly inferred from measurements of gastric pressure, which are more easily made. Gastric and abdominal pressures differ by an amount dependent on the muscle tone of the stomach and the hydrostatic pressure gradient existing between the pleural surface and the point of measurement within the stomach. To an accurate approximation the magnitude of the pressure difference related to these two factors is revealed by the minimum difference between gastric and pleural pressures during relaxation at high lung volumes (Bouhuys et al., 1966). When this difference (an assumed constant) is subtracted from gastric pressure, the residual is the sought after measure of abdominal pressure. Transdiaphragmatic pressure is defined as the difference between pleural and abdominal pressures. Its determination, therefore, depends on the same measurement principles as outlined earlier for these two pressures.

Given the considerations offered in the preceding three paragraphs, the earlier description of the task of any comprehensive approach to the study of chest wall function can now be reworded: it is to specify both the volume displacements and the pressures just considered, as they relate to both the inherent and volitional aspects of the behavior of the different parts of the chest wall.

The inherent contributions of concern can be determined by measuring these volumes and pressures under the condition of voluntary relaxation of the respiratory apparatus against a closed upper airway at various lung volumes throughout the vital capacity. Complete voluntary relaxation brings about one necessary requirement of the measurement situation—namely, that any contribution to pressures developed by contracting muscles is made to be zero. More will be said in later discussion about how adequately this requirement presumably is met. Closure of the upper airway after breathing to various lung volumes brings about a second necessary requirement for measurements in that it provides for static conditions to exist at different volumes during the voluntary relaxations. By suitably combining the various volume and pressure measurements discussed earlier, it is possible to determine precisely the relaxation volume-pressure characteristics for the chest wall, thorax, rib cage, diaphragm (approximately), and abdomen. These characteristics constitute graphic representations of the pressures that always are contributed by the chest wall and its different parts at different volumes. The specific volume-pressure combinations involved in determining such characteristics are considered subsequently under the discussion of "Data Displays: Orientation and Interpretation."

The relevant muscular pressures developed by the chest wall and its parts can be determined by measuring the volumes and pressures discussed previously during typical breathing conditions (including speech), superimposing these data on graphs containing the corresponding relaxation volume-pressure data just mentioned, and graphically analyzing for the differences between relaxation values of the different pressures and those for breathing conditions at corresponding volumes in the different parts. Thus, the pressure developed by contracting muscles in each part of the chest wall is determined by subtraction. Under certain breathing conditions, differences between pressures measured during static conditions and during breathing do not relate solely to muscular pressure differences. This is because of losses due to resistance and mass acceleration in moving the different parts of the chest wall. For speech production, however, the rate of displacement of tissues and the rate of change of the rate of displacement are so low that pressures related to viscance and inertance practically are nil in comparison to other pressures and may be neglected. The reader will better appreciate the specifics of the procedure for determining muscular pressure contributions of the different parts of the chest wall and the possible interpretations from it after reading the discussion under "Data Displays: Orientation and Interpretation."

METHOD

Subjects

Three men served as subjects. Each had normal speech and hearing and had no known abnormalities of the speech apparatus. Subjects were judged to be "excellent relaxers," primarily on the basis of the very high consistency of relaxation pressures generated during repeated voluntary relaxations of the respiratory apparatus against a closed upper airway at different lung volumes.[1] All subjects spoke Standard American English. Pertinent physical characteristics of the subjects are given in Table 4-1.

---

[1]More needs to be said about the term *excellent relaxer*. No one knows the answer to the question of how completely anyone can voluntarily relax the respiratory muscles. Some individuals are known to be able to quiet the electrical activity of the presumed major muscles of respiration completely. Unfortunately, however, it is not possible to sample more than a small fraction of the relevant muscular tissue through electromyographic observations; hence such electromyographic evidence as does exist relative to voluntary relaxation is inadequate. Because excellent relaxers are exceedingly good at producing repeatable relaxation pressures at different lung volumes throughout the vital capacity without any feedback other than the normal sensations associated with the relaxation task, it might be argued that this is good evidence the respiratory muscles

Table 4–1.   *Pertinent Physical Characteristics of the Subjects*

Subject	Age (yr)	Height (cm)	Weight (kg)	Vital Capacity (L)
JM	52	188.0	85.9	6.2
DL	40	186.7	79.0	5.7
MG	36	172.7	86.7	5.1

Equipment

Figure 4–2 portrays schematically the equipment used. Anteroposterior diameters of the rib cage and abdomen were sensed with magnetometers (Mead, Peterson, Grimby, and Mead, 1967). Two generator-sensor coil pairs were used, one to sense rib cage diameter and the other to sense abdominal diameter. Sensing coils in the pairs provided output voltages that were inversely proportional to the cube of the distance between mated coils. Distance changes were small relative to the absolute distance between a coil pair so that each resulting voltage-diameter relationship was essentially linear and provided a continuous measure of anteroposterior diameter change. Signal processing involved amplification, half-wave rectification, filtering, and passage of the signal through a DC amplifier. The component of the output voltage related to the absolute distance between coil mates was zero suppressed at the DC amplifier so that only the voltage equivalent of intercoil distance change remained.

Esophageal and gastric pressures were sensed using catheter-balloon techniques (Bouhuys et al., 1966; Milic-Emili et al., 1964). Each of two units employed consisted of a thin-walled latex balloon (10 and 5 cm long for the esophagus and stomach, respectively) sealed over one end of a polyethylene catheter 100 cm in length. The free end of each catheter was coupled to one

are relaxed. Although it is tempting to lean strongly toward the acceptance of such evidence, the reader should be aware that it does not provide for a completely convincing argument. More fully acceptable evidence might be expected to come from comparisons between measurements made under the condition of voluntary relaxation and the condition following the administration of muscle-relaxing agents. In the case of such human experiments as have been done along these lines, however, it is not clear that the subjects used have met the definition of excellent relaxers. Thus, the occasional observation from such experiments of less than perfect agreement between results from the two conditions may be related solely to inadequate subject selection. Perhaps the best that can be said at present is that data obtained on excellent relaxers correspond well with what would be expected from data obtained in other species during pharmacologically induced relaxation. In any event, one major consideration seems to override many of the concerns relevant to this issue: that is in using excellent relaxers any possible contributions of muscles to the pressures developed during attempted voluntary relaxation, whatever they may be, certainly must be trivial in comparison to the pressures developed by the muscles during breathing. The present method of selecting subjects conforms with the best that the current state of the art allows. Thus, the present investigation surely cannot be far off in attributing measurements during voluntary relaxation to the elasticlike forces of the chest wall and its different parts.

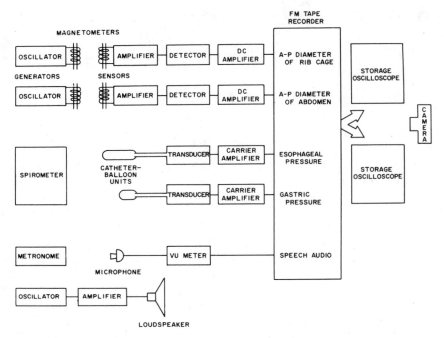

FIGURE 4-2. Diagram of the principal equipment.

side of a differential pressure transducer (the other side was to atmosphere), which in turn was connected to a carrier amplifier.

Outputs from the final-stage amplifiers on the magnetometers and the carrier amplifiers were fed to four channels of an FM tape recorder, where they were stored for playback in various *X-Y* combinations into a pair of storage oscilloscopes. Displays of the oscilloscopes were recorded permanently with a Polaroid camera.

Remaining equipment included a spirometer to measure changes in lung volume and three units to guide subjects in certain utterances. The latter included an air microphone coupled to a VU meter to provide an index of speech intensity (the raw audio signal also was recorded directly), an oscillator-amplifier-loudspeaker to provide pure-tone standards for pitch matching, and a metronome to pace utterance rate.

General Procedure

The subject-equipment interfacing used is portrayed in Figure 4–3. The polyethylene-encased coils were affixed to the body surface with double-sided adhesive tape. Generating coils were positioned at the midline on the anterior torso, one for the rib cage at the level of the nipples, and one for the abdomen immediately above the umbilicus. Sensing coils were attached posteriorly, also

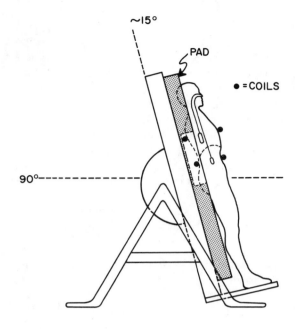

FIGURE 4-3. Subject-tilt table arrangement, magnetometer coil placements, and catheter-balloon positioning.

at the midline, and at the same axial levels as their generator mates. Each coil was oriented with its long axis perpendicular to the sagittal plane.

The catheter-balloon units were passed pernasally and swallowed into the esophagus. The unit with the smaller balloon (5 cm) was passed to the stomach and positioned with its tip approximately 65 cm from an external naris. The end of the larger balloon (10 cm) was located about 45 cm from an external naris. The gastric balloon was inflated with 2 cc of air and 0.2 cc of air was introduced into the esophageal balloon (Milic-Emili et al., 1964).

Measurements were made with subjects in upright and supine body positions. Upright recordings were made with subjects standing on a footplate and leaning backward against a padded tilt table oriented approximately 15 degrees off vertical toward supine. Supine recordings were made with the tilt table adjusted to horizontal. Calibration signals from the magnetometers and pressure transducers were recorded on tape for each investigative session.

RESPIRATORY MANEUVERS.   Recordings were made during vital capacity maneuvers, voluntary relaxations of the respiratory apparatus against a closed upper airway at various lung volumes, and isovolume maneuvers at specified lung volumes. Maneuvers were repeated several times in each body position. Each subject wore a noseclip during performance of the maneuvers.

For vital capacity (VC) measurements, subjects inspired to the total lung capacity (TLC) and then expired completely to the residual volume (RV) into a spirometer.

Voluntary relaxation against a closed glottis was done in repeated passes from TLC to RV at successive descending volume steps (within at least each 5% VC) in which the subject relaxed for 3 to 5 sec. Spot checks on data consistency were provided via closed airway relaxations at TLC, FRC (functional residual capacity), and RV.

Isovolume maneuvers were performed at each even 20% of the vital capacity. Each subject expired from TLC to the 80, 60, 40, and 20% VC levels successively, whereupon he closed his glottis, relaxed, and slowly displaced volume back and forth between the surfaces of the rib cage and abdomen. Spot checks on data consistency were provided by isovolume shifting at FRC. In the upright body position speech does not occur at abdominal diameters exceeding those during relaxation at corresponding lung volumes (see Chapter 3). Therefore, subjects were not required to shift from the relaxed position toward an inspiratory displacement of the abdomen during isovolume maneuvers in that body position.

UTTERANCES. All subjects generated a core of utterances, and randomly chosen subjects performed additional special utterances. All activities were performed twice, each subsequent to standardization of recent volume history. The latter constituted a deep inspiration, a relaxed expiration to FRC, and several resting breathing cycles. Core activities included the following:

1. Sustained production of /ɑ/ throughout most of the vital capacity, at a vocal fundamental frequency of 130 Hz, and at each of three loudness levels—normal, soft, and loud, in that order
2. Repeated utterance of /pɑ/ throughout most of the vital capacity, at a conversational vocal pitch, at a repetition rate of 4 per sec, and at each of three loudness levels—normal, soft, and loud, in that order
3. Spontaneous conversation with an investigator
4. Normal reading of the first paragraph of "The Rainbow Passage" by Fairbanks (1960).

Special activities are described subsequently (see *Discussion*). Subjects were guided in their performances of certain utterances by one or more of the equipment units discussed earlier.

RESULTS

Data Displays: Orientation and Interpretation

The upper part of Figure 4–4 illustrates the form of data displays used to present the results. Anteroposterior diameter is shown on the Y axis,

---

FIGURE 4–4. Illustration of the different charts constructed for data display, together with capsulized statements of the different muscular activity states that could account for positions on each chart relative to the relaxation characteristic.

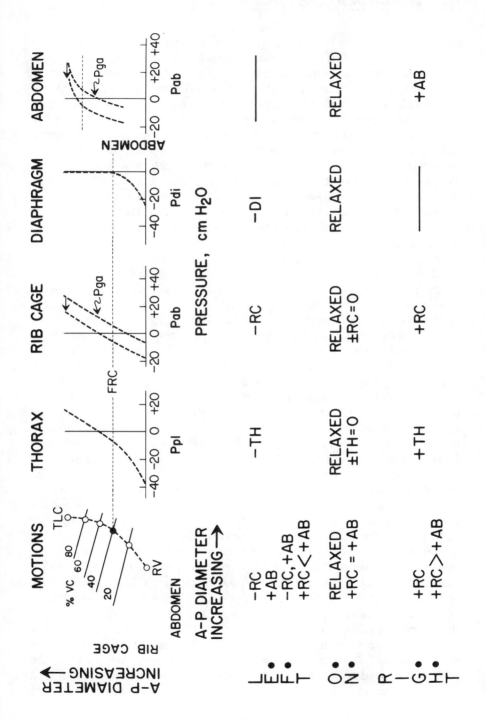

increasing upward for the rib cage in the first four charts and for the abdomen in the fifth. In the first chart, anteroposterior diameter of the abdomen is portrayed on the X axis, increasing to the right. The X axis for the remaining four charts displays pleural (Ppl), abdominal (Pab), transdiaphragmatic (pleural minus abdominal) (Pdi), and again abdominal (Pab) pressures. Zero represents atmospheric pressure in all but the diaphragm data display, where it represents the minimum difference between pleural and abdominal pressures. The curved dashed lines in the charts describe the series of data points generated during voluntary relaxation against a closed glottis at different lung volumes. Presumably they likewise represent the characteristics that would be followed were the respiratory muscles paralyzed and the apparatus driven passively through different volumes by a mechanical respirator. The last feature common to all five charts is the thin dashed line running horizontally across them. This line designates either the rib cage volume (Charts 1 to 4) or abdominal volume (Chart 5) attained during relaxation at FRC (the resting expiratory level).

Interpretation of mechanism from charts like those in Figure 4–4 is based on the position of data tracings on the charts, particularly in relation to the relaxation lines. Muscular activity states that could account for various postions on the five charts are designated in capsule form in the lower part of Figure 4–4. The upper, middle, and lower rows designate, respectively, activities that could prevail when tracings lie to the left, on, and to the right of the different relaxation lines. The symbols TH, RC, DI, and AB refer to the thoracic (rib cage plus diaphragm), rib cage, diaphragmatic, and abdominal muscles. Minus prefixes indicate inspiratory activity by the designated muscle(s) and plus prefixes indicate expiratory activity. The thorax and rib cage prefixes encompass net activities, because both inspiratory and expiratory muscles may be active simultaneously but with one or the other in predominance. Diaphragm and abdomen prefixes do not provide for opposing muscular pressures because each structure can generate pressure in one sign only. The term *relaxed* is self-explanatory, except as is pointed out subsequently for the motions and diaphragm displays. Muscle activity entries are absent for the diaphragm in the "right" row and for the abdomen in the "left" row because no departure alternatives are applicable (also discussed later).

Each chart and its use in interpreting mechanism warrants further individual discussion. The first chart portrays the relative motions of the rib cage and abdomen. Circles on the relaxation characteristic designate each 20% of the vital capacity, the upper and lower extremes being the total lung capacity (TLC) and residual volume (RV), respectively, and the filled circle representing the functional residual capacity (FRC) level. The four solid diagonal lines intersecting the relaxation characteristic at different 20% VC levels are isovolume lines. Movement up and down any isovolume line indicates the pathway followed on the chart during the shifting of volume from the abdomen to the rib cage and vice versa, with lung volume held constant. Difference in lung volume between any two points on the chart is given by the distance between them perpendicular to the isovolume lines. Upward or to the right involves an increasing lung volume, downward or to the left a decreasing lung volume. It is useful to rotate the diagram counterclockwise until the isovolume lines are horizontal. This makes them analogous to a family of X axes, where change in lung volume is given by vertical distance as in a conventional spirogram. Total lung volume change between any two points on the chart can be partitioned into its rib cage and abdominal components by graphic solution. This consists of deriving separate volume-motion relationships for the rib cage and abdomen. For the rib cage such a relationship is obtained graphically by noting rib cage diameter and lung volume changes at constant abdominal diameter, whereas for the abdomen it is achieved analogously by making corresponding comparisons at constant rib cage diameter. As discussed earlier, the separate diameters of the rib cage and abdomen are given by position along the vertical and horizontal axes of the motions chart, respectively. Upward on the chart indicates an increasing rib cage diameter. Toward the right constitutes an increasing abdominal diameter. As portrayed in Figure 4-4, the diameter-volume relationship for each part is nearly linear (revealed in approximately equidistant isovolume lines), so that diameter change of either the rib cage or abdomen can be interpreted directly as volume change. Every point on the chart defines a different chest wall configuration. Thus, any pathway on the chart, because it is a series of points, constitutes a recording of the changing shape of the moving chest wall. For the relative motion relaxation characteristic portrayed, the influence of passive pressures on the shape of the chest wall at different volumes is revealed.

Actual pressures during relaxation or speech cannot be determined from the motions diagram alone. Rather, any interpretation of mechanism from a motions diagram must be based on inferences as to possible muscular actions that could account for chest wall configuration at every instant. Interpretations of this nature depend, for the most part, on comparisons of chest wall shape during speech and relaxation, departures from the relaxed configuration at corresponding lung volumes implying some form of muscular activity. Different combinations of muscular activity can produce a given chest wall shape, so the activity involved cannot be specified unequivocally through use of the motions diagram alone. During moments when data tracings are to the left of the motions relaxation characteristic, pressures are operating to make the rib cage larger and the abdomen correspondingly smaller than they are during relaxation at the prevailing lung volume. Distortion of this nature could be brought about by net inspiratory rib cage activity, abdominal activity, different combinations of these same two, or simultaneous expiratory activity of the rib cage (net) and abdomen, with the latter being predominant. If chest wall shape during speech were identical to that at corresponding lung volumes during relaxation, the muscles of the rib cage and abdomen could be either relaxed or in balanced opposition. Tracings lying to the right of the relaxation characteristic must result from pressures making the rib cage smaller and the abdomen correspondingly larger than they are during relaxation. This type of distortion from relaxation could result from net expiratory rib cage activity alone or in combination with an active but smaller pressure contribution by the muscles of the abdomen.

Note that for the motions diagram, action of the diaphragm is not considered. This is because the diaphragm's action does not cause departure from the relative motions relaxation configuration but merely drives the rib cage and abdomen along their own passive characteristics (i.e., up and down the relaxation line on the chart) (Goldman and Mead, 1973). On the basis of relative motion data alone, therefore, it cannot be specified whether or not the diaphragm is active to any degree. Thus, the "relaxed" alternative listed for the motions diagram applies only to the rib cage and abdomen, with or without relaxation on the part of the diaphragm.

Activities on the remaining four charts can be quantified in terms of net muscular pressures as reflected in the horizontal distance between the various relaxation lines (diaphragm exception to be noted later) and the pressures observed during speech production. The pressures generated can be considered not only directly with reference to the vertical axis plots of either rib cage (Charts 2 to 4) or abdominal (Chart 5) volume, but also with reference to lung volume and the volume of the other part. The latter is done by noting the prevailing volume of the part of interest (either the rib cage or abdomen) and referring it to the motions diagram to determine the other corresponding volumes.

The thorax chart in Figure 4–4 provides a graphic volume-pressure display for determining the function of the entire thorax, defined to include the rib cage wall and the diaphragm together. The relaxation characteristic in the chart portrays the combined influence of the intrinsic elastic properties of the rib cage wall and of diaphragmatic tension on pleural pressure (i.e., transthoracic pressure) at different volumes of the rib cage. The ordinate in the chart shows rib cage volume and not thoracic volume. Although the chart has been labeled *thorax*, actually it is a display for the rib cage as influenced by the diaphragm, the latter not being a part of the rib cage. Departures to the left of the thorax relaxation characteristic result from net inspiratory activity of the thoracic muscles. The particular combination of pressures contributing to this net inspiratory activity cannot be determined from the chart but encompasses the possibilities of net inspiratory rib cage pressure, diaphragmatic pressure, these same two in concert, or a diaphragmatic pressure exceeding a net expiratory pressure by the rib cage muscles. Tracings that fall on the relaxation characteristic itself can be the result of either relaxation of the thoracic muscles or of net balanced opposition among them. Departures to the right of the thorax relaxation characteristic must result from net expiratory activity of the thoracic muscles. The combination of pressures involved cannot be designated unequivocally. Possible alternatives include net expiratory rib cage pressure alone or in combination with a lesser pressure provided by the diaphragm.

The third and fourth charts in Figure 4–4 partition the thorax chart into its rib cage and diaphragm components. The rib cage display differs from that for the thorax in that abdominal pressure rather than pleural pressure is plotted on the abscissa. The influence of diaphragmatic tension on the pressure developed during relaxation is equal to transdiaphragmatic pressure (Goldman and Mead, 1973). The intrinsic contribution of the rib cage wall itself is pleural pressure minus this transdiaphragmatic component, a difference that equals abdominal pressure. Thus, the relaxation line for the rib cage chart describes the intrinsic passive volume-pressure characteristic of the rib cage wall—free from the influence of the diaphragm. There are two characteristics shown in the rib cage chart in Figure 4–4. The one labeled Pga describes what might be actual recorded data, whereas the other is simply an X axis transposition of the same data. This transposition takes into account the difference between gastric and abdominal pressure, which in this sample illustration is taken to be 11 cmH$_2$O. For all subsequent displays, only the transposed characteristic (abdominal pressure) is shown. Departures to the left of the rib cage relaxation characteristic result from net inspiratory activity by the muscles of the rib cage wall. Tracings that fall on the characteristic are the result of either relaxation of the rib cage wall muscles or net balanced opposition among them. Departures to the right of the characteristic result from net expiratory activity of the rib cage muscles.

The chart labeled *diaphragm* is merely a plot of the difference between the thorax and rib cage displays just discussed, transdiaphragmatic pressure being the difference between pleural and abdominal pressures. This display allows a more convenient and direct graphic analysis of the contribution of the diaphragm to function than does visual comparison of the second and third charts. The relaxation characteristic in the diaphragm display reveals the influence of diaphragmatic tension as a contributor to pleural pressure at different rib cage volumes. Departures from the relaxation characteristic in the diaphragm chart cannot be interpreted in the same manner as in the thorax and rib cage charts because the ordinate of the display is rib cage volume and not a measure of diaphragm volume. (Recall that there is no totally satisfactory direct measure of the latter.) Transdiaphragmatic pressure values during utterance must be related to corresponding transdiaphragmatic pressure values during relaxation at the same lung volume for comparison. This is done by referring the rib cage volume on the diaphragm chart to the motions diagram and noting the transdiaphragmatic pressure value associated with relaxation at the same lung volume. The muscular activities listed below the diaphragm chart are meaningful only when rib cage volume is the same for speech as for relaxation at the same lung volume (i.e., when speech data fall on the relaxation characteristic in the motions display). Then it is impossible to be to the right of the relaxation characteristic, possible to be on it only when the diaphragm is relaxed, and possible to be to the left of the characteristic only when the diaphragm is contracting (horizontal distance equaling muscular pressure exerted by the diaphragm).

The abdomen chart in Figure 4–4 depicts the form of volume-pressure display used to evaluate the function of the abdominal wall. As in the third display, relaxation characteristics based on both gastric and abdominal pressures are shown, the latter being an X axis transposition (11 cmH$_2$O) of the former. Only the abdominal pressure line is shown in subsequent charts. This line describes the passive volume-pressure characteristic of the abdominal wall alone. It is impossible to depart to the left of the abdominal relaxation characteristic during speech. Being on the relaxation characteristic itself during speech is possible but only in the event of a relaxed abdominal wall. Tracings falling to the right of the abdominal relaxation characteristic indicate expiratory activity on the part of the abdominal wall muscles.

Respiratory Maneuvers

Figures 4–5 and 4–6 present data obtained during respiratory maneuvers in the upright and supine body positions, respectively. Each chart in each figure reveals data that are qualitatively similar across subjects.

The relative motions relaxation characteristics show both the rib cage and abdomen to decrease in size with decreases in lung volume. For the upright position, relaxation characteristics are concave toward the Y axis with the major part of abdominal volume change occurring below FRC. By contrast, the supine position finds the characteristics to be convex toward the Y axis with the major part of both rib cage and abdominal volume changes occurring above FRC. The 20% VC difference in FRC level between the two body positions is as would be predicted on mechanical grounds. Gravity acts in an expiratory direction on the rib cage in both the upright and supine body positions. Its influence on the abdomen, however, is inspiratory in the upright position and expiratory in the supine position. The expiratory influence in the latter position causes the abdominal mass and diaphragm to be displaced headward and a reduction in lung volume to result relative to that for the upright position. The isovolume tracings are nearly single valued, flat loops or lines, each being linear or roughly so. This character of the isopleths validates the assumption of a single degree of freedom in the "closed" chest

FIGURE 4–5. Relative motion charts and motion-pressure charts for all subjects in the upright body position, showing data obtained during respiratory maneuvers. Heavy dashed lines depict relaxation characteristics; solid lines on the motions charts are configurations assumed during isovolume maneuvers.

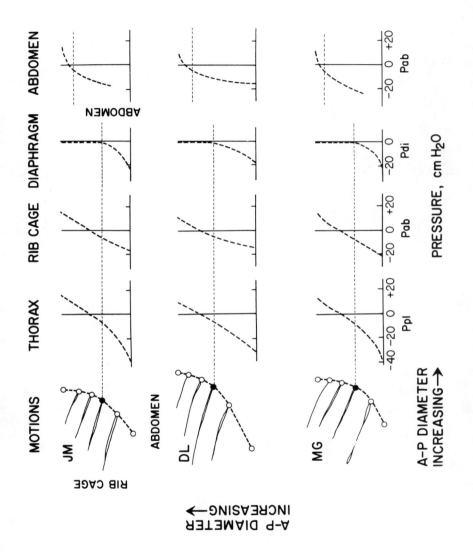

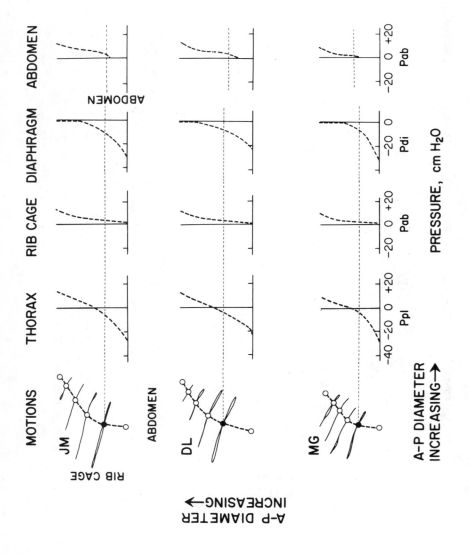

MOTIONS   THORAX   RIB CAGE   DIAPHRAGM   ABDOMEN

JM

DL

MG

RIB CAGE

ABDOMEN

A-P DIAMETER INCREASING→

←A-P DIAMETER INCREASING

Ppl   Pab   Pdi   Pab

−40 −20 0 +20   −20 0 +20   −20 0   −20 0 +20

PRESSURE, cm H₂O

A-P DIAMETER INCREASING→

wall and demonstrates further that the relative motion relationships of the two parts are not influenced significantly by the direction of volume shift between them. Approximate linearity of the isopleths suggests that the ratio of diameter change to volume displacement is similar for the diameters studied in the two parts. The fact that the isopleths are approximately parallel across the different lung volumes indicates that the diameter-volume relationships between the rib cage and abdomen are essentially independent of the configuration of the opposite part. The isopleths for each subject are nearly equidistant for equal volume increments. This means that the relationship between diameter change and volume change is approximately linear for each part. The slopes of the isopleths are substantially less than − 1. This reflects the fact that the diameter change-volume change ratio for the abdomen substantially exceeds that for the rib cage (i.e., the motion of the abdomen exceeds that of the rib cage for an equal volume change).

The thorax relaxation characteristics for each subject are qualitatively similar for the two body positions. Compliance of the thorax is found to be relatively constant at higher volumes and then falls off somewhat at the lower volume extreme in both body positions. At higher volumes, the thorax increasingly opposes expansion and hence operates in the same sense that the lungs do at all volumes. As volume decreases, the thorax becomes mechanically neutral (i.e., pleural pressure is zero) at a level somewhat above FRC. This condition occurs at a higher volume in the upright than in the supine body position. Below this particular volume, pleural pressure is subatmospheric and becomes increasingly more so with volume decreases. Mechanically, this means that the thorax opposes further reductions in volume.

The rib cage relaxation characteristics for each subject are identical to those for the thorax at higher volumes when the diaphragm is not under passive tension (to be discussed subsequently). Otherwise, characteristics for the two body positions are distinctly different. In the upright body position, the situation is analogous to that of the thorax in that at higher volumes the rib cage resists expansion whereas at lower volumes it resists compression. The rib cage curve "tracks" that for the thorax to near FRC in the upright body position. The compliance of the rib cage and thorax are, therefore, identical at higher volumes. At volumes below FRC in the upright position, the compliance increases progressively in two of the three subjects (JM and DL) as the residual volume is approached. For the supine position, the characteristics reveal that the rib cage wall opposes expansion at all volumes and hence operates in the same sense as the lungs do at all volumes. In this

---

FIGURE 4–6. Relative motion charts and motion-pressure charts for all subjects in the supine body position, showing data obtained during respiratory maneuvers. Heavy dashed lines depict relaxation characteristics; solid lines on the motions charts are configurations assumed during isovolume maneuvers.

body position, the rib cage curve tracks that for the thorax only at the upper volume extreme. Throughout the remainder of the volume range the compliance of the rib cage is relatively constant and greater than that typical of the upper volume extreme.

The diaphragm relaxation characteristics for each subject reveal the passive tension developed by the inactive diaphragmatic structure at different volumes. In both body positions, this tension is zero at high lung volumes (i.e., where the thorax and rib cage curves track one another) and increases with decreases in volume. Tension within the structure increases relatively rapidly as volume is decreased below FRC in the upright position and from well above FRC in the supine position. Once the diaphragm comes under passive tension in either body position it increasingly opposes further distention as lung volume decreases such that the compliance of the diaphragm is gradually and continuously reduced with decreases in volume.

Relaxation characteristics for the abdominal wall reflect major differences between the two body positions. In both body positions, compliance of the abdominal wall is relatively constant through the lower volume range. As higher and higher volumes are attained, compliance decreases, more so in the upright than in the supine body position. In the upright position the abdominal wall increasingly opposes outward displacement at volumes somewhat above the FRC level, whereas at volumes below this particular volume it increasingly opposes reductions in volume; the latter is reflected in the increasingly more subatmospheric abdominal pressure accompanying volume decrease. For the supine position, the abdominal wall opposes outward displacement at all volumes except the residual volume, where its mechanical behavior is neutral.

Sustained Vowel and Syllable Repetition Utterances

Figures 4–7 and 4–8 show data for the sustained /ɑ/ task performed in the upright and supine body positions. Data were highly similar for repeated performances of the same tasks, so only the tracing for the first utterance of each activity is presented. The numbers 1, 2, and 3 on the different charts designate tracings for successively louder phonations. Analogous data for syllable repetitions were deemed equivalent to those presented and, therefore, are not displayed.

UPRIGHT BODY POSITION. For the upright position, tracings on the motions charts extend through most of the vital capacity range and involve less of the lung volume extremes for DL than for the other two subjects.

FIGURE 4–7. Relative motion charts and motion-pressure charts for subjects in the upright body position, showing data obtained during production of a sustained vowel at three loudnesses throughout most of the vital capacity. Numbers 1, 2, and 3 denote pathways for successive increases in loudness (soft, normal, and loud). Relaxation characteristics and isopleths are repeated from Figure 4–5.

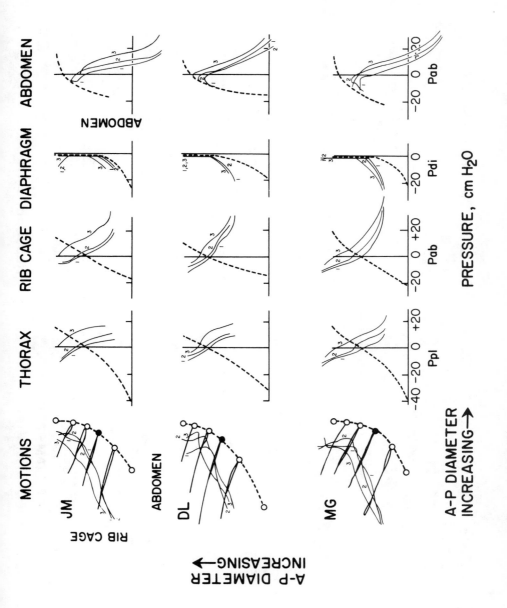

MOTIONS   THORAX   RIB CAGE   DIAPHRAGM   ABDOMEN

PRESSURE, cm H₂O

A-P DIAMETER
INCREASING→

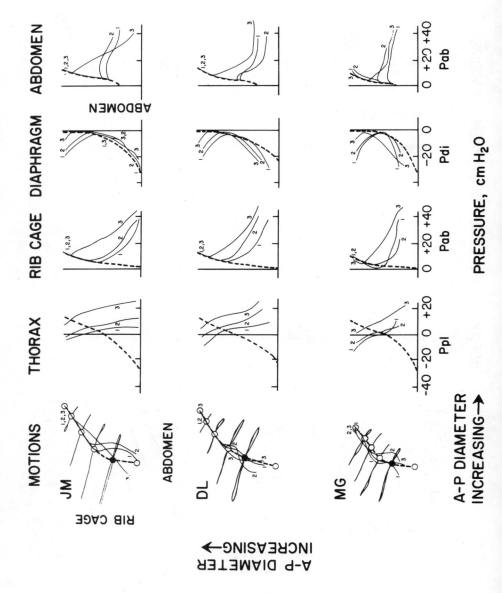

MOTIONS   THORAX   RIB CAGE   DIAPHRAGM   ABDOMEN

PRESSURE, cm H₂O

A-P DIAMETER INCREASING →

156

Tracings generally are concave toward the Y axis and involve a wide range of relative volume displacements by the rib cage and abdomen. A predominant expiratory rib cage displacement is demonstrated to various degrees at high lung volumes. This predominance is associated at times with an expiratory abdominal contribution (JM, 3), with no abdominal displacement (MG, 1), and with simultaneous paradoxical inspiratory displacement of the abdomen (DL, 1–3; JM and MG, 2). From the upper midvolume range downward, tracings for most utterances show roughly equal volume displacements by the rib cage and abdomen. The partitioning of volume change between the rib cage and abdomen depends on utterance loudness, particularly in the midvolume range and higher. At high lung volumes, patterns across loudness are idiosyncratic, the only common feature among subjects being abdominal paradoxing for utterances of normal loudness. The most consistent and striking loudness influence across subjects is found in the midvolume range. Marked shifts occur there from rib cage predominance to roughly equal contributions by the rib cage and abdomen at successively higher lung volumes with successive increases in loudness.

A large range of rib cage volumes is covered. JM and DL initiate utterances at rib cage sizes equal to those attained on relaxation between TLC and 90% VC, whereas MG begins his utterances at rib cage volumes larger than those at relaxed TLC. In nearly all cases, the size of the rib cage decreases continuously. Volumes equivalent to those measured during relaxation near 20% to 30% VC are attained ultimately.

Volume excursions of the abdomen also are substantial. Subjects differ as to the largest abdominal size used. The sizes are the same as those attained on relaxation at FRC, 60% and 30% VC for JM, DL, and MG. The smallest abdominal size reached by DL is near that for relaxed RV, whereas for JM and MG markedly smaller sizes are reached for utterances than for relaxed RV. The abdomen does not decrease in size continuously. For more utterances than not, it either moves outward or maintains a constant position for some segment through the higher lung volume range. For example, DL's abdomen always gets larger in the midvolume range than it is at the beginning of each utterance.

Chest wall configuration during the utterances is markedly different from that for relaxation. Utterances take place well to the left of the motions relaxation characteristic. Thus, the rib cage is relatively more and the abdomen relatively less expanded for all phonations than they are in the relaxed state

FIGURE 4–8. Relative motion charts and motion-pressure charts for subjects in the supine body position, showing data obtained during production of a sustained vowel at three loudnesses throughout most of the vital capacity. Numbers 1, 2, and 3 denote pathways for successive increases in loudness (soft, normal, and loud). Relaxation characteristics and isopleths are repeated from Figure 4–6.

at the prevailing lung volume. A loudness effect also can be seen in this configurational adjustment from relaxation. This is found at lower lung volumes, at which a trend exists for more leftward positioning on the diagram of all (JM) or a large part (DL and MG) of each tracing for loud phonation as compared with the other two phonations. Thus, the abdomen is smaller and the rib cage is correspondingly larger for the loud utterances than they are for the soft and normal phonations at the same lung volumes.

Those mechanisms responsible for the motions of the chest wall during the utterances can be determined through consideration of data in the remaining four displays. Here, and in discussion of other utterances, the data in each display will be considered separately, followed by a composite review of the entire data set.

Pleural pressure covers a wide range of values on the thorax chart (e.g., in MG from -15 to $+25$ cmH$_2$O) and increases with decreases in both lung volume and rib cage volume. It is higher at each lung volume and rib cage volume across successively louder utterances. Tracings depart nearly continuously from the relaxation characteristic, indicating that the thorax is active nearly continuously. This activity is net inspiratory at high volumes (e.g., -20 cmH$_2$O or more in muscular pressure at the start of soft phonations), where tracings fall to the left of the relaxation characteristic. The inspiratory muscular pressure applied is less for successively louder utterances and gradually decreases to zero where tracings intersect the relaxation characteristic, points of intersection being at higher volumes for successively louder phonations. Also, these points of intersection occur at the approximate volume levels where, on the motions chart, abrupt change takes place from a predominant rib cage displacement to essentially equal volume displacements by the rib cage and abdomen. It cannot be determined from the thorax chart alone whether the muscles of the thorax are relaxed completely or whether opposing pressures are balanced at these points of intersection. It can merely be stated that if in balance, only muscles of the rib cage wall are involved because the diaphragm is inactive at these moments. As phonation continues through lower volumes, a net expiratory pressure is provided by the thoracic muscles. This pressure gradually increases with decreasing volume and is of greater magnitude for successively louder utterances at corresponding lung volumes and rib cage volumes. Near the end of loud utterances, the positive muscular pressure applied to the thorax reaches magnitudes of near 30 cmH$_2$O.

The rib cage chart reveals the contribution of the intrinsic rib cage muscles to the total muscular pressure provided by the thorax. A large range of abdominal pressure is encompassed for the utterances in the rib cage display (e.g., in MG from -15 to $+45$ cmH$_2$O). This pressure increases continuously during the phonations, except for JM on soft and normal loudness utterances above approximately the 80% VC level, where it remains relatively constant.

Tracings show higher pressures at corresponding lung volumes and rib cage volumes for successively louder phonations and nearly continuous departure from the relaxation characteristic. Qualitatively, the derived muscular pressure data from the rib cage chart are highly similar to those for the thorax. Net inspiratory muscular pressure is provided by the rib cage at higher lung volumes and rib cage volumes, this pressure being less at corresponding volumes across increasing loudnesses. As phonation proceeds, the inspiratory effort of the rib cage decreases gradually to zero, with the data tracings intersecting the relaxation characteristic at the same volume levels at which intersections occur on the thorax diagram. Thereafter, each phonation is accompanied by rib cage efforts that are net expiratory and increasing continuously in magnitude until utterance termination. When the muscular pressures derived from the rib cage and thorax charts are compared at corresponding volumes, they are found to be equal for all or a major part of each phonation. This means that, for most of each utterance, the intrinsic rib cage muscles alone account for the muscular pressure being applied to the thorax. Exceptions are confined to one or the other of the volume extremes for each subject. At the upper end of the vital capacity the rib cage muscles provide less inspiratory pressure than that which is supplied to the thorax by JM for soft and normal phonation and by MG for soft utterance (e.g., the rib cage provides about 8 cmH$_2$O less inspiratory muscular pressure than the entire thorax provides at the start of JM's two utterances). At the other extreme of the vital capacity, DL's utterances show the rib cage muscles providing a greater positive muscular pressure than that which is supplied by the thorax from the 30% VC level through utterance termination. Toward the end of utterance, for example, the intrinsic rib cage muscles at times generate in excess of 10 cmH$_2$O of muscular pressure more than that which is supplied by the thorax. Differences between the thorax and rib cage data at the volume extremes must, by definition, be attributed to coactivity of the diaphragm.

The pressure developed across the diaphragm during the utterances ranges from -25 to 0 cmH$_2$O (see MG). Conveniently, the relaxation transdiaphragmatic pressure value is the same as the reference zero through the upper 60% of the vital capacity so that segments of the tracings that lie above FRC can be read directly for muscular pressure as the transdiaphragmatic pressure indicated in the displays. When the display is read in this way, it is readily apparent that the diaphragm is relaxed above FRC for all but three of the nine utterances of the subjects—the same three in which the thorax and rib cage muscular pressures differ. For MG the diaphragm is active a negligible amount down to the 90% VC level during soft phonation. For JM it is contracting a moderate amount at the initiation of his soft and normal utterances, diminishing its pressure contribution gradually to zero near the 80% VC level. The maximum pressure contributed by the diaphragm during the three utterances noted is -8 cmH$_2$O near 90% VC for JM's phonations. This constitutes less than a third of the total negative muscular pressure that is exerted on the thorax; the remainder is generated by the intrinsic muscles of the rib cage. Whereas transdiaphragmatic pressure either becomes less negative or remains constant at high volumes, it becomes continuously more negative from the vicinity of FRC downward. This latter increase in negativity occurs in the same general range of lung volumes through which transdiaphragmatic pressure changes similarly as a result of passive stretch of the diaphragm. Comparing transdiaphragmatic pressure values for phonations and relaxation at corresponding lung volumes, no differences are found for either JM or MG at these lower volumes, indicating that the diaphragm continues to be relaxed. For DL, however, transdiaphragmatic pressure is more negative for phonations than for relaxation from about the 30% VC level on. This indicates that his diaphragm is active at low volumes, an activity that increases gradually until utterance termination. At times near the termination of DL's phonations, the counteracting muscular pressure provided by the diaphragm is a third or more of the magnitude of the expiratory effort being generated by the intrinsic rib cage muscles.

In the chart for the abdomen, abdominal pressure generally is found to increase as lung volume decreases but not necessarily as abdominal volume decreases. The latter can be noted, for example, from the tracings for DL at high lung volumes, at which abdominal volume changes are paradoxical to total lung volume changes. Higher abdominal pressure prevails at corresponding lung volumes for successively louder phonations. The same is not always the case with respect to abdominal volume, however, as can be noted from DL's soft and normal phonations through lower volumes. The pathways traced for the different utterances fall either on or to the right of the abdominal relaxation characteristic, indicating relaxation and the generation of a positive muscular pressure, respectively. At high lung volumes muscular pressure patterns differ for the different subjects. DL's abdominal muscles are relaxed until near the 65%, 70%, and 76% VC levels across increasing loudnesses. MG, however, shows abdominal activity immediately on utterance initiation, and JM's abdomen is active at the start of loud phonation and becomes active shortly after the start of soft and normal phonations. In most instances in which abdominal paradoxing occurs (see DL's tracings and JM, 2), abdominal pressure increases slightly, but tracings do not depart from the relaxation characteristic; this indicates that the abdominal wall itself is relaxed during its outward movement. Such paradoxing is not confined to circumstances involving a relaxed abdomen. This can be seen in MG's normal-loudness utterance at high volumes at which the tracing grossly parallels the relaxation characteristic to the right. This shows an abdominal paradoxing in the face of an appreciable abdominal muscle tone. Once active for a given subject, the abdomen exerts a continuously increasing effort. This effort generally is greater at corresponding lung volumes for successively louder phonations. The magnitude of the muscular pressure generated is substantial and at times exceeds 40 cmH$_2$O (see DL, 3, near utterance termination).

Figure 4–9 presents a graphic summary of the muscular pressure events just discussed for the different charts. This summary incorporates binary statements of muscular events by showing where in the vital capacity each part of the chest wall is active (solid bars) or inactive during the three sustained vowels. Also indicated is the sign of the net muscular pressure being produced in the cases of the thorax and rib cage (i.e., minus for inspiratory and plus for expiratory). Even though only binary information is presented, a relatively comprehensive picture of function is contained in Figure 4–9 when it is remembered that inspiratory efforts generally are found to decrease with volume decrease through high lung volumes and to increase with volume decrease through low lung volumes, whereas expiratory efforts generally increase with volume decrease at all levels of the vital capacity. Vertical arrows running through the data sets designate the levels in the vital capacity at which changeover occurs from the exertion of a net negative to a net positive muscular pressure by the chest wall. The method for determining these levels and their importance to a description of function are considered later.

SUPINE BODY POSITION. For the supine position, relative motion tracings for utterances extend over most of the vital capacity range, except for the lowest 10% VC in DL and MG.

A wide range of relative volume displacements of the rib cage and abdomen is involved, with several tracings characterized as generally convex toward the *Y* axis. Expiratory rib cage displacement generally predominates

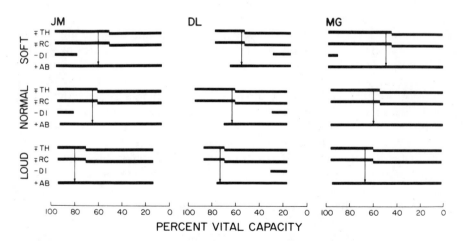

FIGURE 4–9. Graphic summary of data for subjects in the upright body position, showing where in the vital capacity each part of the chest wall is active (solid bars) or inactive during production of a sustained vowel at three loudnesses throughout most of the vital capacity. The symbols TH, RC, DI, and AB represent the thorax, rib cage, diaphragm, and abdomen. Minus and plus signs denote inspiratory and expiratory activities, respectively. Arrows mark points where the net muscular pressure of the chest wall is zero.

during the utterances. The exceptions are a low volume segment for DL, 2 and an upper-to-midvolume segment for MG, 1. The degree of rib cage predominance varies both between and within utterances. In the upper half of the vital capacity, a considerable expiratory abdominal displacement accompanies the predominant displacement of the rib cage. Idiosyncratic tracings are found in the lower half of the vital capacity for the different subjects, with the abdomen at times showing no concomitant displacement (see DL, 3, below FRC), an expiratory displacement (see JM, 3), or a paradoxical inspiratory displacement (e.g., see segments between 40% and 20% VC for JM, 1 and 2, and MG, 2). Tracings for the supine position do not reveal any systematic across-subject influence of utterance loudness on the relative contributions of the rib cage and abdomen. Only JM shows relative contribution changes at successively higher lung volumes with successively higher loudnesses. The direction of change is toward more rib cage contribution.

The range of rib cage volumes encompassed for the utterances nearly equals that covered during relaxation over the vital capacity range. All phonations begin at rib cage sizes close to those attained on relaxation at TLC and end at sizes equal to those associated with relaxation at 10% VC or lower. During the course of the phonations, the size of the rib cage decreases continuously.

Abdominal excursions also are large during the utterances. At the start of utterance, the abdomen is near the size it assumes on relaxation at TLC. It moves inward markedly during phonation to sizes near those for relaxation at very low lung volumes. The volume history of the abdomen is not one of continuous decrease. For some segment of all but one data tracing (JM, 3), abdominal size remains nearly constant or increases somewhat as lung volume decreases.

With regard to chest wall configuration during the utterances in relation to relaxation, the tracings are found to lie on, to the left, and to the right sides of the relaxation characteristic, crossing it variously. Systematic across-subject trends are not apparent. The only common feature for subjects JM and DL is that tracings for the soft and normal loudness utterances follow the characteristic until the midvolume range before departing to the right. Configurational adjustment is not seen to bear any systematic relationship to loudness changes for the different subjects. At higher lung volumes, tracings follow similar pathways, whereas at lower volumes they are idiosyncratic for the different subjects.

As seen in the thorax chart, a large range of pleural pressure is covered during the utterances (DL and MG cover over 35 cmH$_2$O). This pressure increases with decreases in lung volume and rib cage volume and typically is higher at the same volumes for successively louder phonations. Tracings depart nearly continuously from the relaxation characteristic, meaning that the thorax essentially is active continuously during the utterances. Muscular pressure is initially net inspiratory at high volumes (e.g., greater than -20 cmH$_2$O at the start of MG's soft utterance), decreases gradually to zero, and then becomes increasingly net expiratory through the remainder of each phonation. Near the end of utterance, the thoracic muscular pressure is sometimes found to exceed 40 cmH$_2$O (see JM, 3). During moments of inspiratory effort, less pressure is provided at corresponding volumes for successively louder phonations, whereas for nearly all moments involving expiratory effort, greater pressure is provided for increasingly louder phonations. The changeover from net inspiratory to net expiratory thoracic pressure occurs at higher lung volumes for louder utterances. For a number of utterances (see JM, 1 to 3; DL, 1 and 2; and MG, 2) the moments of changeover from net inspiratory to net expiratory activity are tied closely to changes in relative volume contributions of the rib cage and abdomen. In these cases the motions charts reveal marked increases in rib cage contribution.

The rib cage chart shows abdominal pressure to be positive continuously during the utterances and to cover a wide range of values (e.g., in MG from 2 to 48 cmH$_2$O). During the course of each phonation, the magnitude of abdominal pressure decreases moderately from its value at the start of utterance and then increases substantially thereafter. Typical tracings do not show continuous departure from the relaxation characteristic, nor is pressure always higher at corresponding volumes for successively louder phonations. At the start of phonation, all but one of the tracings lie on the relaxation characteristic, indicating that the intrinsic rib cage muscles either are relaxed or in antagonistic inspiratory-expiratory balance. The single exception is MG's loud utterance, for which a negative muscular pressure of a few cmH$_2$O is exerted to the 78% VC level. The only other instance of inspiratory rib cage effort occurs between the 80% and 34% VC levels during the course of MG's soft utterance. For this segment, the muscular pressure becomes increasingly negative to about -3 cmH$_2$O and then returns to zero. Each of the tracings departs to the right of the relaxation characteristic at some point during the course of utterance, indicating that a net expiratory pressure is being provided. These points of departure occur at the same rib cage and lung volumes at which the net thoracic muscular pressure first becomes positive. Thus, the rib cage muscles begin to generate a positive muscular pressure at higher rib cage volumes and lung volumes for successively louder phonations and then increase continuously the magnitude of this effort throughout each phonation. When comparisons can be made, the derived muscular pressure typically is higher at corresponding rib cage volumes and lung volumes for successively louder phonations. The muscular pressures generated by the intrinsic rib cage muscles and by the thorax are disparate at corresponding volumes, for much of each phonation. This means that the intrinsic rib cage muscles are not themselves providing the total thoracic muscular pressure. During moments when a net negative pressure is being supplied, the contribution of the rib cage muscles is zero (see JM and DL on all utterances and MG, 2) or only a fraction of the total inspiratory effort of the thorax (see MG, 3 and MG, 1). As an example of the latter, the inspiratory effort of the rib cage at the start of MG's loud phonation is less than one third of the total effort of the thorax. During moments when the net activity of the thorax is expiratory, the effort of the rib cage at times exceeds that of the thorax. This is the case toward the end of all of DL's phonations and for MG's soft and normal utterances, in which the rib cage drive sometimes exceeds that for the thorax by 10 cmH$_2$O or more. MG's loud phonation is unique for the various utterances in that the rib cage effort exceeds that of the thorax over the entire range of volumes through which a net expiratory thoracic muscular pressure is exerted (i.e., from 78% VC to utterance termination). By definition, the muscular pressure disparity between the rib cage and thorax is the result of diaphragmatic activity.

A range of -30 to 0 cmH$_2$O of transdiaphragmatic pressure is developed during the supine phonations. From its negative value at the start of each phonation, this pressure first becomes less negative and then later returns to more negative values. Figure 4–8 reveals the diaphragm to be active at the start of every utterance and to continue its activity to the same (JM and DL) or approximate (MG) volumes at which the negative muscular effort of the thorax ceases. Its effort is greatest at the start of utterance (e.g., about -20 cmH$_2$O or more for the soft condition) and diminishes gradually until relaxation. When different loudnesses are contrasted it is found that the diaphragm exerts less muscular pressure at corresponding volumes for successively louder phonations. For all of JM's and DL's utterances and for MG's normal-loudness phonation, the inspiratory pressure of the diaphragm alone accounts for the inspiratory pressure of the thorax. The only two phonations in which the negative thoracic effort is not equaled by the diaphragm's effort are those for soft and loud utterances by MG, which were noted previously to involve inspiratory rib cage activity. For these two utterances, the inspiratory effort of the diaphragm generally exceeds that of the rib cage muscles, making the diaphragm the more important contributor to the total negative thoracic effort. For example, MG, 3 shows diaphragmatic effort that is triple that of his rib cage muscles at the start of phonation (i.e., -6 of the total of -8 cmH$_2$O). From the first moment of total relaxation of the diaphragm, only JM maintains his diaphragm in a relaxed state throughout the remainder of each utterance. DL shows reactivation of the diaphragm at low volumes near the end of each of his utterances, whereas MG presents a similar pattern for his soft and normal phonations. For MG's loud utterance, the diaphragm reactivates almost immediately after it is fully relaxed. All of these returns of diaphragmatic activity after relaxation take the form of gradual increases in inspiratory effort to a maximum at the end of phonation. The muscular pressure provided by the diaphragm during such moments is in counteraction to the expiratory exertion of the rib cage muscles and at times constitutes approximately a third of the magnitude of effort being produced by the rib cage (see DL, 1).

Pressure in the abdomen chart first goes through a moderate decrease, followed by a marked increase. At the start of phonation, seven of the nine tracings lie on the relaxation characteristic, indicating that the abdominal muscles are relaxed. The remaining two tracings (i.e., MG, 1 and 2) show a moderate abdominal contraction (e.g., 4 cmH$_2$O of muscular pressure for normal loudness) at the beginning of utterance. For soft phonation this activity lasts only briefly, whereas for normal loudness it continues at a relatively constant magnitude to near 50% of the vital capacity, at which the abdomen relaxes momentarily. Each of the nine tracings departs from the relaxation characteristic at some point during the course of phonation, indicating the moment of activation of the abdominal muscles or, in the case of MG, 1 and 2, reactivation of the abdomen. These departures are exactly or approximately coincident with the first moments of net expiratory thorax and rib cage activity. For successively louder utterances the abdomen becomes active at higher lung volumes and abdominal volumes and thereafter increases continuously the magnitude of its effort. Contrasted across increasing loudnesses, muscular pressure generally is greater at corresponding lung volumes but not abdominal volumes. At times near the end of utterance (see MG, 1 and 3) the abdominal contribution exceeds 40 cmH$_2$O of muscular pressure.

A graphic summary of the overall muscular pressure events for the different displays is presented in Figure 4–10. As with Figure 4–9, this is a binary statement that disregards the magnitudes of muscular pressures being exerted and indicates only their signs and presence or absence. Vertical arrows indicate changeover levels from net negative to net positive chest wall muscular pressures.

Spontaneous Conversation and Normal Reading

For each body position, the data for spontaneous conversation and normal reading were judged to be highly similar. Data were pooled within each position and treated as a single task, henceforth designated as conversational speech. Figures 4–11 and 4–12 show data tracings for such conversational speech produced first in the upright and then in the supine body positions. Data included are representative of the variety of tracings obtained from each subject. Only a few of the expiratory limbs (breathing phrases) of the data loops are shown to avoid cluttering the charts. Numbers on the figures designate corresponding tracings across the different charts for each subject. The discussion that follows characterizes the entire data pool from which these tracings were selected.

UPRIGHT BODY POSITION. From the motions chart for the upright position, it can be seen that lung volume is limited to the midrange of the

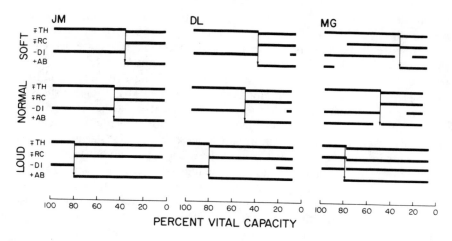

FIGURE 4–10. Graphic summary of data for subjects in the supine body position, showing where in the vital capacity each part of the chest wall is active (solid bars) or inactive during production of a sustained vowel at three loudnesses throughout most of the vital capacity. The symbols TH, RC, DI, and AB represent the thorax, rib cage, diaphragm, and abdomen. Minus and plus signs denote inspiratory and expiratory activities, respectively. Arrows mark points where the net muscular pressure of the chest wall is zero.

vital capacity for conversational speech. All expiratory limbs are initiated from well above FRC, typically from between the 60% and 50% VC levels. Limbs extend over 10% to 20% of the vital capacity and terminate above or in the near vicinity of FRC, there being an occasional encroachment upon the expiratory reserve volume (see MG, 3).

Changes in lung volume during the utterances result from expiratory displacement by both the rib cage and abdomen, the relative contribution of the two differing among the subjects. JM and DL show a predominance of rib cage displacement for all of their utterances. MG, on the other hand, typically uses a predominance of abdominal displacement or occasionally equal volume displacements of the rib cage and abdomen.

All conversational speech occurs at larger rib cage volumes than those measured on relaxation at FRC. Limbs are initiated from within a narrow range

FIGURE 4–11. Relative motion charts and motion-pressure charts for subjects in the upright body position, showing data obtained during conversational speech of normal loudness. Numbers 1, 2, and 3 denote pathways for corresponding tracings across the different charts for different subjects. Partial relaxation characteristics and isopleths are repeated from Figure 4–5.

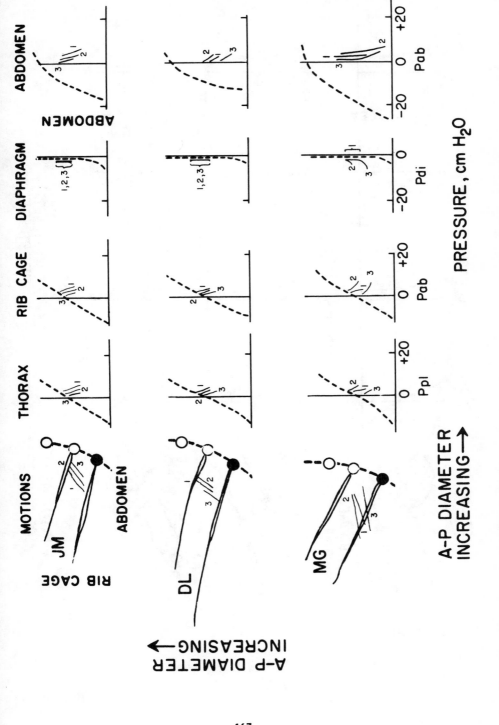

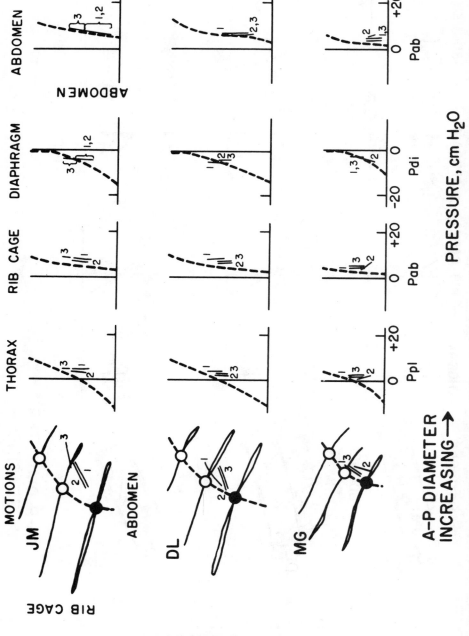

of rib cage volumes, encompassing sizes comparable to those attained during relaxation between 65% and 55% VC. Typical rib cage excursions cover the equivalent of 10% VC changes or less in relaxed rib cage volumes. Limbs end at rib cage sizes the equivalent of those attained by the relaxed rib cage beween the 60% and 50% VC levels.

The abdomen is confined to smaller volumes during conversational speech than those attained at relaxed FRC. At the initiation of limbs, the abdomen is found within a range of sizes usually equal to those recorded during relaxation between the 40% and 30% VC levels. Typical limbs for JM and DL involve abdominal excursions similar in magnitude to those associated with 10% to 20% VC changes on relaxation, whereas those for MG are greater. The size of the abdomen at the termination of limbs ranges between sizes equal to those attained between the 30 and 10% VC levels during relaxation.

Conversational speech takes places well to the left of the motions relaxation configuration on the chart. Thus, the rib cage is relatively more and the abdomen is correspondingly less expanded than they are in the relaxed state at the same lung volume.

Examination of the remaining four charts allows determination of the pressures responsible for the displacements observed on the motions chart.

In the thorax chart, pleural pressure is seen to be positive continuously and to cover a relatively small range of values (e.g., in JM from 2 to 7 cmH_2O). Pressure increases with decreases in lung volume and rib cage volume and differs only a small amount from limb to limb. Tracings start on or slightly to the right of the thorax relaxation characteristic and depart farther from the characteristic as utterance proceeds. (On a few occasions subjects took deeper than normal breaths prior to utterance. Then the upper part of tracings extended slightly to the left of the characteristic during speech.) Thus, the thorax essentially is active continuously in the expiratory direction during conversational speech, with the exertion of net thoracic muscular pressure increasing gradually throughout each expiratory limb. At the end of JM's No. 1 limb, for example, the thoracic muscular pressure is near 10 cmH_2O.

Abdominal pressure in the rib cage display is found to be positive continuously and to cover a relatively small range of values. This pressure increases with decreases in lung volume and rib cage volume and differs a small amount from limb to limb. Tracings begin on or slightly to the right of the rib cage relaxation characteristic and gradually depart farther from the

FIGURE 4–12. Relative motion charts and motion-pressure charts for subjects in the supine body position, showing data obtained during conversational speech of normal loudness. Numbers 1, 2, and 3 denote pathways for corresponding tracings across the different charts for different subjects. Partial relaxation characteristics and isopleths are repeated from Figure 4–6.

characteristic as utterance proceeds. Accordingly, the rib cage is active nearly continuously in the expiratory direction and increasingly so as volume decreases. Muscular pressures derived from the rib cage and thorax charts at corresponding volumes are found to be equal for all or a major part of each expiratory limb. This indicates that the intrinsic rib cage muscles alone are responsible for the muscular pressure being applied by the thorax. Only toward the end of MG's No. 2 and No. 3 limbs does abdominal pressure exceed slightly the corresponding value of pleural pressure, an observation that is attributable to the behavior of the diaphragm.

Transdiaphragmatic pressure is zero throughout all of JM's and DL's conversational speech. For MG, it ranges from 0 to -4 cmH$_2$O, departing from zero only near the end of expiratory limbs No. 2 and No. 3. Transdiaphragmatic pressure values for the various utterances are found to be equal to their relaxation values at corresponding lung volumes. Development of a small transdiaphragmatic pressure near the end of some expiratory limbs in MG's case reflects a passive stretch placed on the diaphragm below FRC and not a volitional contraction of the diaphragm. Thus, the diaphragm is inactive during conversational speech for all of the subjects.

The abdomen chart shows abdominal pressure to increase continuously with decreases in lung volume and abdominal volume. Tracings begin substantially to the right of the relaxation characteristic of the abdomen and depart from it increasingly as utterance proceeds. This means that the abdomen is continuously and quite forcefully active during speech. The magnitude of this activity increases during the course of utterance until by the end of some utterances, it is in the neighborhood of 35 cmH$_2$O of muscular pressure (see MG, 2).

Figure 4–13 presents a summary of the muscular pressure events just described. The magnitudes of the muscular pressures exerted are disregarded and only their signs and presence or absence are indicated, as in other previous analogous displays.

SUPINE BODY POSITION. As is revealed in the motions chart in Figure 4–12, conversational speech occurs at relatively low lung volumes in the supine position. All expiratory limbs begin well above the FRC level, typically in the neighborhood of the 50% to 40% VC levels. Limbs usually cover between 10% and 15% of the vital capacity and terminate above the FRC level. For subject MG, some breathing phrases extend into the expiratory reserve volume.

Both the rib cage and abdomen contribute to the volume displacement of the chest wall during the utterances. For JM and DL, relative contributions of the two parts are approximately equal or slightly in favor of the rib cage. By contrast, tracings for MG reveal a marked rib cage predominance.

Nearly all conversational speech occurs at larger rib cage volumes than those recorded during relaxation at FRC. Limbs start from within a range of

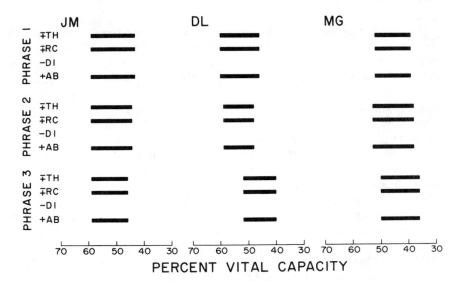

FIGURE 4–13. Graphic summary of data for subjects in the upright body position, showing the activity (solid bars) or inactivity of each part of the chest wall at various lung volumes during conversational speech production. The symbols TH, RC, DI, and AB represent the thorax, rib cage, diaphragm, and abdomen. Minus and plus signs denote inspiratory and expiratory activities, respectively.

rib cage volumes comparable to those achieved for relaxation between the 40% and 30% VC levels. Typical rib cage excursions cover the equivalent of about 5% to 15% VC changes in relaxed rib cage volume, exceptions being confined to an occasional larger excursion by subject MG. The majority of limbs are terminated at rib cage volumes comparable to those measured for the relaxed rib cage between the 30% and 20% VC levels.

The abdomen is maintained at a larger size during conversational speech in the supine position than the size it assumes at relaxed FRC. Most limbs start within a range of abdominal sizes encompassing those measured during relaxation between the 60% and 50% VC levels. Abdominal excursions typically cover the equivalent of 10% to 20% VC changes on relaxation, with the size of the abdomen at the termination of expiratory phrases usually falling between the range of sizes attained between the 40% and 20% VC levels.

In all cases for the supine position, conversational speech occurs to the right of the motions relaxation characteristic. This means that the rib cage is relatively less and the abdomen relatively more expanded than they are in the relaxed state at the prevailing lung volume.

The pressures responsible for the kinematic observations just discussed are revealed in the remaining four charts in Figure 4–12.

In the thorax chart, pleural pressure is found to be positive continuously and to encompass a very small range of values. The magnitude of this pressure differs slightly from limb to limb and changes only minimally, if at all, during the breathing phrases. Tracings start just to the right of the thorax relaxation characteristic. During the course of utterance, the tracings and relaxation characteristic gradually diverge. The thorax is, therefore, expiring continuously during conversational speech, with its level of effort increasing gradually throughout each expiratory limb.

In the rib cage chart, abdominal pressure is positive continuously, encompasses a very small range of values, differs slightly from limb to limb, and changes only a small amount, if at all, during the course of each breathing phrase. Tracings begin slightly to the right of the rib cage relaxation characteristic and remain to the right of the characteristic through the duration of each utterance. Thus, the rib cage is active continuously in the expiratory direction during the utterances. Muscular pressures derived from the rib cage and thorax charts are identical or nearly so, indicating that the activity of the rib cage wall alone is responsible for the effort of the thorax. Differences between pleural and abdominal pressures in the two charts are attributable to the passive behavior of the diaphragm, as revealed in the fourth chart.

Transdiaphragmatic pressure is negative and in the neighborhood of -5 cmH_2O during each of the conversational speech limbs. This pressure either remains constant or becomes slightly more negative during the course of each limb. When utterance values of pressure are compared to those for relaxation at corresponding lung volumes, the two are found to be identical or highly similar. This is interpreted to mean that the diaphragm's activity is zero during conversational speech in the supine position for all of the subjects. The small transdiaphragmatic pressures developed during the utterances are attributable to passive stretch of the diaphragm.

Data tracings for JM and DL follow the abdominal relaxation characteristic, indicating that the abdominal muscles are relaxed during the speech task. For MG, tracings fall slightly to the right of the relaxation characteristic, meaning that his abdomen is contracting. Muscular pressures generated are relatively small and build slowly in each breathing phrase as utterance proceeds.

A summary graph indicating which parts of the chest wall are active at different lung volumes during supine conversational speech is given in Figure 4–14. As before, this constitutes a binary statement for each part, indicating the sign and presence or absence of activity.

DISCUSSION

Muscular Pressure Adjustments of the Chest Wall

The problem solved by the respiratory apparatus during speech production is that of regulating alveolar pressure in accordance with the demands of utterance. This is accomplished by adding muscular pressure to

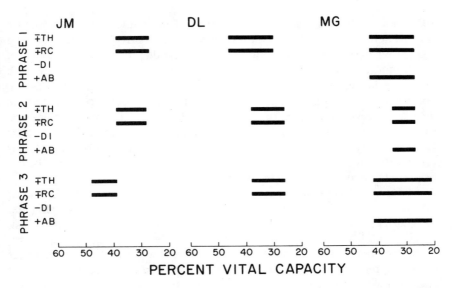

FIGURE 4–14. Graphic summary of data for subjects in the supine body position, showing the activity (solid bars) or inactivity of each part of the chest wall at various lung volumes during conversational speech production. The symbols TH, RC, DI, and AB represent the thorax, rib cage, diaphragm, and abdomen. Minus and plus signs denote inspiratory and expiratory activities, respectively.

the relaxation pressure of the respiratory apparatus, the sign and magnitude of the effort required at any instant depending on the alveolar pressure needed and the relaxation pressure available at the prevailing lung volume. The muscular pressure provided by the chest wall can be derived from motions and thorax charts by plotting the relaxation characteristic of the chest wall and noting departures therefrom during utterance. This can be accomplished graphically by displaying pleural pressure against lung volume, the latter determined by referring rib cage volume in the thorax chart to the motions chart and noting the corresponding lung volume. Chest wall muscular pressure adjustments constitute the collective goal-directed behavior of the different parts of the chest wall. Therefore, it is both important and instructive to consider the present data relative to such adjustments. Such an analysis demonstrates that function of the chest wall and its parts depends on lung volume, utterance loudness, body position, and utterance task.

EFFECT OF LUNG VOLUME. For all utterances, the chest wall exerted increasingly more positive efforts (i.e., either less inspiratory or more expiratory) as lung volume decreased. This finding agrees with previous observations on utterances produced in the upright position (Bouhuys et al.,

1966; Hixon, Siebens, and Ewanowski, 1968). During utterances of the nature studied here, the alveolar pressure requirement is relatively steady, hovering around whatever level is specified by the demands (principally loudness) of the utterance. Because the available relaxation pressure decreases with decreases in lung volume, it is necessary to increase the muscular pressure contribution of the chest wall continuously in an amount proportional to the decrease in relaxation pressure. The magnitudes of muscular pressure exerted by different subjects differed somewhat on similar utterances. This is to be expected on the basis of subjects' different relaxation characteristics and their use of different alveolar pressures to achieve what they each judged to be the prescribed speech loudness levels (Kunze, 1964).

For sustained utterances, increasingly more positive chest wall efforts were manifested through higher lung volumes by continuously decreasing net inspiratory muscular pressures (i.e., diminishing braking or checking efforts), and through lower lung volumes by continuously increasing net expiratory muscular pressures (i.e., increasing supplementary efforts). Zero muscular pressure points for the sustained utterances studied are marked by vertical arrows along the percent vital capacity dimensions in Figures 4–9 and 4–10. Volumes falling to the left and right of the arrows are accompanied by net inspiratory and net expiratory chest wall muscular pressures. Net inspiratory efforts are used when the relaxation pressure exceeds the necessary alveolar pressure. Net expiratory efforts are used when the relaxation pressure is insufficient to provide the needed alveolar pressure.

Chest wall efforts during conversational speech typically were positive and increasing continuously. When subjects occasionally took a deeper breath than usual before utterance, a small inspiratory chest wall effort occurred during the early moments of the ensuing utterance. Conversational speech occurs only through the midrange of the vital capacity. This is a range of volumes in which the relaxation pressure of the respiratory apparatus is less than the needed alveolar pressure (see Chapter 1). Therefore, only expiratory chest wall efforts are required to supplement the decreasing relaxation pressure as utterance proceeds. There generally is no need for a chest wall braking or checking effort of any magnitude at any of the lung volumes of concern.

Just as the muscular pressure exerted by the chest wall became relatively more positive as lung volume decreased, so did the muscular pressure exerted by the individual parts of the chest wall (i.e., the rib cage, diaphragm, and abdomen). During activity of the rib cage wall, lung volume dependency typically was manifested through either decreasing net inspiratory efforts or increasing net expiratory efforts. Inspiratory efforts were restricted mainly to higher lung volumes, and expiratory efforts were restricted to lower lung volumes. When the diaphragm was active, it provided decreasingly negative efforts through the higher lung volume range and in some cases an increasingly negative effort at low lung volumes. When the abdominal wall was active, it increased its expiratory effort as lung volume decreased, regardless of the volume range at which the activity occurred. Thus, to the extent that the different parts of the chest wall demonstrated effort adjustments in the expiratory direction (i.e., becoming either less negative or more positive), these parts may be thought of as working in concert to raise the overall muscular pressure of the chest wall gradually and in systematic relationship to the decreasing relaxation pressure that accompanies decreasing lung volume. A noteworthy departure from such increasingly positive efforts with decreases in lung volume was the behavior of the diaphragm at times at low lung volumes. At these times, the diaphragm generated an increasingly negative effort as lung volume decreased, an activity seemingly counter to the goal-directed muscular pressure adjustment of the chest wall.

EFFECT OF UTTERANCE LOUDNESS. The analysis reveals chest wall muscular pressure to be relatively more positive at each lung volume for successively louder utterances in each body position. Stated otherwise, the inspiratory braking or checking efforts exerted through the higher lung volume range were less forceful at each lung volume and the expiratory supplementing efforts exerted through the lower lung volume range were more forceful at each lung volume for successively louder utterances. The finding of relatively more positive chest wall efforts for louder utterances is in agreement with previous observations on comparable utterances in the upright body position (Bouhuys et al., 1966; Hixon, Siebens, and Ewanowski, 1968). Because successively louder vowel and syllable productions require higher alveolar pressures to drive the speech production apparatus (Isshiki, 1964; Kunze, 1964), the subject must adjust the chest wall effort in a more positive direction at each lung volume for louder utterances. Thus, at higher volumes when the relaxation pressure exceeds the pressure needed in various amounts, more of the relaxation pressure is permitted to operate on the speech apparatus for the louder utterances via the subject's use of less braking with the chest wall. At lower lung volumes when the relaxation pressure is less in various amounts than the pressure required, more positive expiratory effort is provided via the subject's chest wall for louder utterances.

It is clear from the analysis that each of the three chest wall parts behaved in ways dependent on lung volume. In the case of the rib cage wall, this dependency was manifested by adjustments that involved less forceful inspiratory braking at higher lung volumes and more forceful expiratory supplementing at lower lung volumes for successively louder utterances. Cessation of inspiratory and onset of expiratory efforts by the rib cage occurred at higher lung volumes for successively louder sustained utterances. In addition, when rib cage wall activity began after the initiation of utterance, this activity was found to begin earlier for successively louder utterances. When the diaphragm was active, it provided less forceful inspiratory braking efforts through the high lung volume range for successively louder utterances and terminated these efforts at higher lung volumes for louder speech. The occasional return of diaphragmatic activity at low lung volumes did not appear to relate to utterance loudness in any systematic way. As for moments when the abdominal wall was active, the data reveal that the abdomen generated more positive efforts at corresponding lung volumes for successively louder utterances. In cases in which abdominal activity began after the initiation of utterance, earlier onsets of activity were demonstrated for successively louder utterances. Thus, analysis reveals patterns of function wherein negative and positive pressure generators make adjustments singularly or in combination to provide relatively more positive muscular input to the chest wall for louder utterances.

Although the required heightened alveolar pressure for louder speech was often achieved through a cooperative effort of different parts of the chest wall, it is important to consider that the sharing of this effort was not always done equally in terms of muscular pressure increments from the different parts. Several examples of such nonequal increments can be seen in Figures 4–7 and 4–8. A systematic example is found in the upright body position from the midvolume range on for the expiratory adjustments of the rib cage wall and the abdominal wall. In going from either the soft or normal-loudness condition to the loud condition, the abdominal wall muscular pressure contribution is increased much more than the simultaneous contribution of the rib cage wall. This can be seen in quantitative terms in the motion-pressure charts for the rib cage and abdomen and also is reflected in the motions chart by the fact that the tracing for the loudest utterance is displaced prominently leftward on the chart relative to the other two tracings for each subject. These motions data reveal that the predominant increase in abdominal drive served to distort the chest wall relatively further toward an increased rib cage size and a smaller abdominal size even though the rib cage heightened its activity in the expiratory direction.

The formal design of this investigation did not include utterance loudness as a variable under the conversational speech condition. To compensate for this lack, additional observations were made on a randomly selected subject (JM) as he spoke spontaneously at normal loudness and at a loudness he judged to be twice as loud in both upright and supine body positions. Typical results for the twice normal loudness condition are presented in the lower portions of Figures 4–15 and 4–16 for the upright and supine body positions. Results for the normal-loudness condition proved comparable to those obtained for JM in the major investigation. The earlier results, therefore, taken from Figures 4–5 and 4–6, are repeated in the upper portions of the figures to permit convenient comparisons of the two loudness conditions. Positive and continuously increasing chest wall efforts occurred during the utterances of twice normal loudness. These efforts were of greater magnitude than the

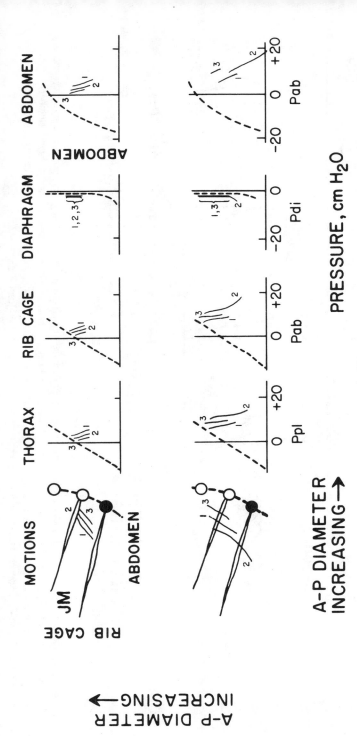

Figure 4–15. Relative motion charts and motion-pressure charts for Subject JM in the upright body position, showing data obtained during conversational speech of normal loudness (upper portion of figure) and data obtained during loud conversational speech (lower portion of figure). Numbers 1, 2, and 3 denote pathways for corresponding tracings across the different charts in each utterance condition. Partial relaxation characteristics and isopleths are repeated from Figure 4–11. Speech data in the upper portion of the figure are repeated from Figure 4–5.

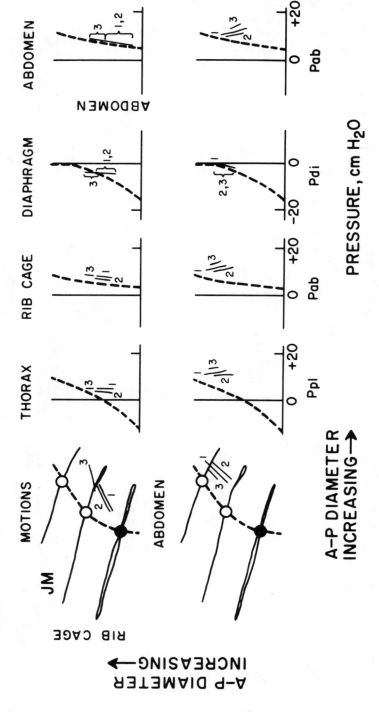

FIGURE 4–16. Relative motion charts and motion-pressure charts for Subject JM in the supine body position, showing data obtained during conversational speech of normal loudness (upper portion of figure) and data obtained during loud conversational speech (lower portion of figure). Numbers 1, 2, and 3 denote pathways for corresponding tracings across the different charts in each utterance condition. Partial relaxation characteristics and isopleths are repeated from Figure 4–6. Speech data in the upper portion of the figure are repeated from Figure 4–12.

analogous ones that occurred during speech of normal loudness in each body position. Although it is apparent that the heightened expiratory muscular pressure exerted by the chest wall for the louder utterances serves to raise alveolar pressure above its value for normal loudness utterances, it also is apparent that this increased volitional drive does not constitute the complete mechanism responsible for raising the magnitude of alveolar pressure for louder conversational speech. The motions charts in Figures 4–15 and 4–16 reveal that loud speech is initiated from higher lung volumes than is speech of normal loudness. This observation is consistent with observations on six subjects in the companion investigation of chest wall kinematics reported in Chapter 3. Deeper pre-utterance inspirations for loud than for normal conversational speech mean that greater inspiratory muscular pressures are exerted by the chest wall during the inspiratory side of the breathing cycle for the loud utterances, just as greater expiratory muscular pressures are exerted during the expiratory side of the same cycle. By preceding each loud utterance with a deeper inspiration, greater relaxation pressure is made available for use in providing a heightened alveolar pressure for the ensuing utterance. This inspiratory adjustment brings about the storage of increased potential energy within the respiratory apparatus by stretching its "spring" to a greater length. The release of this energy and its supplementation by a voluntarily increased expiratory drive combine during the ensuing expiratory phase of breathing to raise alveolar pressure above its value for speech of normal loudness. The strategy involved, then, is to make adjustments during both sides of the respiratory cycle when increasing the loudness of conversational speech. The adjustment made on the inspiratory side of the cycle in effect partially offsets the need for increased expiratory muscular pressure in the upcoming phase of the cycle. Having the potential to achieve louder speech by going to very high lung volumes or simply increasing chest wall drive through the same lung volume range as is used for normal-loudness conversational speech, humans appear to adopt a compromise strategy that takes advantage of both capabilities to some degree. Such a compromise solution may be employed to avoid two undesirable aspects of adopting either of the other strategies solely: (1) inspiratory breaks do not have to be prolonged during the attainment of much higher lung volumes, and (2) expiratory muscular pressures do not have to be increased markedly and thereby require further major shortening of the expiratory muscles involved. With respect to the first of these, going to substantially higher lung volumes for louder conversational speech also would present the subject with a far more costly inspiratory task in having to operate against a much stiffer (less compliant) respiratory apparatus as the upper volume extreme is approached.

Activities of individual parts of the chest wall changed with the change from normal to loud conversational speech just as the effort of the chest wall did. For the upright position, data are analogous to those for sustained utterances produced at increased loudness through the same lung volume range. That is, expiratory efforts of both the rib cage wall and the abdominal wall were increased for utterance, with the predominant increase occurring in the abdominal wall. For the supine position, the subject increased his rib cage effort for loud conversational speech and in addition recruited an expiratory drive from his abdominal wall, a part of the apparatus that had been inactive during his normal-loudness speech. As in the upright position, both expiratory parts of the chest wall worked in concert to raise chest wall muscular pressure and alveolar pressure. In the supine position, however, the heightened contribution of the chest wall was shared more equally by the rib cage wall and the abdominal wall than it was in the upright position. Later consideration is given to the probable mechanism involved in recruitment of the abdomen for participation in loud supine utterances.

EFFECT OF BODY POSITION

Sustained Vowel and Syllable Repetition Utterances.   Findings show that for each of the subjects, the passive pressure contributed by the chest wall is greater in the supine position than in the upright position at corresponding lung volumes. Thus, utterances involving identical alveolar pressure would demand less positive chest wall muscular pressure in the supine position than in the upright position at corresponding lung volumes. It might be expected, therefore, that the sustained utterances of the subjects would have required less positive chest wall efforts for the supine than for the upright condition. This is the case for the soft and normal-loudness utterances, but not for the loud utterances. Changeover levels from negative to positive chest wall muscular pressures (see Figs. 4–9 and 4–10) reveal this for one point in the lung volume for each utterance. Rather than changeover occurring at a lower lung volume supine than upright for the loud utterances, it occurs at the same lung volume in both body positions for one subject (JM) and at a higher lung volume for supine than for upright in the remaining two subjects. The discrepancy of loud utterances involving the same or greater muscular pressures supine than upright merely reflects the subjects' use of a slightly higher alveolar pressure supine than upright. This is not surprising because no attempt was made to equate precisely the sound pressure levels of the utterances between the two investigative conditions.

Even though muscular pressure values differed somewhat between body positions, these differences were of a small magnitude. It might be thought, therefore, that the solution to the problem of providing utterances of comparable loudness in the two body positions would be similar and would involve the same parts of the chest wall. The findings reveal, to the contrary, that markedly different adjustments are made by the different parts of the chest wall for comparable utterances in the two body positions. This is considered conveniently relative to inspiratory, zero, and expiratory efforts of the chest wall.

Net Inspiratory Efforts of the Chest Wall: In the upright position, net inspiratory efforts of the chest wall were provided through net inspiratory activity of the rib cage wall muscles alone or, in the case of one subject, with the rib cage wall muscles aided secondarily by the diaphragm at very high lung volumes for some utterances. By contrast, in the supine position, net inspiratory chest wall efforts were provided through diaphragmatic activity alone or, in the case of one subject, through diaphragmatic effort aided secondarily by a small inspiratory effort of the rib cage wall muscles.

It is apparent from the findings that the concerted inspiratory actions of the rib cage wall and diaphragm that characterize tidal breathing (see Chapter 1) become dissociated during negative chest wall efforts involving utterance. This dissociation takes different forms in the two body positions studied: the upright position involving action of the rib cage wall muscles with little or no recourse to use of the diaphragm, and the supine position involving action of the diaphragm with little or no recourse to use of the rib cage wall muscles. Thus, subjects did not take advantage of the simultaneous two-structure inspiratory capabilities of the chest wall in either body position, and with respect to the upright position they did not employ what usually is regarded as the major muscle of inspiration—the diaphragm. It would appear that the different control strategies used by the subjects in the two body positions were adopted because of certain design features of the chest wall and because of the differential influence of gravity on the chest wall in the two positions.

Considering first the upright position, the observation of inspiratory action by the chest wall in the absence of diaphragmatic activity is consistent with earlier observations on subjects singing (Bouhuys et al., 1966) and speaking (Hixon, Minifie, Peyrot, and Siebens, 1968) in the upright position. This earlier work involved measurements of the muscular pressures generated by the chest wall and the diaphragm. From these two measurements, accounts previously have been constructed of respiratory function for singing and speaking at high lung volumes in the upright position in which the rib cage wall was inferentially ascribed a major inspiratory role in governing chest wall behavior. The present findings clearly support these earlier inferences and beyond that enable the development of a detailed account of the underlying dynamics. The analyses offered here reveal that the rib cage wall muscles generate a major inspiratory effort of gradually decreasing magnitude as utterance proceeds through the range of lung volumes at which negative muscular pressures are required of the chest wall. This effort operates on the rib cage wall such that, at each lung volume, the rib cage is expanded substantially relative to the size it assumes during relaxation at the same lung volume. Such expansion in turn causes pleural pressure to be lower at each lung volume than it would be during the relaxed state of the chest wall at corresponding lung volumes. This lowered pleural pressure acts as a major upward lifting force on the diaphragm-abdomen, its magnitude being sufficient to suck the diaphragm headward, to assume partial support of the abdominal contents from the abdominal wall, and to pull the abdominal wall inward. To the extent that the diaphragm is essentially inactive during these adjustments, it behaves as a tensionless partition between the air-filled thoracic cavity and the liquid-filled abdominal cavity. Thus, any lowering of pleural pressure as a result of rib cage wall activity is transmitted across the diaphragm and is manifested in a corresponding lowering of pressure at all points throughout the abdomen. Direct evidence of such an influence on abdominal pressure is found in both the rib cage and abdomen charts in Figure 4–7. Abdominal pressure values for the utterances of the subjects are found to be lower than those for relaxation at corresponding lung volumes throughout the entire range of volumes for which the effort of the chest wall is net inspiratory.

The functional consequence of a lower abdominal pressure during utterance than during relaxation at the same lung volume is that the liquid-filled abdomen places a hydraulic pull on the undersurface of the diaphragm, the pressure in the abdomen exactly balancing that of the pleural space. This pull supplants the need to contract the diaphragm actively during the generation of a negative chest wall muscular pressure. The pull achieves the same purpose as would active contraction of the diaphragm. A situation exists, then, in which the muscular contribution of one part of the chest wall—namely the rib cage wall—is realized in the remaining two parts, the diaphragm and the abdominal wall. By virtue of (1) the parallel mechanical arrangement of the rib cage wall and the diaphragm-abdomen and (2) the hydraulic nature of the abdominal system, the pressure developed by the inspiratory rib cage wall muscles is manifested not only as an upward and outward pull on the rib cage but also as an equivalent downward pull on the diaphragm and inward pull on the abdominal wall. Without the abdomen's hydraulic pull or active contraction of the diaphragm, the rib cage wall muscles acting alone would be only moderately effective in accomplishing the task of generating a negative chest wall effort. This is because the tensionless diaphragm would tend to ride axially headward during rib cage elevation (i.e., the inactive base of the thorax—the diaphragm—would tend to move upward along with the vertical walls to a considerable degree), thus significantly compromising the net thoracic volume change. In effect, the hydraulic behavior of the abdominal contents provides a mechanism for the rib cage wall inspiratory muscles to "pull against" so as not to spend an appreciable part of their effort in displacing the entire thorax upward within the torso.

Use of the overall strategy described here is limited by the strength of the rib cage wall inspiratory muscles or by the maximum hydraulic pull of the abdominal contents, whichever is smaller. Limitation can be demonstrated by having subjects phonate into substantial artificial negative loads at the airway opening (i.e., with different magnitudes of subatmospheric pressure at the mouth) and noting changes in chest wall dynamics during moments when the lung volume is high and the overall effort of the chest wall is negative.

Under these circumstances, a subject who normally does not use the diaphragm will adopt a strategy involving diaphragmatic activity. In general, as progressively greater negative loads are applied, subjects provide progressively greater inspiratory contributions from the diaphragm and continue these contributions to successively lower lung volumes (Bouhuys et al., 1966; Hixon, Siebens, and Ewanowski, 1968).

In the upright body position, the mechanism of chest wall control by the rib cage wall alone is dependent on the fact that the influence of gravity in that body position is expiratory on the rib cage wall and inspiratory on the diaphragm and abdomen (contents and wall). In the supine body position a very different situation prevails. Gravity continues to have an expiratory influence on the rib cage wall; however, unlike the upright body position, it operates in the expiratory direction on the diaphragm and abdomen (contents and wall) in the supine position. The major influence of gravity in this position causes the abdominal wall to be displaced inward and the abdominal contents and diaphragm to be driven headward. Owing to this adjustment, humans find themselves with a very different respiratory control problem when it comes to generating inspiratory muscular pressures than they face in the upright body position. The present analyses reveal that the diaphragm generates a major inspiratory effort of gradually decreasing magnitude as utterance proceeds through the range of lung volumes for which negative muscular pressures are required of the chest wall. This effort operates on the expanded and typically relaxed rib cage wall and abdominal wall to govern their passive inward displacements. Through its activity, the diaphragm causes pleural pressure to be lower at each lung volume than it would be during the relaxed state of the chest wall at corresponding lung volumes. This lower pleural pressure is generated in the presence of a higher abdominal pressure, the difference between the two reflecting, by definition, the magnitude of diaphragmatic activity. Control of the chest wall via the diaphragm in this circumstance confirms the earlier presumption that any efficient strategy for lowering pleural pressure below relaxation values at high lung volumes in the supine body position during singing (Bouhuys et al., 1966; Hixon, 1974) or speaking (see Chapter 1) would require use of the diaphragm. Of foremost importance to the selection of a control strategy in this body position is the fact that relaxation values for abdominal pressure are positive throughout the entire vital capacity range. Higher values for abdominal pressure in this body position than in the upright position are attributable to the major influence of gravity on the abdominal components of the chest wall. In the absence of a significant hydraulic pull on the undersurface of the diaphragm in the supine body position, the inspiratory rib cage wall muscles contribute significantly and efficiently only to a lowering of pleural pressure as long as significant simultaneous active contraction of the diaphragm is occurring. Otherwise, the rib cage wall inspiratory muscle activity tends to pull the diaphragm and abdomen (contents and wall) further in the expiratory direction than they are driven by relaxation forces alone, such that the bulk of the chest wall is in effect pulled up the table (axially) with little resulting net lung volume change. Because the major increment in relaxation pressure obtained in shifting from the upright to the supine body position comes from the diaphragm-abdomen pathway of the chest wall, the most mechanically efficient strategy to counteract such pressure is through use of the major inspiratory muscle of the pathway—the diaphragm. Although the option of simultaneous diaphragmatic and rib cage wall activity was available for use by the subjects, it was not selected (unless, of course, the rib cage wall's zero activity represents an unlikely net zero activity). Thus there exists a circumstance in which the inspiratory control problem was again solved by a single part of the system, but this time in contrast to the upright body position, by the diaphragm instead of the rib cage wall.

By involving an approximately 90 degree reorientation of the body within the earth's gravity field, control of the chest wall during moments when the effort of the system had to be net inspiratory switched dramatically from one inspiratory force generating component to the other (i.e., from the rib cage wall to the diaphragm). In each case, the change occurred so as to actively involve the pathway in which the primary gravitational influence on the system was solely expiratory or more forcefully expiratory than on the remaining pathway.

In addition to the predominant inspiratory thoracic efforts provided during inspiratory chest wall efforts, at times various degrees of expiratory abdominal wall muscle effort were provided concurrently. In the supine body position such efforts were restricted to one subject, occurred only during a portion of the time when negative chest wall efforts were exerted, were of a very small magnitude, and constituted what seemed to be relatively insignificant idiosyncratic behavior. In the upright body position, however, these abdominal efforts were of major magnitude in all subjects and constituted a significant portion of the solution to the chest wall control problem.[2] Two subjects generated such expiratory abdominal efforts throughout the entire range of lung volumes at which negative chest wall muscular pressures were

---

[2]Previous work on singing (Bouhuys et al., 1966; Hixon, 1974) and speech (Hixon, Minifie, Peyrot, and Siebens, 1968; Hixon, Siebens, and Ewanowski, 1968) did not allow partitioning of the muscular pressure contributions of the rib cage wall and the abdominal wall, but only of the chest wall and the diaphragm. Faced with a circumstance in which chest wall effort was inspiratory and unaccounted for fully or at all by diaphragmatic activity, the residual inspiratory activity was ascribed to solely "inspiratory" possibilities, namely the inspiratory rib cage wall muscles. Later kinematic observations (see Chapter 3) led to the belief that the inspiratory rib cage wall muscles alone were responsible for control because outward movements of the abdominal wall often were observed through the range of lung volumes for which inspiratory chest wall efforts presumably were required. In this case, it was reasoned that outward movement of the abdomen reflected a passive displacement of the relaxed structure, its movement being regulated by action of the rib cage wall. Clearly, these earlier inferences about mechanism were incorrect.

required. The third subject brought his abdomen into play later on, but still during the continuing exertion of negative chest wall effort. Such findings initially may seem counterintuitive and as if the subjects adopted strategies for generating inspiratory chest wall efforts that involved greater than needed inspiratory thoracic efforts that simultaneously were partially offset by an expiratory contribution from the abdominal wall. There appear to be no major chest wall configuration advantages in activating the abdominal wall under these circumstances. For example, it is clear that often during the generation of negative chest wall effort the position of the abdominal wall is influenced mainly through the predominant inspiratory activity of the rib cage wall muscles rather than the expiratory activity of the abdominal wall itself. This obviously is the case during moments when the abdominal wall's displacement is in the inspiratory direction (outward) even though the wall itself is active significantly in the expiratory direction. It is believed, rather, that the use of simultaneous inspiratory and expiratory activity in this manner enables the subject to gain more economical control over the chest wall than would otherwise be possible through use of the rib cage wall muscles alone.

With the rib cage wall and the diaphragm-abdomen mechanically arranged in parallel and the diaphragm under no tension, both the rib cage wall and the abdominal wall are subjected to identical changes in transmural pressure. Accordingly, motion (flow) in each branch of the chest wall depends on the impedance offered by that branch. In a system such as the chest wall, the most economical strategy for achieving adjustments in alveolar pressure in the face of a small leak from the system (i.e., flow across the larynx and upper airway) is to maintain simultaneous muscular activity of a significant magnitude in the two parallel branches. This results in the establishment of a relatively high impedance pathway in each branch so that paradoxical inspiratory motion (flow) will not decrease the efficiency of operation of either the rib cage wall or the abdominal wall. In the case of concern here, not to maintain some activity in the abdominal wall would cause the rib cage wall inspiratory muscles to have to decrease their checking activity substantially more for each desired pressure increment because an outwardly moving abdominal wall would partially offset the decreasing force adjustment of the rib cage wall. Viewed from another perspective, not to have activity in the diaphragm-abdomen branch of the chest wall under these utterance circumstances would result in the inspiratory rib cage wall activity being resolved into regulating a shape change of the chest wall much akin to that involved during the inward motion of the rib cage wall and the outward motion of the abdominal wall during an isovolume maneuver. That is, the configuration of the chest wall would change as a result of the consistent decrease in inspiratory rib cage wall activity, but alveolar pressure would not increase efficiently without the rib cage wall muscles having something (abdominal wall stiffness in this case) to develop the pressure against. The generation of an increasingly more forceful abdominal effort as utterance proceeds is consistent with the mechanism discussed in that an increasingly less negative rib cage wall effort demands a greater abdominal effort to resist paradoxing of the abdomen. The strategy chosen by subjects in the upright position clearly is related to the inspiratory influence of gravity on the abdominal system (contents and wall). There is no need to adopt such a strategy in the supine position under these circumstances because the system is regulated mainly by the diaphragm. Gravity is operating in the expiratory direction on the rib cage wall pathway in the supine position so that its influence and that of the muscular effort of the rib cage are operating in the right sign for the decreasing activity of the diaphragm to be efficiently resolved into changes in alveolar pressure.

A very crude analogy to the mechanism discussed earlier for the upright position is found in the performance of some simple manual maneuvers on a long inflated balloon containing a squeaker in its neck. If the half of the balloon nearest the squeaker is squeezed manually (to simulate an increasingly less negative rib cage wall effort) pressure inside the balloon will increase and simultaneously cause the other half of the balloon to expand outwardly. If both halves of the balloon are squeezed simultaneously, however, the motion required of the one half of the balloon needs to be less to raise the pressure the same amount desired and the motion of neither half of the balloon is partially offset, in terms of raising pressure, by driving the other half of the balloon to a larger size paradoxically.

Net Zero Efforts of the Chest Wall: Net zero efforts of the chest wall occurred only for an instant during each of the sustained vowel and syllable repetition utterances of the subjects. In the upright position, control was maintained in the same fashion as during preceding moments when negative chest wall efforts were generated, but in this instance the inspiratory effort of the rib cage wall and the expiratory effort of the abdominal wall were in balanced opposition and cancelled to a net zero chest wall effort. Thus, moments of zero chest wall effort in the upright position did not involve relaxation forces alone, but, as with other moments during utterance, involved active muscular control by the chest wall. This finding is in sharp contrast to the suggestions of others (Draper, Ladefoged, and Whitteridge, 1959; Ladefoged, 1968) that muscles of the chest wall are relaxed completely during moments of zero muscular pressure in the upright position. It seems likely that this discrepancy can be accounted for on the basis of several inadequacies of the electromyographic observations on which this alternate conclusion is based.

The supine position showed moments of zero muscular pressure for utterances, these moments involving zero muscular pressure contributions from each of the three parts of the chest wall. It is not certain whether this means a complete relaxation of the chest wall during such moments or whether the rib cage wall, the only part of the system capable of generating pressure in two signs, could have been exhibiting a net zero effort as a result of a balanced cocontraction of its inspiratory and expiratory muscles. It seems unlikely that an inspiratory-expiratory balanced tonus would exist for this instant because the rib cage wall muscles typically were inactive during inspiratory chest wall efforts immediately preceding. Thus, the interpretation is favored that the chest wall was exhibiting a momentary lack of muscular activity at the instant the chest wall muscular pressure was zero. This, then, constitutes the only circumstance in this investigation for which the chest wall was not actively governed by muscular effort but was solely under the influence of relaxation forces.

Net Expiratory Efforts of the Chest Wall: For the most part, net expiratory efforts of the chest wall were controlled by simultaneous expiratory activity of the rib cage wall and the abdominal wall. The relative magnitude of the muscular pressure contribution from the two parts differed between body positions, being predominantely abdominal in the upright position and shared roughly equally in the supine position. In terms of muscular pressure increments for given decreases in lung volume, however, these two parts of the chest wall demonstrated comparable changes. The mechanism observed for net expiratory efforts of the chest wall, then, capitalizes on the efficiency gained by keeping the two parallel branches of the system active, as discussed earlier.

Two other characteristics of chest wall behavior during expiratory efforts are especially noteworthy. First, in the upright position, regulation of the chest wall during early moments of net expiratory activity involved simultaneous inspiratory rib cage wall and expiratory abdominal wall activity in which the latter predominated. Thus, there were brief periods during which the rib cage wall was operating in the inspiratory direction while the net effort of the chest wall was expiratory. This seemingly paradoxical inspiratory-expiratory activity is explainable along the lines of the earlier discussion under the section on "Net Inspiratory Efforts of the Chest Wall." Second, diaphragmatic activity was found to occur during certain moments of utterances at lower lung volumes. Such was the case for subject DL in both body positions and for subject MG in the supine position. This seems to be a paradoxical behavior because at such times expiratory muscular pressure of a very large positive magnitude was involved. Previous investigators of diaphragmatic behavior during speech have noted the occurrence of diaphragmatic activity at lower lung volumes during sustained utterances (Draper et al., 1959; Hixon, Siebens, and Ewanowski, 1968). Activity also has been shown to be characteristic of loud trumpet playing when subjects are proceeding toward the residual volume (Draper, Ladefoged, and Whitteridge, 1960) and to be observed during forced expirations, during moments toward the end of maximal expirations (near RV), and during expulsive maneuvers (Agostoni, Sant'Ambrogio, and del Portillo Carrasco, 1960). For each of these activities muscles of the abdominal wall often are observed to contract in excess of the pressure that the muscles of the rib cage wall can exert at a given lung volume and the diaphragm contracts in a seemingly counteractive maneuver to the excess abdominal drive. Adoption of a strategy by certain subjects whereby a higher than needed magnitude of abdominal drive is opposed somewhat with diaphragmatic activity may reflect these subjects' attempts to gain better graded control over the diaphragm-abdomen under the utterance conditions studied. That is, given that the abdominal drive is operating in substantial magnitudes at such times and that the muscles of the abdominal wall are shortened majorly, subjects may be able to realize a more finite control through the diaphragm-abdomen pathway of the system by opposing this drive with a less forceful diaphragmatic contraction. Thus, the strategy is to use the abdominal wall and diaphragm as agonist-antagonist along one of the system's pathways, the diaphragm being in an excellent mechanical position to finely tune the abdominal drive by virtue of the fact that at lower lung volumes it is highly domed and can efficiently bring about a graded control over the input provided by the abdominal wall.

Conversational Speech.   The analysis reveals the muscular pressure contribution of the chest wall to be of roughly the same magnitude for the two body positions studied. Comparable chest wall muscular pressure for similar speech events in the two body positions may at first seem incongruent with the fact that the relaxation pressure of the chest wall is greater in the supine than in the upright body position at corresponding lung volumes. Supine conversational speech occurs at lower lung volumes than similar speech in the upright position, however. This effect has been accounted for previously by the observation that speech events are tied closely to the prevailing equilibrium level (FRC) of the respiratory apparatus (see Chapter 3). The principal contributor to equilibrium level differences between the two body positions studied here is axial displacement of the diaphragm brought about by the influence of gravity on the abdominal contents. In shifting from upright to supine positions, for example, the influence of gravity changes from being inspiratory to being expiratory on the diaphragm-abdomen, the latter manifested in the diaphragm's being driven headward by the abdominal mass and a quantity of gas equalling 20% of the vital capacity being driven out of the lung. The shift to lower lung volumes for supine conversational speech is accompanied by a reduction in relaxation pressure to levels equivalent to those that prevail during upright conversational speech. The net result is that the subject is faced with a task of having to meet similar overall muscular pressure demands with the chest wall in both body positions, even though speech is occurring at quite different lung volumes.

There were marked differences between the two body positions with respect to the control strategies used to provide this similar chest wall muscular pressure. In the case of the upright position, analysis revealed control by simultaneous expiratory activity of the rib cage wall and abdominal wall. Specifically, the rib cage wall contributed a small to moderate magnitude of muscular pressure relative to that of which it was capable, whereas the abdominal wall contributed a muscular pressure of major magnitude relative to its potential, this magnitude far exceeding, often by several-fold, the rib cage wall's effort. By contrast, in the supine position control was found to be vested in expiratory rib cage wall activity alone in two subjects and in a combined rib cage wall and abdominal wall effort in the third subject. The muscular pressure provided by the rib cage wall in the supine position was essentially the same in magnitude as that used by subjects in the upright position. In the lone subject who demonstrated an abdominal wall effort during supine conversational speech, the magnitude of such effort was far less than that observed in the upright position and more closely approximated the contribution of the rib cage wall in both body positions. When instructed to do so under the guidance of biofeedback (i.e., observing various motion-motion and motion-pressure charts), the subjects easily were able to produce normal speech utterances using a wide variety of combinations of muscular pressure contributions from the three parts of the chest wall. Why then under the condition of natural running conversational speech production do speakers adopt the specific strategies they do in the two body positions?

Use of the rib cage wall under these circumstances in both body positions seems an obviously favorable mechanical choice by the subjects. Because the rib cage wall is in contact with approximately three fourths of the lung's surface, it can very effectively contribute to the adjustment of alveolar pressure for conversational speech production. In comparison to the abdominal wall, for example, the rib cage wall needs to move only about one fourth the distance that the abdominal wall does to achieve the same change in alveolar pressure. Beyond this significant advantage there is the advantage that the rib cage wall contains the smallest and fastest acting muscles in the chest wall. This means that the rib cage wall offers distinct control advantages for speech events in which discrete and brief pressure variations of respiratory origin are called for, such as in lexical stressing (see Chapter 1).

But, what of the marked differences in abdominal wall function between the two body positions studied; that is, why do speakers keep the abdominal wall so forcefully active during speech in the upright body position and typically not use the abdominal wall at all in the supine position? It would appear that the answer to this question has to do with the fact that during running conversational speech production significant changes are imposed on the entire breathing cycle relative to those which prevail during tidal breathing. These changes are embodied in differences with regard to timing, volume events, pressure events, and muscular control. Most importantly here is that, compared with tidal breathing, speech breathing consists of extremely abrupt inspirations and considerably prolonged expirations. Running conversational speech constitutes a circumstance in which the speaker desires to transmit information in as continuous a fashion as possible. The inspiratory refills required in running speech are undesirable and in a linguistic sense represent inherent performance constraints. It is reasonable, therefore, that speakers would design their chest wall control strategies to minimize the durations of such interruptions and thereby facilitate the continued transmission of information. The methods of function chosen by the present subjects clearly take into account the optimizing of such inspiratory function (i.e., improving its efficiency) and have to do specifically with the mechanical advantage of the diaphragm that obtains in the two body positions, as now discussed.

In the upright position, the subjects adopted a strategy in which the muscular pressure contributed by the abdominal wall was far greater than that contributed by the rib cage wall. This predominant expiratory contribution from the abdominal wall distorted the shape of the chest wall markedly from that which it would assume during relaxation at corresponding lung volumes. The adjustment involved is somewhat analogous to an isovolume maneuver in which the major abdominal effort serves to displace the abdominal wall inward and the rib cage wall outward in the face of a lesser expiratory effort by the rib cage wall. The reason for performing such a costly muscular maneuver with the abdominal wall is hypothesized as having to do with the consequence it has on the opposite surface of the diaphragm-abdomen part of the chest wall—namely, the diaphragm. Because of inward displacement of the abdominal wall, the diaphragm is displaced axially headward such that its principal muscular fibers (costal) become substantially elongated and its radius of curvature is increased. The significance of this externally imposed adjustment is that the diaphragm is in effect "mechanically tuned" to a configuration that tends to optimize its potential for producing rapid and forceful inspiratory efforts. The costly effort on the expiratory side of the breathing cycle during conversational speech may be viewed as an investment to enable the subject to meet rapidly and effectively the important inspiratory demands that running conversational speech imposes.

Strong evidence in support of such an hypothesis is contained in events within the inspiratory side of the breathing cycles interspersed in running conversational speech production. In replaying the FM data tape recordings, it was observed that the abdominal wall invariably maintained a major muscular pressure activity during both the expiratory (utterance) and inspiratory (refill) sides of the breathing cycle. The use of abdominal wall activity of this magnitude throughout both phases of the speech breathing cycle suggests that the abdominal wall muscles are involved in providing a form of "speech-specific posturing" of the chest wall. Use of abdominal wall activity during the expiratory side of the breathing cycle is necessary to prevent rib cage wall expiratory activity from driving the diaphragm footward and flattening it so as to compromise the diaphragm's mechanical advantage. Adjustment of the abdominal wall's activity during utterance segments was such that the abdomen provided muscular pressure increments of similar magnitude to those provided by the expiring rib cage wall, a finding in keeping with the foregoing hypothesis, because a lesser input change from the abdomen than from the rib cage would work against diaphragmatic tuning. It would be possible to leave the abdominal wall off during the expiratory side of the breathing cycle and then to activate it for diaphragmatic tuning just before the inspiratory side of the cycle. Such a strategy would be extremely costly in the upright body position, however, because the shape of the chest wall would change dramatically between the two phases of respiration. The rib cage wall typically was not found to participate in the inspiratory direction during the rapid inspirations interspersed in conversational speech. Rather, analysis indicated that it was relaxed or maintaining a small expiratory tone. The diaphragm, then, must be credited with providing all of the inspiratory drive during the inspiratory portion of the breathing cycle of running conversational speech.

To recapitulate for the upright position, it seems that during actual sound production in running conversational speech the rib cage wall and abdominal wall exert expiratory pressures to drive the chest wall at a speech-specific configuration that is determined largely by abdominal wall activity. When utterance needs to be interrupted abruptly for a refilling of the respiratory apparatus, the rib cage wall reduces its expiratory activity to zero or in such a way as to maintain a minimal expiratory tone. The abdominal wall muscles, however, continue to maintain their major input in the expiratory direction and thereby keep the diaphragm mechanically tuned so that when it activates majorly it works against the taught abdominal wall to elevate the relaxed (or nearly so) rib cage wall. In the typical case in which both the rib cage wall and abdominal wall remain active during inspiration, the powerful inspiratory activity of the diaphragm seemingly overpowers the expiratory efforts of the rib cage wall and abdominal wall and restores the apparatus to a higher lung volume, rib cage volume, and abdominal volume. The diaphragm in this circumstance constitutes an agonist with the rib cage wall and abdominal wall as combined antagonists.

A further economy of function is apparent in the strategy of maintaining an expiratory activity in the two expiratory pressure generators of the chest wall during the inspiratory phase of the breathing cycle of running conversational speech production. That economy is that the expiratory muscles are in a state of readiness for their continued expiratory activity for speech once the diaphragmatic activity is terminated. Because the expiratory muscles already are under tone, there is no time lost in activating them from a slack state, a circumstance that would increase delays between utterances.

In the case of the supine body position, analysis reveals an absence of abdominal drive during running conversational speech. From the viewpoint just discussed for the upright body position's function, it is apparent that an abdominal drive is not needed to tune the diaphragm mechanically in this particular body position. Because of the gravitational influence in the supine position, the diaphragm is forced headward axially and its radius of curvature is increased in a manner akin to that achieved voluntarily through abdominal wall activity in the upright body position. Thus, in the supine position, the diaphragm is once again optimally mechanically tuned, but in this case passively and naturally via the displacement of the abdominal mass headward under the influence of gravity. Unlike the upright body position in which gravity tends to compromise the mechanical advantage of the diaphragm by driving it footward and decreasing its radius of curvature, in the supine position just the opposite occurs and to the advantage of function.

As in the case of the upright body position, evidence is found during the inspiratory phase of the breathing cycle for running conversational speech in the supine body position that is supportive of the general notions about function discussed earlier. Playback of the FM tapes revealed that during the inspiratory phase of the breathing cycle the diaphragm is the sole inspiratory generator for the chest wall. Activity of the diaphragm was sometimes accompanied by a continued absence of abdominal muscle tone, as in the expiratory phase of the breathing cycle, and in some instances by a slight activity of the abdominal wall. The latter observation is interpreted as representing the subjects' attempts to provide a firmer base for the diaphragm to operate against in resolving the main of its force into elevation of the rib cage wall and not into displacement of the abdominal wall outward. The sole subject who used his abdomen during the expiratory phase of the cycle during supine conversational speech also continued the activity of his abdominal wall during the inspiratory phase of the cycle, as all of the subjects did in the upright body position. The rib cage wall continued to be active in the expiratory direction during the inspiratory phase of the breathing cycle despite the fact that the entire thorax was operating in the inspiratory direction due to the predominating drive of the diaphragm. In one sense, then, the rib cage wall behaved somewhat analogously to the way the abdominal wall behaved for the upright body position. That is, the rib cage wall activity tended to maintain a posturing of the chest wall off its relaxation configuration, in this case toward smaller rib cage and larger abdominal sizes than those attained during relaxation at corresponding lung volumes.

To recapitulate events for the supine body position, there exists a circumstance in running conversational speech in which the rib cage wall alone or aided slightly by the abdominal wall (in one subject) exerts the expiratory pressures needed to drive the chest wall. The configuration of the chest wall in this circumstance is determined largely by the activity of the rib cage wall. When utterance needs to be interrupted abruptly for a refilling of the respiratory apparatus, the rib cage wall (and the abdominal wall in the case of one subject) continues its expiratory activity but is overpowered by the forcefully contracting inspiratory effort of the diaphragm. The diaphragm and those expiratory muscles that are active during the inspiratory phase of the cycle, therefore, can be viewed as in an agonist-antagonist relationship during the inspiratory phase of the cycle. Once again, as with the upright body position, the continued expiratory activity by the rib cage wall (and in the one subject for the abdominal wall also) constitutes an economical strategy because the muscles of importance to the expiratory side of the cycle already are under tone and somewhat shortened once the inspiratory gesture of the respiratory apparatus is terminated.

In conclusion, then, it has been seen that the rib cage wall assumed basically a similar function in the two body positions for running conversational speech, that the diaphragm likewise assumed a similar function in the two body positions, but that the abdominal wall muscles and the influence of gravity interchanged functional roles in the two body positions. Although one of the subjects used his abdominal wall in the supine body position, the magnitude of the activity was relatively small compared to that for the upright body position and may be viewed as an insignificant idiosyncrasy of the particular speaker.

Other observations are consistent with the mechanism proposed to account for differences in chest wall behavior in the two body positions during running conversational speech. First, in the subject who spoke loudly in the upright position (JM), a large increase in abdominal wall activity was found to accompany a similar increase in rib cage drive. This abdominal increase probably was supplied not only to contribute to an increased chest wall drive for utterance but also to maintain the chest wall in its speech-specific configuration. A heightened drive from the rib cage without an equivalent heightening of abdominal drive would result in a footward displacement of the diaphragm and a diminution of the mechanical advantage discussed. Second, when the same subject spoke at a high loudness level in the supine position, he recruited his abdominal wall to work in conjunction with his rib cage instead of incrementing solely with his already active rib cage. This action is interpreted as being consistent with preserving the mechanical advantage of the diaphragm. Third, further observations on TH in a wide variety of body positions revealed the rib cage to be similarly active in different positions but the abdomen to be active only in those positions in which a footward displacement and flattening of the diaphragm would be predicted to result because of the influence of gravity on the abdominal system (Agostoni and Mead, 1964). If, as is believed, the primary role of the abdominal wall muscles in conversational speech is to maintain an optimal "tuning" of the diaphragm, then any gravitational influence that would compromise the diaphragm's mechanical advantage could be counteracted by using the abdominal muscles to regain an appropriate chest wall configuration for which rapid inspirations would be mechanically less costly. Fourth, there is also clinical evidence in support of the foregoing hypothesis. This evidence is found in clients whose abdominal muscles are paralyzed or show significant paresis. Studies on more than a dozen of such clients have revealed that when they are placed in an upright position they demonstrate difficulty with diaphragm inspiratory function unless the abdominal wall is supported against gravity via girdling or other mechanical means. Diaphragmatic difficulty of this nature generally is not found in the supine position, in which the diaphragm is naturally tuned for function through gravity. Perhaps the most significant clinical observation in support of the hypothesis is that inspiratory durations in the running conversational speech of such clients are substantially longer in the upright than supine position if the abdominal wall is not aided mechanically in the former. A binding of the abdominal wall will often lead to an immediate and dramatic reduction in inspiratory pause times in the upright position for clients with abdominal muscle involvement. Althought not relevant to the test of the hypothesis, such binding also often improves the client's chest wall control on the expiratory (speech) side of the breathing cycle. This improvement seems related to the removal of one degree of freedom in the involved chest wall and thereby enables the client to effectively use whatever rib cage wall expiratory potential there is rather than partially wasting it in driving against an abdominal wall that paradoxes outward because of a lack of tautness.

EFFECT OF UTTERANCE TASK.   Within each body position the muscular pressure demands of conversational speech and the sustained normal-loudness utterances of the subjects were comparable through the range of lung volumes common to the two activities. In the case of the upright body position, both the general deformation of the chest wall and the pressures applied by its different parts also were roughly comparable for the two activities. In fact, the marked similarity in mechanism observed between the two activities through their common range of lung volumes makes it tempting to view the sustained utterance data as extrapolations of those for conversational speech production. In the case of the supine body position, sustained utterances involved simultaneous expiratory activity by the rib cage wall and the abdominal wall through the same range of lung volumes in which the rib cage wall alone generally prevailed during conversational speech utterances. Such a clear effect of utterance task on the behavior of the chest wall in the supine position shows that muscular pressure demands alone do not determine the specific adjustments to be made by the respiratory apparatus. Apparently the control strategies used through the common range of lung volumes covered in the two types of activities differed because the problems under solution are quite different. In the case of the sustained utterance tasks, the chest wall is set into goal-specific motion well before entering the range of lung volumes characteristic of conversational speech production, continues that motion through the common range of lung volumes for the two types of activities, and proceeds beyond that range of volumes to utterance termination. In the case of supine conversational speech utterances, however, the function of the chest wall involves repeated adjustments at the points bounding the lung volume range common to the two types of activities.

Prediction of Dynamics from Kinematics Alone: Clinical Significance

In earlier work (Chapter 3) relative motions data alone (rib cage diameter versus abdominal diameter) were used to infer underlying muscular mechanism associated with various utterances. Inferences were based on possible muscular actions that could account for instantaneous chest wall configuration (and its history) during utterance. Interpretations depended largely on comparisons of chest wall configuration during speech and relaxation, with departures from the relaxed configuration at corresponding lung volumes being ascribed to a small number of possible combinations of muscular actions among the different parts of the chest wall. These possible actions have been detailed previously (see Chapter 3) and have been reviewed further here (see pages 146 to 148 and Figure 4–4). Unequivocal designation of the precise combination of actions could not be made in the earlier work because more than a single combination can maintain any specified configuration of the chest wall. It was necessary to reason, therefore, as to the more likely of the different possible combinations (excluding consideration of possible diaphragmatic activity) by taking account of what was believed to be reasonable estimates of the sign and magnitude of the chest wall effort required for various utterances. These estimates were derived from knowledge of the relaxation pressure of the respiratory apparatus at prevailing lung volumes for normal subjects and from estimates of alveolar pressure requirements for various utterances.

Considering previous findings (Chapter 3) in combination with those of the present investigation, it is apparent that the mechanism involved can be predicted with considerable certainty by using kinematics observations alone. There is substantial, practical clinical interest in this capability. Given the potential of predicting the mechanism from observations of thoraco-abdominal surface motions alone, there is available a relatively powerful clinical tool for the analysis of respiratory-based speech problems. This potential is particularly encouraging in light of the simplicity of kinematics measurements and in view of the great deal of information that can be obtained very quickly and with little inconvenience to the client through their use. Further encouragement in this regard comes from the confirmation of equally good predictions of dynamics from kinematics in studies of more than a dozen clients with various degrees of respiratory muscle involvement as sequela to poliomyelitis and cervical spinal cord lesions. Thus, although dynamics observations are more definitive and precise, kinematics observations show much promise in and of themselves as clinical procedures for specifying possible dysfunctions of the rib cage and abdomen. This promise currently is being realized in the study of two populations of speakers, the hearing impaired (see Chapter 5) and the neuromuscularly impaired (Hixon, 1976).

Other Considerations

Much of this chapter has dealt with the major background adjustments of the chest wall during speech production. Of greater linguistic interest, perhaps, are the relatively minute chest wall adjustments that are superimposed on these background adjustments during utterance segments of varying linguistic content (Stetson, 1951). The remaining problem of precisely quantifying these minute adjustments is under study using the volume-pressure approach developed here.

Finally, the present results are substantially at odds with accounts of speech breathing physiology based on electromyographic observations (Draper et al., 1959, 1960; Eblen, 1963; Hixon, Siebens, and Ewanowski, 1968). Because the differences are major and raise questions concerning current notions about the nature of speech breathing function that have stood unchallenged for over two and a half decades, they have been judged suitable for consideration in an expanded account dealing with inadequacies in the use of electromyographic procedures in studies of speech breathing mechanics (Hixon and colleagues, in preparation).

ACKNOWLEDGMENT

The preparation of this manuscript was supported by Research Grant NS-09656 and Research Career Development Award NS-1 K4, 41,350 from the National Institute of Neurological Diseases and Stroke.

REFERENCES

Agostoni, E., and Mead, J. (1964). Statics of the respiratory system (pp. 387–409). *In* W. Fenn and H. Rahn (Eds.): *Handbook of physiology. Respiration 1, Sect. 3.* Washington, DC: American Physiological Society.

Agostoni, E., Sant'Ambrogio, G., and del Portillo Carrasco, H. (1960). Electromyography of the diaphragm in man and transdiaphragmatic pressures. *Journal of Applied Physiology,* 15, 1093–1097.

Bouhuys, A., Proctor, D., and Mead, J. (1966). Kinetic aspects of singing. *Journal of Applied Physiology,* 21, 483–496.

Draper, M., Ladefoged, P., and Whitteridge, D. (1959). Respiratory muscles in speech. *Journal of Speech and Hearing Research,* 2, 16–27.

Draper, M., Ladefoged, P., and Whitteridge, D. (1960). Expiratory pressures and air flow during speech. *British Medical Journal,* 1, 1837–1843.

Eblen, R. (1963). Limitations of the use of surface electromyography in studies of speech breathing. *Journal of Speech and Hearing Research,* 6, 3–18.

Fairbanks, G. (1960). *Voice and articulation drillbook* (2nd ed.). New York: Harper and Row.

Goldman, M., and Mead, J. (1973). Mechanical interaction between the diaphragm and rib cage. *Journal of Applied Physiology,* **35**, 197–204.

Hixon, T. (1974). *Role of the diaphragm in singing: Myth and reality*. Paper presented at the Voice Foundation Annual Symposium on Care of the Professional Voice, New York.

Hixon, T. (1976). *The mechanical bases of so-called "reversed breathing" in cerebral palsy*. Progress Report of Research Grant NS-09656 from the National Institute of Neurological Diseases and Stroke.

Hixon, T., Minifie, F., Peyrot, A., and Siebens, A. (1968). *Mechanical behavior of the diaphragm during speech production*. Paper presented at the fall meeting of the Acoustical Society of America, Cleveland.

Hixon, T., Siebens, A., and Ewanowski, S. (1968). *Respiratory mechanics during speech production*. Paper presented at the spring meeting of the Acoustical Society of America, Ottawa.

Isshiki, N. (1964). Regulatory mechanism of voice intensity variation. *Journal of Speech and Hearing Research,* 7, 17–29.

Kunze, L. (1964). Evaluation of methods of estimating sub-glottal air pressure. *Journal of Speech Hearing Research,* 7, 151–164.

Ladefoged, P. (1968). Linguistic aspects of respiratory phenomena. *Annals of the New York Academy of Science,* **155**, 141–151.

Mead, J., Peterson, N., Grimby, G., and Mead, J. (1967). Pulmonary ventilation measured from body surface movements. *Science,* **156**, 1383–1384.

Milic-Emili, J., Mead, J., Turner, J., and Glauser, E. (1964). Improved technique for estimating pleural pressure from esophageal balloons. *Journal of Applied Physiology,* **19**, 207–211.

Stetson, R. (1951). *Motor phonetics*. Amsterdam: North-Holland.

CHAPTER 5

Respiratory Kinematics in Profoundly Hearing-Impaired Speakers

Linda L. Forner
Thomas J. Hixon

I nappropriate use of the respiratory apparatus long has been suspected of being one of the major factors contributing to the abnormal speech of individuals with major hearing impairment (Hudgins and Numbers, 1942). Presumably, such individuals demonstrate problems in regulating the behavior of different parts of the respiratory pump and in regulating the output of the pump in conjunction with other parts of the speech apparatus. This is because they lack normal auditory sensation concerning the acoustic consequences of motions of the speech apparatus. The precise nature of these problems of regulation is not well known. Speech-language pathologists seem convinced that the problems are substantial, complex, of a variety, and contribute in a major way to the abnormal speech. The few research attempts that have been

Reprinted by permission of the publisher from the *Journal of Speech and Hearing Research*, *20*, pp. 373–408, © American Speech-Language-Hearing Association, Rockville, MD.

made in an effort to delineate such problems and to determine their underlying bases (Hudgins, 1934; Rawlings, 1935, 1936; Woldring, 1968) have been somewhat limited in focus and carry minimal conviction owing to their use of equipment systems that are considered suspect by current research methodology standards (see Chapter 2).

The present investigation sought to apply modern research techniques to the study of speech breathing in a sizable group of profoundly hearing-impaired individuals. The intent was that the investigation be useful in several respects. Most importantly it would provide insights into the bases of respiratory regulation problems in speakers with major hearing impairment and would offer inroads toward improved methodologies for the evaluation and management of the speech abnormalities exhibited by hearing-impaired speakers. It seems reasonable to assume that a wide range of abnormal respiratory signs and severity of dysfunction is to be found across the wide spectrum of hearing impairment that humans manifest. Attention was focused on profoundly hearing-impaired individuals because they constitute the subgroup of the hearing-impaired population that speech-language pathologists consider most likely to have speech abnormalities that are partially respiratory based. They also may well be the subgroup that manifests the widest range of respiratory dysfunctions for observation.

Function was explored using a measurement approach that incorporates a kinematic procedure for studying the behavior of the respiratory apparatus (see Chapter 3). This approach has the advantages over other available approaches of enabling systematic investigation of the respiratory behavior of a sizable number of subjects while requiring little investigative sophistication on their part. Recent investigations have demonstrated that relatively comprehensive accounts of respiratory behavior can be developed using this approach, and that reasonably accurate predictions can be made as to the inherent and volitional forces involved (see Chapters 3 and 4). The theoretical bases for the approach are discussed in detail elsewhere (see Chapter 3 and Konno and Mead, 1967). Some of these bases are essential to the present work and are summarized in the next section.

MEASUREMENT FRAMEWORK

The respiratory apparatus is composed of two concentric parts, the pulmonary system and chest wall. Included in the latter are the rib cage wall, diaphragm, and abdominal wall. The rib cage and diaphragm delimit the thoracic cavity, whereas the abdominal cavity is bounded by the diaphragm and abdominal wall. The contents of the abdominal cavity are an essentially incompressible mass. The diaphragm, abdominal contents, and abdominal wall can be conceptualized as a single thick structure, having the diaphragm and abdominal wall as its inner and outer surfaces. The three-structure anatomical

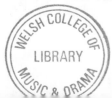

arrangement of the chest wall (i.e., the rib cage wall, diaphragm, and abdominal wall) then reduces to a simpler two-structure arrangement consisting of the rib cage wall and the diaphragm-abdomen.

The rib cage and diaphragm-abdomen displace volume during their movements and their combined displacement equals the displacement of the lungs. Each of the two chest wall parts moves as a unit during breathing, the movement of each being functionally separate from that of the other part. This can be demonstrated through paradoxical movements in which the displacement of either of the parts is opposite in sign to lung volume change (e.g., an expiration where the rib cage is moving inward and the abdomen is moving outward).

Each of the two parts of the chest wall has a single degree of freedom of motion. That is, each has only one way to move and exhibits a fixed shape at any particular volume. The chest wall presents either one or two degrees of freedom depending on whether the respiratory apparatus is open or closed. When the larynx and upper airway are open to atmosphere, the chest wall can exchange volume with its surroundings and has two degrees of freedom, one for each of its two parts. Under this circumstance, changes in lung volume can be accomplished with either part of the chest wall, or with any combination of displacements of the two parts. By contrast, when the respiratory apparatus is closed, the chest wall cannot exchange volume with its surroundings and volume change can only take place between the chest wall's two parts. The chest wall has only one degree of freedom under this circumstance. It follows that the volumes displaced by the rib cage wall and abdominal wall are interdependent, with the volume displaced by either being equal and opposite to that displaced by the other. Figure 5–1 illustrates this interdependence with reference to chest wall configuration. The three conditions illustrated are at the same lung volume. Panel (A) shows a relaxed chest wall, whereas in panels (B) and (C) volume is shifted into and out of the rib cage, respectively. Displacement of volume back and forth between the two parts of the chest wall at constant lung volume is termed an *isovolume maneuver*. An appreciation for the maneuver can be gained by alternately contracting and relaxing the abdominal muscles with the larynx closed.

Recall that each part of the chest wall exhibits a fixed shape at a given volume. Accordingly, volume displacement can be determined by measuring the motion of any point within a part, once the calibration between the volume displaced by that part and the motion of the point selected for measurement has been established. The simplest means of establishing this calibration is to displace volume into and out of a part through an isovolume maneuver while simultaneously measuring change in the part's anteroposterior diameter. By doing this at different known lung volumes, a family of data can be generated that reveals the functional relationships between the relative motion of the rib cage wall and abdominal wall. From these data, the volume-motion

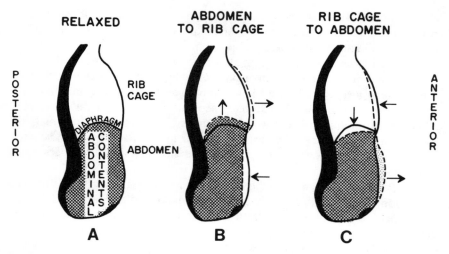

FIGURE 5-1. Chest wall configuration under conditions of relaxation (A), and distortion by muscle activity (B) and (C) toward maximal displacements of volume into the rib cage and abdomen, respectively.

relations for each part can be derived through any procedure that graphically removes one part (i.e., reduces the number of degrees of freedom to one). An additional means of solving for volume in real time is described subsequently and involves adjusting analogues of anteroposterior diameter change for the rib cage and abdomen so that they are equal during the equal and opposite volume displacements accompanying isovolume maneuvers. By displaying the data from isovolume maneuvers together with those obtained during speech, it is possible to specify the separate volume contributions of the rib cage and abdomen to changes in lung volume during the latter.

METHOD

Subjects

Subjects were 10 male students from the National Technical Institute for the Deaf (NTID), Rochester, New York. Each was of normal intelligence and had a normal speech apparatus. Their ages ranged from 19 to 24 years, the mean being 20 years.

HEARING CHARACTERISTICS. Each subject had a congenital, bilateral sensorineural hearing loss. Nine demonstrated an unaided better ear average loss for the octave frequencies from 500 to 2000 Hz that was greater than 96 dB (American National Standards Institute, 1969); one demonstrated an unaided better ear average loss of 83 dB. The former subjects are in the profound hearing-impairment range and the latter is in the severe range. Pure-tone thresholds for each frequency for each subject are given in Table 5–1.

Unaided speech discrimination ability of each subject was determined via Central Institute for the Deaf (CID) Everyday Sentence lists and spondee words. Ability ratings ranged from an inability to understand any of the message to an understanding of about half of the message. The typical subject understood little of the message but did understand a few words or phrases. An NTID-scored rating for each subject is given in Table 5–1.

The approximate number of years each subject had worn a hearing aid ranged from never having worn an aid to having worn one throughout most of his life. The majority were in the latter group. The average number of hours of daily use ranged from no use to 10 hours. The typical subject wore his aid a large portion of his awake hours. Information about each subject's use of aids is included in Table 5–1.

No subject wore his aid during this investigation. Pilot study on four profoundly hearing-impaired individuals revealed no differences in speech breathing between aided and unaided conditions.

SPEECH CHARACTERISTICS. No subject used oral communication exclusively in daily life, five used manual communication almost entirely, and five used oral and manual communication simultaneously. The second column in Table 5–2 presents this information for each subject.

To characterize the speech performance skills of each subject, three experienced speech-language pathologists evaluated tape recordings of the subject's normal reading. Initially, two global judgments were made: speech defectiveness and speech intelligibility. All subjects were judged severely speech defective and highly unintelligible. Isolated words were rarely understood even though the listeners knew the story read. Recordings also were considered relative to 10 separate aspects of production: voice quality, vocal pitch, utterance loudness, nasal resonance, articulation, intonation, rhythm, stress, linguistic phrasing, and utterance rate. The majority of subjects were judged deviant in voice quality. A minority demonstrated deviance in vocal pitch or utterance loudness, or both, and none showed deviant nasal resonance. The remaining six aspects were judged to be deviant in all subjects. Table 5–2 presents descriptors for each subject's performance on each of the 10 aspects. Interclinician agreement was nearly perfect. In discrepancies, tapes were replayed until a consensus was met. Reevaluations of three randomly selected tapes resulted in congruent descriptors for all aspects.

OTHER CHARACTERISTICS. At NTID, a standard four-point scale is used to specify the clinician's judgment as to the magnitude of the contribution of respiratory dysfunction to each student's speech abnormality. This scale

Table 5-1. *Unaided Better Ear Pure-Tone Thresholds, Speech Discrimination Profile Ratings, and Information Concerning Use of Hearing Aids for Each Subject*

Subject	Unaided Better Ear Pure-Tone Thresholds (dB) (ANSI, 1969)			Profile Rating for Speech Discrimination Ability	Use of Hearing Aids	
	500 Hz	*1000 Hz*	*2000 Hz*		Approximate Number of Years	Current Average Hours Daily
WL	80	105	105	2	14	7–10
RB	90	NR	NR	1	9	0
TK	80	110	115	2	13	10
JR	100	115	NR	2	1	4
DC	85	110	NR	1	11	10
MO	75	75	100	3	16	8
JM	90	105	NR	2	13	7–8
DW	100	100	95	3	4	10
HV	90	NR	NR	2	0	0
RR	100	100	90	2	1	4

NR = No Response. 1 = Cannot understand any of the message. 2 = Understands little of the content of the message, but does understand a few isolated words or phrases. 3 = Understands about half of the message.

Table 5-2. Mode of Expressive Communication Used Most Often in Daily Life by Each Subject, and Descriptors of Each Subject's Speech Performance on 10 Aspects of Production

Subject	Mode of Communication	Voice Quality	Vocal Pitch	Utterance Loudness	Nasal Resonance	Articulation	Intonation	Rhythm	Stress	Linguistic Phrasing	Utterance Rate
WL	Simultaneous oral and manual	Breathy	High	Soft	Normal	Severely deviant	Monotonous and inappropriate variation	Severely deviant	Severely deviant	Severely deviant	Slow
RB	Manual	Breathy	Normal	Normal	Normal	Severely deviant	Monotonous	Severely deviant	Severely deviant	Severely deviant	Slow
TK	Simultaneous oral and manual	Breathy	High	Soft	Normal	Severely deviant	Monotonous	Severely deviant	Severely deviant	Severely deviant	Slow
JR	Manual	Breathy	Normal	Soft	Normal	Severely deviant	Inappropriate variation	Severely deviant	Severely deviant	Severely deviant	Slow
DC	Simultaneous oral and manual	Normal	Normal	Normal	Normal	Severely deviant	Inappropriate variation	Severely deviant	Severely deviant	Severely deviant	Slow
MO	Simultaneous oral and manual	Normal	Normal	Normal	Normal	Severely deviant	Monotonous and inappropriate variation	Moderately deviant	Moderately deviant	Moderately deviant	Slow
JM	Simultaneous oral and manual	Normal	Normal	Normal	Normal	Severely deviant	Monotonous and inappropriate variation	Severely deviant	Severely deviant	Severely deviant	Slow
DW	Manual	Normal	Normal	Normal	Normal	Severely deviant	Inappropriate variation	Moderately deviant	Severely deviant	Moderately deviant	Slow
HV	Manual	Harsh	Normal	Normal	Normal	Severely deviant	Inappropriate variation	Severely deviant	Severely deviant	Mild to moderately deviant	Slow
RR	Manual	Harsh	Normal	Normal	Normal	Severely deviant	Monotonous	Severely deviant	Severely deviant	Severely deviant	Slow

205

covers a category of speech performance designated as "control of air expenditure during speech." Ratings within this category are assigned on the basis of the examining speech-language pathologist's perceptual judgment of the student's speech, with special reference given to what the clinician considers to be "heard" cues to a partially respiratory-based speech disorder. Scale designations range from normal respiratory function to function judged to have a severe effect on speech. Only those male students demonstrating problems rated moderate or severe were included in this investigation. Approximately 10% of the current NTID male students are so labeled. From this group, 10 were chosen randomly for paid participation in this investigation.

Equipment

Figure 5–2 diagrams the equipment used. Anteroposterior diameter changes of the rib cage and abdomen were sensed with magnetometers (Mead, Peterson, Grimby, and Mead, 1967). Two generator-sensor coil pairs were used, one for each part of the chest wall. The functional characteristics of these electromagnetic transducers and the theory underlying their use in the study of speech breathing function have been detailed elsewhere (see Chapter 3).

Magnetometer signals were fed to two channels of an FM tape recorder for subsequent playback into a storage oscilloscope. Displays on the oscilloscope were traced onto translucent paper.

Utterances were sensed with two microphones—an air microphone and a throat microphone. Signals from each were fed to separate amplifiers and from their outputs to different tape recorders—the throat signal to an FM

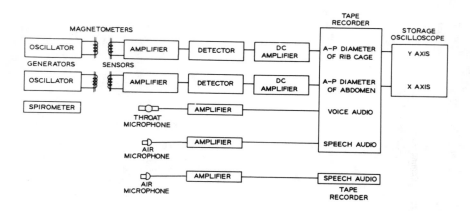

FIGURE 5–2. Diagram of equipment used.

recorder and the air signal to another recorder. A second air microphone and amplifier were used with a direct record channel on the FM recorder to provide a banter channel for the investigators.

General Procedure

Each polyethylene-encased magnetometer coil was attached to the body with double-sided adhesive tape. Generating coils were positioned at the midline on the anterior surface of the chest wall, one for the rib cage at the level of the nipples and one for the abdomen immediately above the umbilicus. Sensing coils were positioned posteriorly, also at the midline, and at the same axial levels as their generator mates (see Fig. 5–3).

Tasks were performed in a standing position with subjects leaning backward against a foam pad placed against a wall. A segment of the pad had a rectangular indentation running vertically at the midline to provide a space within which the coils on the subject's back were free to move. Subjects were

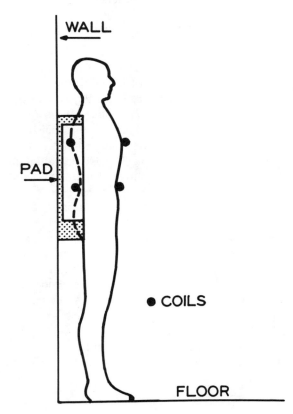

FIGURE 5–3. Illustration of subject positioning and magnetometer coil placements.

told to avoid raising their arms, using sign language, or shifting their position during recordings.

Two types of activities were performed: respiratory activities and utterances.

RESPIRATORY ACTIVITIES. Recordings were made during two non-speech activities: resting breathing and isovolume maneuvers. The former was recorded while subjects breathed quietly for 1 minute. Before performing the latter, each subject breathed quietly into a spirometer. At tidal end-expiratory level, functional residual capacity (FRC), the subject closed his glottis, relaxed, and slowly displaced volume back and forth between the rib cage and abdomen. He then inspired to a level 1 L above FRC and did the same maneuver.

UTTERANCES. Utterance tasks consisted of two groups of activities. The first group involved four tasks, each performed twice:

1. Two minutes of spontaneous conversation
2. Normal reading of a short story
3. Normal reading of numerical strings in a paragraph array
4. Loud reading of the same story as in 2 above.

Spontaneous conversation was elicited by having the subject describe several action pictures of his choosing.

To study respiratory behavior as it varied during reading, a story was adapted from the *Reader's Digest Skill Builder* (Moore and Mastrotto, 1958). The story had high level interest material and was within the reading ability of all subjects. Structure of 46 sentences was altered to provide short (five syllables or less), medium (10 syllables), and long (20 syllables) sentence forms with both rising and falling intonation and a large variety of rhythm, stress, and phrasing patterns. Sentence types were ordered so that no sentence was followed by another of the same number of syllables or intonation contour.

To allow study of respiratory behavior as it varied with prosodic features apart from normal linguistic context, an exact duplicate of the number of syllables per sentence and a close approximation of the prosodic patterns contained in the adapted story were prepared using numerical strings in a paragraph array. For example, the sentence "It was a warm day" contains five syllables and the approximate prosodic pattern as the number "77." Using the numbers one through 100, each sentence in the story was assigned a numerical sequence containing from one to 11 numbers. Numerical sequences were separated by a period and two spaces, and the subject was instructed to read the sequences as he would any paragraph.

The second group of activities was sustained vowel and syllable repetition tasks, each performed twice. Subjects were instructed to inspire to the total lung capacity and then do the tasks on a single expiration until they could no longer perform. The tasks included the following:

1. Sustained production of /ɑ/ at normal pitch and at two loudness levels—normal and loud
2. Repetition of /pɑ/ at a rate of approximately 4 per sec, at normal pitch, and at two loudness levels—normal and loud
3. Repetition of /hɑ/ at a rate of approximately 4 per sec, at normal pitch, and at two loudness levels—normal and loud.

RESULTS

Data Displays: Orientation and Interpretation

Figure 5–4 illustrates the display used to present the results. Anteroposterior diameter of the rib cage is shown on the Y axis, increasing upward. Abdominal anteroposterior diameter is displayed on the X axis, increasing rightward.

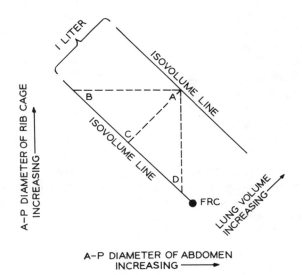

FIGURE 5–4. Relative motion chart (rib cage versus abdomen) illustrative of those constructed for data display.

The long diagonals are isovolume lines. Each traces the relative motion pathway followed during the shifting of volume back and forth between the rib cage and abdomen at a fixed lung volume. The lower line is at FRC and the upper line is 1 L higher. Both lines have − 1 slopes, meaning that for any shift in volume between the rib cage and abdomen, equal diameter changes occur. Charts displaying absolute diameters of the rib cage and abdomen have isovolume slopes of less than − 1. Such charts can be interpreted by graphically solving the relationship between diameter change and volume change for each part (Konno and Mead, 1967). A more direct and convenient procedure is to adjust the gains of the rib cage and abdominal diameter signals to make the slopes of the isovolume lines − 1 (see Chapter 3). Thus modified, the chart provides a direct display of changes in lung volume, of the relative volume contributions of the rib cage and abdomen to changes in lung volume, and of the separate volume displacements of the rib cage and abdomen.

Change in lung volume between any two points is indicated by the distance between them perpendicular to the isovolume lines. Increasing volume is upward and to the right. Decreasing volume is downward and to the left. The pathways AB, AC, and AD in Figure 5–4 each track 1 L changes in lung volume. The specification of volume change often is aided by rotating the chart 45 degrees counterclockwise so that the isovolume lines become analogous to the X axes in a conventional spirogram.

The slope of the line between any two points gives the relative volume contributions of the rib cage and abdomen to lung volume change. For the horizontal pathway (AB), total volume change is accomplished by displacement of the abdomen. The vertical pathway (AD) shows the converse, with rib cage displacement alone accounting for the total volume change. Slopes between these two extremes result from different relative contributions, the magnitude of the slope being proportional to the percentage contribution of each part. Pathway AC shows equal rib cage and abdominal contributions.

The separate volumes of the rib cage and abdomen are indicated by position along the vertical and horizontal axes of the chart, respectively. Upward on the chart indicates an increasing rib cage volume. Toward the right constitutes an increasing abdominal volume. Every point on the chart defines a different chest wall configuration. A record of the changing shape of the moving chest wall is provided by any series of points forming a pathway.

Respiratory Activities

Respiratory activities data are contained in Figures 5–5 and 5–6. Resting breathing and isovolume pathways are represented by straight lines. Tracings were flat loops or single lines, each being linear or approximately so. Isovolume lines have been adjusted to − 1 slopes. Lower and upper isopleths are at FRC and 1 L above, respectively. A single-valued character for the isopleths demonstrates that the relative motion relationships of the two parts are without

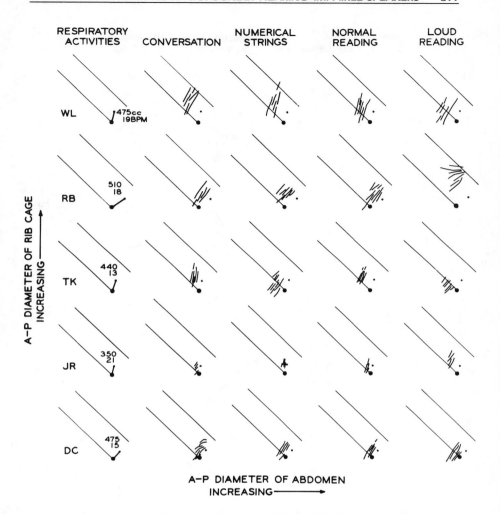

FIGURE 5–5. Relative motion charts for subjects WL, RB, TK, JR, and DC, showing data obtained during respiratory activities, conversation, numerical strings, normal reading, and loud reading. Long sloping lines (– 1 slopes) depict configurations assumed during isovolume maneuvers. Short lines bounded by filled circles in column 1 depict resting breathing patterns. Associated numbers indicate resting breathing excursion and rate. Resting breathing extremes are indicated in the remaining columns by filled circles. Utterance data are shown as thin solid lines.

hysteresis. Isopleth linearity suggests that the diameter change-volume displacement ratio is similar for the two parts. Parallel isopleths mean that the diameter-volume relationships between the rib cage and abdomen are independent of the opposite part's configuration.

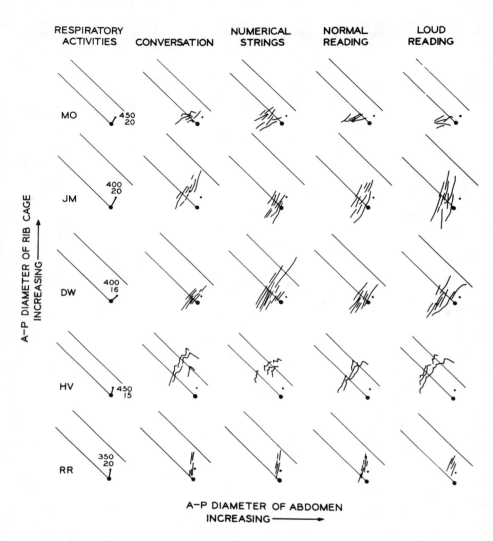

FIGURE 5-6. Relative motion charts for subjects MO, JM, DW, HV, and RR, showing data obtained during respiratory activities, conversation, numerical strings, normal reading, and loud reading (details same as for Figure 5-5).

Two filled circles bound the resting breathing tracings, the larger at FRC and the smaller at the tidal end-inspiratory level. Tidal volume and breathing rate (average of 10 consecutive cycles) are indicated in each chart. Tidal volume ranged between 350 and 510 cc. The average was 430 cc. Breathing rates ranged between 13 and 21 breaths per minute (BPM). The average was approximately 18 BPM. Lung volume change resulted from combined rib cage and abdominal displacements. The contribution of the rib cage exceeded that of the abdomen for nine subjects, ranging from essentially all rib cage displacement (RR) to a slight rib cage predominance (DC and DW). In RB the abdomen displaced greater volumes than the rib cage.

Configuration of the chest wall was qualitatively the same for all subjects and in the neighborhood of the configuration assumed at the right-most extreme of the FRC isovolume line. Thus, breathing occurred with the abdominal wall far outward along its potential range of positions and the rib cage wall at about midrange along its potential assumable positions. A configuration of this nature approximates those attained during relaxation at corresponding lung volumes (see Chapter 3.)

Conversation, Numerical Strings, Normal Reading, and Loud Reading

Figures 5–5 and 5–6 contain data for conversation, numerical strings, normal reading, and loud reading. The tracings shown are representative of the variety of expiratory limbs recorded for each task.

LUNG VOLUME. Lung volume typically was restricted to the midrange of the vital capacity. Initiation levels encompassed a range from more than 1 L above FRC (HV) to well below FRC (MO) and differed among subjects, among tasks, and within tasks. The majority of limbs were initiated above FRC, one half being initiated within the tidal volume range. Limbs initiated below FRC were confined mainly to a few subjects (MO, JM, and DW). Initiation levels were maintained across conversation, numerical strings, and normal reading by seven subjects. TK and JM frequently started numerical strings at lower levels than for the other activities, whereas DW did just the converse. For loud reading, five subjects (DC, JM, DW, HV, and RR) generally used starting levels the equivalent of those for other utterances; three (WL, TK, and MO) typically started at lower volumes; and two (RB and JR) characteristically started at higher volumes. Within-task differences were sometimes major, as with subjects JM, DW, and HV who generated limbs differing in starting level by as much as 1 L or more.

Most limbs were terminated below FRC. Marked encroachments on the expiratory reserve volume were displayed mainly by four subjects (MO, JM, DW, and HV). Of those limbs terminated at or above FRC, most ended within the tidal volume range. Termination levels were maintained across the different normal-loudness tasks by seven subjects. Three terminated limbs at different volumes for one of the tasks (WL lower for normal reading, TK lower for numerical strings, and JR higher for numerical strings). Loud reading was terminated at approximately the same level as was characteristic of normal-loudness tasks for seven subjects, at a lower level for two (WL and TK), and at a higher level for one (RB).

Volume excursions differed among subjects, among tasks, and within tasks. At one extreme were excursions smaller than those for tidal breathing (JR), whereas at the other extreme were excursions covering as much as 2 L (DW, numerical strings). The different excursions were maintained across the normal-loudness tasks by eight subjects. One subject (HV) used smaller excursions during numerical strings than during other tasks, and another (DW) changed from small excursions to large excursions during the numerical strings task. Excursions for loud reading were similar to those for normal-loudness tasks for seven subjects. One (TK) demonstrated smaller excursions and two (JR and JM) demonstrated larger excursions for most loud-reading limbs.

Certain features of lung volume events are not discernible readily in the charts. Time is not designated along the pathways, nor are they marked for linguistic segmentation. Thus, the volume expenditures accompanying various events cannot be specified. This can be achieved only in these unsegmented tracings by replaying the FM tapes to relive data gathering and noting the correspondence between volume change and speech performance.

During such a playback, it was noted that segments of many tracings were not accompanied by utterance. These nonutterance volume expenditures constitute a form of air wastage. Such behavior is shown for one limb in JM's conversational speech data. For that limb, JM initiated utterance, stopped after a few seconds but continued to expire (dashed segment), and then resumed utterance. Segments like this occurred occasionally in the midportion of limbs for subjects TK, JM, HV, and RR, and at the end of limbs for DC and HV. The magnitude of air wastage varied considerably within and between subjects, utterance tasks, and expiratory limbs. Frequently it was as great as 250 cc.

It also was noted during tape playback that widely differing volumes were expended during comparable utterance segments of different subjects. A determination of the average expenditure per syllable for each subject's normal reading revealed extremes of 30 cc/syllable (JR) and 200 cc/syllable (HV). The group average proved to be approximately 100 cc/syllable with subjects being relatively evenly distributed around this mean and within the range. Not only was a wide range of expenditures characteristic of the group, it also was characteristic of comparisons from syllable to syllable within single limbs produced by subjects. Differences within limbs often were manyfold and did not appear related in any systematic fashion to phonetic content of the utterances.

It further was noted during tape playback that volume phrasing differed among numerical strings, normal reading, and loud reading tasks. Phrasing could not be determined for conversational speech because utterances were highly unintelligible. All subjects paused to breathe at most sentence boundaries and at many points of within-sentence punctuation. Most subjects also inspired frequently during nonpunctuated word sequences. The average number of syllables uttered per breath varied over a wide range within subjects and tasks. The smallest average number, 1.8, was demonstrated by RB for numerical strings and the largest, 7.9, by DC and DW for loud reading. The group average varied from 5.2 for numerical strings to 4.5 for normal reading and 4.9 for loud reading. Half of the subjects used more syllables per breath during loud reading than normal reading. Numerical strings involved a greater number of syllables per breath than both normal reading and loud reading for most of the subjects.

RELATIVE VOLUME DISPLACEMENTS OF THE RIB CAGE AND ABDOMEN.   Relative contributions of the two parts differed among subjects, among tasks, within tasks, and within expiratory limbs. Extremes occurred in subjects MO and RR, who typically showed a marked predominance of abdominal displacement and a marked predominance of rib cage displacement, respectively, during their utterances. Remaining subjects showed various degrees of rib cage predominance, abdominal predominance being rare.

Six subjects showed no appreciable relative contribution change across conversation, numerical strings, and normal reading. Two (WL and DC) showed less rib cage predominance for conversation than for the other tasks, and two (RB and TK) showed less predominance for numerical strings than for the other tasks. Six subjects showed no relative contribution differences between normal and loud utterance. JM used a greater rib cage contribution for loud utterance than for normal utterance. WL demonstrated a rib cage predominance for loud reading that was less than that for other tasks except conversational speech, and TK demonstrated a rib cage predominance for loud reading that was less than that for other tasks except numerical strings. RB demonstrated a marked shift from rib cage to abdominal predominance in changing from normal to loud reading.

The majority of limbs did not change slope. When changes were involved, they were of different magnitudes and forms. Many tracings for DC (conversation) tended convex toward the Y axis, showing a decreasing abdominal and increasing rib cage contribution with decreasing lung volume. JM (normal reading) often showed the converse, with tracings that tended concave toward the Y axis. HV frequently demonstrated abrupt and extensive relative contribution changes.

Paradoxical displacements of the rib cage and abdomen were reflected in tracings in which the sign of volume displacement of one or the other of the parts was opposite to that of lung volume change. The most common paradoxing showed decreases in both lung volume and abdominal volume while rib cage volume increased (see certain tracings for RB, loud reading; DC, conversation; MO, conversation and loud reading; and HV, all tasks). Only one subject (HV) demonstrated paradoxing in the opposite sense. This subject frequently showed an alternation between rib cage and abdominal paradoxing. Rib cage paradoxing accompanied the production of discrete syllables or words whereas abdominal paradoxing occurred between such utterances.

SEPARATE VOLUMES OF THE RIB CAGE AND ABDOMEN: CHEST WALL CONFIGURATION. A vast majority of limbs were initiated at rib cage volumes greater than those at the tidal end-expiratory level. In fact, well over half of the limbs were initiated at rib cage sizes larger than those at the tidal end-inspiratory level. Different initiation levels were maintained across conversation, numerical strings, and normal reading by seven subjects. Three often initiated speech at different rib cage sizes for numerical strings than for the other two activities (TK and JM at lower rib cage volumes and DW at higher rib cage volumes). Six subjects initiated loud reading at roughly the same rib cage volume they used for normal-loudness tasks. Two (RB and JR) initiated loud reading at higher rib cage volumes than normal reading, and two (TK and MO) did just the opposite.

The majority of limbs were terminated at rib cage volumes in excess of those at tidal end-expiration. Some limbs terminated at rib cage volumes even in excess of those for tidal end-inspiration. Termination levels were maintained across conversation, numerical strings, and normal reading by subjects WL, JR, DC, MO, and RR. RB and HV terminated numerical strings at higher rib cage volumes than those for the other two tasks, and TK terminated numerical strings at lower volumes. JM and DW demonstrated major within-task differences in termination levels. These ranged from rib cage volumes well in excess of those at tidal end-inspiration to volumes considerably smaller than those attained at tidal end-expiration. Seven subjects terminated loud reading at approximately the same rib cage levels as those for normal reading. Two (RB and JR) terminated loud utterances at higher rib cage levels, and one (TK) at lower levels.

Rib cage excursions differed among subjects, among tasks, and within tasks. Extremes were demonstrated by JR and HV and ranged from a change appreciably less than that for tidal breathing to a change of 1.6 L. Excursion magnitudes were maintained across conversation, numerical strings, and normal reading by eight subjects. DW changed from small to large excursions during the numerical strings task, and HV used smaller excursions for numerical strings than during other normal-loudness tasks. Excursions for loud reading were similar to those for other tasks for seven subjects, whereas one (TK) demonstrated smaller excursions and two (JR and JM) showed larger excursions for most loud reading.

The majority of limbs were initiated at abdominal volumes smaller than those at tidal end-expiration. Limbs initiated at larger abdominal volumes were confined mainly to four subjects (RB, DC, JM, and DW) and rarely were initiated at abdominal sizes larger than those at tidal end-inspiration. No appreciable differences in initiation levels were observed across conversation, numerical strings, and normal reading. Eight subjects initiated loud reading at roughly the same abdominal volume as that used for normal-loudness tasks. One (WL) initiated limbs at a generally smaller abdominal size and one (RR) often started from slightly larger abdominal sizes for loud reading than for normal-loudness tasks.

Nine subjects terminated most utterances at smaller abdominal volumes than those at tidal end-expiration. RB terminated some normal-loudness limbs at abdominal sizes larger than those at tidal end-expiration but smaller than those at tidal end-inspiration.

Abdominal excursions differed among subjects, among tasks, and within tasks. Extremes were demonstrated by RR and MO and involved changes from .03 to .85 L, respectively. Abdominal excursions remained similar across conversation, numerical strings, and normal reading for six subjects. Two (WL and DC) demonstrated slightly larger excursions during conversation than the other two tasks, and two (RB and TK) used somewhat larger excursions during numerical strings than during the other tasks. Six subjects showed no difference in excursions between normal and loud utterances. JM showed smaller excursions for loud than normal-loudness utterance. WL demonstrated excursions for loud reading that were greater than those for all tasks except conversational speech, and TK demonstrated excursions for loud reading that were greater than those for all tasks except numerical strings. RB showed a marked shift from small to large excursions with the change from normal to loud reading.

Utterances took place to the left of the chest wall configuration assumed on the charts for tidal breathing. Thus, the rib cage was more, and the abdomen was less expanded than they were for tidal breathing in the same lung volume range. Although utterances for two subjects (RB and DC) took place to the left of the configuration assumed at tidal end-inspiration, those for eight subjects typically took place well to the left of the tidal end-expiration configuration. The most extreme of this latter group was subject HV.

Sustained Vowel and Syllable
Repetition Utterances

Figure 5–7 and 5–8 contain data for sustained vowel and syllable repetition utterances. Only one tracing is shown for each activity, repeat performances having been comparable. Numbers 1 and 2 designate normal and loud utterances, respectively.

LUNG VOLUME. The majority of subjects began utterances far above FRC and ended them far below FRC, expiring through a large portion of the vital capacity. Two subjects (TK and RR) did not initiate utterance at high lung volumes, and one (JR) frequently did not continue below FRC. Initiation and

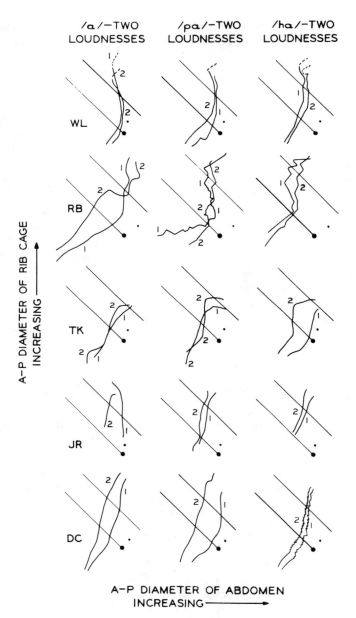

FIGURE 5-7. Relative motion charts for subjects WL, RB, TK, JR, and DC, showing data obtained during a sustained vowel and two syllable repetition activities, each performed at two loudnesses and throughout most of the vital capacity. Numbers 1 and 2 denote normal and loud utterances, respectively. Isovolume lines and resting breathing extremes are repeated from Figure 5–5.

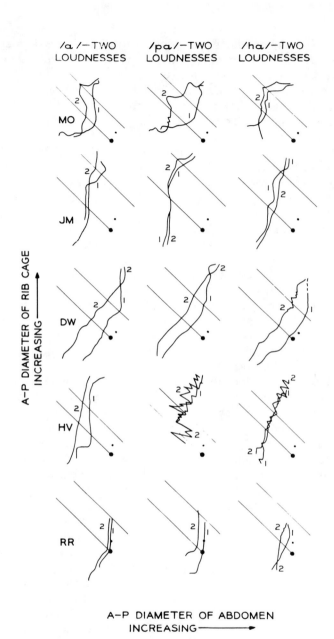

FIGURE 5-8. Relative motion charts for subjects MO, JM, DW, HV, and RR, showing data obtained during a sustained vowel and two syllable repetition activities, each performed throughout most of the vital capacity (details same as for Figure 5-7 with repeated data coming from Figure 5-6).

termination levels did not differ significantly across loudnesses or tasks except for HV, who terminated /pɑ/ at higher volumes, and RR, who initiated /hɑ/ at lower lung volumes than for other utterances.

Volume excursions were approximately the same across tasks and loudnesses. They covered from under 2 L (JR and RR) to over 3 L (HV). Average excursions were approximately 2.5 L.

RELATIVE VOLUME DISPLACEMENTS OF THE RIB CAGE AND ABDOMEN. Pathway slopes were relatively constant for some utterances (see loud /ɑ/ productions for JR, DC, and HV), whereas for others they differed markedly with lung volume (JM, /ɑ/ 1; DW, /hɑ/ 2). The range of relative contributions was reflected within a single tracing for MO (/pɑ/ 2). Changes in slope ranged from gradual (WL, /pɑ/ 2) to abrupt (HV, /pɑ/).

Most subjects used a predominant rib cage displacement at very high lung volumes. This included instances of slight rib cage predominance (JR, /pɑ/ 1), displacement attributable to motion of the rib cage entirely (DW, /ɑ/ 1), and rib cage displacement accompanied by abdominal paradoxing (JM, /ɑ/ 1). Abdominal predominance was confined mainly to certain utterances of three subjects (RB, TK, and MO). Contributions ranged from slight abdominal predominance (HV, /ɑ/ 1), to displacement almost entirely by the abdomen (RB, /hɑ/ 1), to abdominal displacement accompanied by rib cage paradoxing (MO, /hɑ/ 2). Dashed portions of limbs for two subjects (WL, most tasks; DW, /hɑ/ 1) indicate segments of the high lung volume range in which air was expended prior to utterance. The rib cage also typically predominated in the midvolume range. In fact, several expiratory limbs showing predominantly abdominal displacements at high volumes showed predominantly rib cage displacements in the midvolume range (see MO, /ɑ/ 2; HV, /ɑ/ 1). Instances of abdominal predominance in midvolumes were confined mainly to two subjects (RB, /ɑ/ 2; MO, /pɑ/ 2). The low lung volume range included rib cage predominance (JM, /pɑ/; RR, /hɑ/ 2), almost equal contributions by the two parts (WL, /pɑ/ 2), and abdominal predominance (MO, /pɑ/ 1; RR, /pɑ/1). Many subjects showed a gradual shift toward more abdominal and less rib cage contribution at low lung volumes (see MO, normal loudness for all tasks).

Loudness did not systematically influence the relative displacements of the rib cage and abdomen. Also, no appreciable differences occurred in relative contributions for seven subjects across tasks. One subject (JR) used relatively more abdominal contribution from /ɑ/ to /pɑ/ to /hɑ/ (especially normal loudness). Task differences occurred for the remaining two subjects in the form of abrupt slope changes (i.e., "relative motion jogs") accompanying individual syllables. DC showed these changes during /hɑ/ productions. HV demonstrated them during normal and loud productions of /pɑ/ and /hɑ/. Paradoxical displacements of the rib cage and abdomen were frequent. Abdominal paradoxing was restricted mainly to the high and midvolume ranges (e.g., see WL, all utterances except /hɑ/ 2; RB, all utterances; JR, /ɑ/ 1; MO, all utterances; JM, /ɑ/ 1; HV, all utterances except /ɑ/ 2; RR, /hɑ/ 1). Rib cage paradoxing occurred at widely differing volumes (see WL, /pɑ/ 1; RB, /ɑ/ 2 and /pɑ/ 1; TK, /pɑ/; DC, /hɑ/; MO, all utterances; HV, /hɑ/ and /pɑ/).

SEPARATE VOLUME DISPLACEMENTS OF THE RIB CAGE AND ABDOMEN: CHEST WALL CONFIGURATION. All vowel and syllable utterances were initiated at very high rib cage volumes. A majority of limbs terminated at rib cage volumes smaller than at the tidal end-expiratory level (see JR and MO for exceptions). Rib cage excursions covered a wide range, some typically averaging between 1 and 2 L (TK, JR, and RR), others typically averaging between 2 and 3 L (WL, RB, DC, MO, JM, and DW), and still others often averaging as much as 3 to 4 L (HV).

Approximately one half of the vowel and syllable utterances were initiated at smaller abdominal volumes than those for tidal end-expiration. Of those remaining, approximately one half were initiated at volumes typical of the tidal breathing range (e.g., see RB /ɑ/) and one half were initiated at volumes larger or approximately the same as those at tidal end-inspiration (see DW). Utterances terminated at substantially smaller volumes than those at FRC with the exception of one utterance by JR (/ɑ/ 1). Abdominal excursions typically averaged less than 1 L for some subjects (WL, JR, JM, HV, and RR), and from 1 to 2 L for others (RB, TK, DC, MO, and DW).

Chest wall configuration differed with loudness and utterance task for some subjects. Limbs for a majority of subjects shifted more leftward on the chart when changing from normal to loud utterance (see JR). Thus, the abdomen was smaller and the rib cage larger for the loud utterances than they were for the normal utterances at the same lung volume. Occasionally, loudness did not influence the tracings appreciably (e.g., see WL, /ɑ/) or the influence was in the opposite direction to that observed usually (see WL and RB on /hɑ/). Limbs for four subjects (WL; RB, except /ɑ/ 2; TK, except /hɑ/ 1; and RR) shifted more leftward on the chart from /ɑ/ to /pɑ/ to /hɑ/. Limbs for three subjects remained at about the same configuration with one exception across tasks (JR /ɑ/ 1, more to the right; DW, /hɑ/ 1 and 2, more to the right; HV, /ɑ/ 2, more to the left). Three subjects (DC, MO, and JM) demonstrated unsystematic differences in configuration across tasks.

DISCUSSION

The respiratory behaviors of the subjects were abnormal in some regards and normal in others. These behaviors are considered subsequently with respect to the following topics: resting breathing, utterances of a continuous discourse nature, sustained vowel and syllable repetition utterances, muscular mechanisms of the chest wall, and clinical implications.

Resting Breathing

Resting tidal volumes ranged between 350 and 510 cc. The average was 430 cc. Breathing rates encompassed a range of 13 to 21 BPM and averaged 18 BPM. Excursions and rates of these magnitudes approximate those for normal individuals (see Chapter 3 and Comroe, 1974). Several of the subjects tended toward the low side of the normal tidal volume range and the high side of the normal breathing rate range. No particular significance is attached to these tendencies. They may reflect nothing more than certain subjects' initial anxieties over the testing situation (Mead and Agostoni, 1964). For all but one subject, the volume contribution of the rib cage exceeded that of the abdomen. This finding is consistent with observations on normal individuals in the upright body position (see Chapter 3 and Fugl-Meyer, 1974). One subject demonstrated a slight abdominal predominance. A small number of normal subjects also are known to demonstrate a slight abdominal predominance during resting tidal breathing in the upright position (Fugl-Meyer, 1974). The configuration of the chest wall during resting tidal breathing approximated what is presumed to be the configuration obtained for relaxation at corresponding lung volumes. This is likewise the configuration at which normal individuals typically rest breathe when instructed to do so in as relaxed a manner as possible (see Chapter 3). In summary, the observations on resting breathing reveal function within normal limits.

Utterances of a Continuous Discourse Nature

The present data on continous discourse utterances reveal frequent deviances in three factors governing respiratory function in profoundly hearing-impaired individuals: (1) linguistic programming, (2) mechanical adjustments of respiratory origin, and (3) mechanical adjustments of the larynx and upper airway. It appears that what clinicians designate variously as problems of "respiratory control" are manifestations of deviances in one or more of these factors—more often than not, in more than one.

Deviances in linguistic programming are manifested in the data mainly as subjects' failure to follow normal conventions of phrasing. The kinematic task in continuous discourse utterances is to provide relatively continuous expiration, halted occasionally for inspiratory refills or breath holdings. In normal speakers, these refills or holdings occur inconspicuously at sentence or phrase boundaries or other appropriate linguistic points interspersed within the flow of speech (see Chapter 1). By contrast, typical of the present findings were short stretches of speech containing only a few syllables and broken by inappropriate pauses. For normal reading, for example, the subjects averaged less than one third the number of syllables per breath than do normal individuals.[1] Instead of halting only at appropriate lingusitic points within utterances, the subjects included many unnecessary and seemingly unlawful interruptions for breaths and holdings at points other than those known to be linguistically appropriate (e.g., in nonpunctuated word sequences). The haltings themselves often were inappropriately long, both between syllables within expiratory excursions and between separate expiratory excursions. Finally, it is noteworthy, from the perspective of linguistic programming, that the majority of the subjects averaged more syllables for numerical strings, in which linguistic cues were substantially removed, than for either normal or loud continous discourse utterances. Just the opposite occurs in individuals with normal hearing.[2]

Deviances in mechanical adjustments of respiratory origin are manifested in a variety of ways in the data. For example, whereas those haltings that involved inspirations served to return the respiratory apparatus to higher lung volumes, the returns for many subjects showed a considerable inconsistency in attainment of similar starting levels for successive expiratory excursions. This is in contrast to a rather high consistency in starting level from limb to limb for normal speakers (see Chapter 3). Those haltings that did not involve inspiration often were not the usual form of breath holdings seen in normal individuals. Rather, major quantities of air often were expended during these pauses such that the available air supply was diminished further unnecessarily. In many instances, relatively wide variations in the magnitudes of expiratory excursions occurred from breath to breath during continuous discourse utterances. Instead of encompassing the 10% to 20% VC magnitude of excursion typical of the speech of individuals with normal hearing (see Chapter 3), the subjects' excursions often were considerably smaller or considerably larger. Such excursions are, of course, determined by two factors: the length of utterance and the average rate of volume expenditure associated with the utterance. The range of lung volumes used by the subjects also was considerably different from that which normal speakers employ. Rather than inspiring to nearly twice normal depth for speech purposes as normal individuals do (see Chapter 1), many subjects initiated their expiratory limbs

---

[1]Ten subjects with normal hearing read the reading passage aloud to provide data for this comparison. Average number of syllables per breath ranged from 12 to 15.8 for individual subjects, with an overall mean of 13.6.

[2]The same 10 subjects with normal hearing mentioned in footnote 1 also read the paragraph of numerical strings aloud to provide data for comparison. Average number of syllables per breath ranged from 9.8 to 12.8 for individual subjects, with an overall mean of 10.7. Examination of individual data revealed that each normal speaker used fewer syllables per breath for numerical strings than for normal reading.

within the tidal breathing range or lower. This means that their utterances often carried them to lung volume levels well below FRC, a level only occasionally reached by normal speakers (see Chapter 1). Initiating utterances from lower than normal levels and carrying speech through lower than normal levels undoubtedly was costly for the subjects. First, they had to use higher than normal muscular pressures to achieve speech at lower lung volumes. And second, they had to work against inspiratory recoil forces after they passed below FRC. The present subjects typically did not go to higher lung volumes for loud speech, as normal-hearing subjects do (see Chapter 4). Thus, they required of themselves additional major increases in expiratory muscular pressure that could have been offset partially through attainable respiratory recoil forces. Normal speakers take advantage of such forces.

Other mechanical adjustments of respiratory origin were, for the most part, normal. This was somewhat surprising in view of frequent clinical statements and some research reports (Hudgins, 1934; Woldring, 1968) alluding to major abnormalities in certain of these adjustments. The relative volume contributions of the rib cage and abdomen in the subjects were found to fall within the range of observations made previously on individuals with normal hearing (see Chapter 3). Rib cage contributions usually predominated for the subjects, as they do for normal subjects in the upright body position. Major dysynchronies between the actions of the rib cage and abdomen during speech generally were not observed. In addition, the relative volume contributions of the rib cage and abdomen did not change abruptly for most subjects. Rather, they typically showed changes of a gradual nature that presumably reflected the use of an economical coordination between the rib cage and abdomen. Only in one of the subjects (HV) were rib cage–abdomen synchronization problems seen. In his case, the inward motion of the abdomen often was accompanied by an outward motion of the rib cage wall, or vice versa. It is possible that the subject group was not characteristic of other groups observed clinically or in other research studies, although this is believed to be quite unlikely. The more probable reason for the frequent report of rib cage–abdomen dysynchronies has to do with the fact that some of the paradoxical motions noted previously in hearing-impaired speakers may have been labeled inappropriately as abnormal. This is due to the observers' lack of knowledge of normal function, normative data having been unavailable until relatively recently (see Chapters 3 and 4). A second somewhat surprising normalcy observed in the subjects, given clinical and research accounts of function, was that the chest wall configurations they assumed during utterances of a continous discourse nature were similar to those found for normal speakers under similar utterance conditions (see Chapter 3). Each subject took on a torso shape that involved a larger rib cage size and a smaller abdominal size than those accompanying relaxation at the prevailing lung volumes. Thus, the subjects assumed configurations that optimized diaphragmatic function along the lines observed previously for normal individuals (see Chapter 4); the major mechanical advantage gained served to place the diaphragm in an optimal position for action during inspiratory segments interspersed in running speech.

Deviances in mechanical adjustments of the larynx and upper airway are manifested in the data by the very high volume expenditures that accompanied syllable production. These averaged approximately 100 cc/syllable, a value that is severalfold greater than the average observed in normal speakers and at least twice as great as the average observed for speakers with dysarthria (Hardy, 1961). Assuming that the respiratory drive reasonably approximates that for normal speakers, it would appear that these extremely high volume expenditures per syllable reflect low average resistive mechanical loads in the larynx and upper airway. Stated otherwise, it would appear that the subjects valved the speech airstream very inefficiently during their articulatory performances. This observation and the one noted previously of large air wastages during moments when breath holding is called for, combine to suggest a picture of abnormal function in which the air supply is relatively rapidly depleted during continuous discourse. This can be contrasted with the speech of normal individuals, in which the respiratory apparatus operates into high resistive mechanical loads that serve in conjunction with the respiratory drive to govern a low rate of lung volume change during utterance and frugal control of the air supply during breath holding.

The individual contributions of linguistic programming, mechanical respiratory adjustments, and larynx and upper airway mechanical adjustments to the abnormal respiratory kinematics of the subjects have been stressed here. It is important to note the interactive nature of these different deviances, because they occur in constellation during the speech act. Numerous examples could be cited from the data to make this point. The following is illustrative: Because of his abnormal linguistic programming, the speaker does not realize that he must produce a fairly large number of syllables on one expiratory excursion to maintain the phrasing dictated by the punctuation of a sentence. Accordingly, he realizes no need to take a deeper than normal inspiration prior to the beginning of his utterance. Further, he does not take into account the fact that he will run out of air rapidly because of his inefficient valving of the expiratory output during the ensuing utterance and because of his air wastage during pauses. An adjustment in any of the three factors would help the situation. The optimal solution would be an adjustment in all three.

Obviously, the respiratory dysfunctions of the subjects are related to their congenital, profound, bilateral sensorineural hearing impairments. Lacking normal auditory sensation, they did not have appropriate acoutic cues available to them that are needed for the development of normal oral language or for contributing to the monitoring of the respiratory apparatus and its interactions with other speech subsystems. It might seem logical to ascribe the present observations entirely to the subjects' hearing impairments and thus believe that the findings would have significant implications for understanding the role of auditory sensation in speech control. It seems reasonable, however, to suppose that a substantial part of their kinematic behavior may be related to instructional methodologies employed with some of the subjects in the early stages of speech skill development. According to individual subject reports, many were instructed in ways that stressed sound and syllable-by-syllable speech production. This may have encouraged them to break their speech into equally stressed segments lacking natural prosodic characteristics over long stretches of utterance. Such instructional situations do not require the development of normal respiratory control strategies, nor the development of normal speech apparatus control strategies for coodinating the actions of the various apparatus subsystems. For example, the subject taught to produce individual short utterances may not perceive the need to breathe outside his tidal volume range or to plan ahead to produce a large number of syllables without stopping for an inspiratory refill. It is encouraging that present-day instructional methodologies for the hearing impaired emphasize natural speech and language development with an aim toward a strong prosodic underpinning (e.g., see, Calvert and Silverman, 1975; Connor, 1971; Ling, 1976; Moog, 1973; Pollack, 1970; Simmons-Martin, 1974). Training of this nature may well aid the development of more efficient respiratory behavior in coordination with the actions of other speech apparatus subsystems.

Sustained Vowel and
Syllable Repetition Utterances

Two areas are important for consideration in discussion of the data on sustained vowels and syllable repetitions: (1) mechanical adjustments of respiratory origin and (2) mechanical adjustments of the larynx and upper airway.

With respect to the first of these, the subjects demonstrated performances comparable to normal subjects (see Chapter 3) in the following ways: Their tracings revealed a wide variety of relative volume contributions, being relatively constant for some utterances and differing markedly with lung volume for others; their tracings generally were characterized by a rib cage predominance, particularly through higher lung volume segments; their chest wall configurations involved leftward departures from the presumed relaxation configuration of the chest wall on the motions chart; and their tracings frequently included the normal pattern of more leftward positions on the motions chart for louder utterances. By contrast, performance differences between the present subjects and normal subjects are manifested in three major ways: First, several subjects often expended substantial volumes of air prior to the initiation of utterance, an observation rarely made in normal individuals; second, gradual relative contribution changes occurred quite frequently during a substantial number of the expiratory excursions of the subjects, whereas a characteristic small number of such changes is found in normal individuals; and third, small abrupt relative volume contribution changes occurred in the case of several subjects (i.e., motion jogs appeared on the charts). This is an observation made in normal subjects only in instances of major linguistic stressing.

The three observations just mentioned are interpreted to reveal deviances in the subjects' abilities to regulate the output of the respiratory apparatus and to regulate its different parts in an economically coordinated fashion, such as is observed in the individual with normal hearing. Note that the most prominent deviances for the subject group had to do with the two-part regulation of the chest wall. This is in contrast to utterances of a continuous discourse nature in which few problems in two-part regulation were manifested. Perhaps the task of producing speech well outside the tidal breathing range is especially difficult for the hearing-impaired speaker. Reasons for this could be many, including the possibility of different sensory cues at different lung volumes, little practice through this range such as normals would get through singing, and so on, and the problem of not having an acoustic cue for loudness, to know if the respiratory adjustments for alveolar pressure are near target. It would be informative to know whether the observations reported by speech-language pathologists are made for utterances produced in the tidal breathing range or outside of it. The present data for utterances of a continuous discourse nature and of a sustained vowel and syllable repetition nature suggest that somewhat different pictures of kinematic function would be portrayed for the profoundly hearing-impaired individual, depending upon the type of utterance observed.

Mechanical adjustments of the larynx and upper airway presumably also were frequently deviant during the sustained vowel and syllable repetition utterances of the subjects. Most prominent for the vowel utterances were instances in which subjects phonated throughout nearly their entire vital capacity, but the utterances were of short duration (sometimes less than 5 secs). This observation is accounted for by the fact that the rate of volume expenditure (i.e., flow) was abnormally high, and presumably it reflects the fact that the resistive mechanical load offered by the larynx was lower than is found for normal individuals. Voice quality for many such instances was breathy. At the other extreme was an occasional sustained vowel that was prolonged inordinately long relative to the duration anticipated for normal individuals. This was interpreted to indicate an abnormally high resistive mechanical load offered by the larynx. Such behavior appeared to be linked to the perception of harsh voice quality in particular subjects. In the case of the syllable repetition tasks, each usually involved a smaller number of syllables per expiratory excursion than would be expected from normal individuals covering the same volume range. This suggests that mechanical valving of the larynx or upper airway, or both, was inefficient for such utterances, a finding congruent with the observations for utterances of a continuous discourse nature. These observations on sustained vowels and syllable repetitions may be taken to further document the profoundly hearing-impaired speaker's difficulty in coordinating the actions of various subsystems (respiratory, larngeal, and upper airway) of the speech apparatus.

Muscular Mechanisms of the Chest Wall

It is possible to use the present data to infer what muscular mechanisms may underlie chest wall behavior during utterance. Inferences of this nature are based, for the most part, on chest wall configuration and its changes during speech in comparison to configurations associated with a relaxed chest wall. Departures from the relaxed configuration are taken to imply some form of muscular activity. On the basis of relative motion data alone, the precise muscular activity cannot be specified unequivocally, there being more than a single way to attain a configuration or to change a configuration.

The protocol used in this investigation did not require the generation of relative motion relaxation data. To obtain such data on even a small number of individuals would have required a substantial amount of subject screening and training (see Chapter 4). Rather, the fact was taken into account that data obtained from known good relaxers (see Chapter 3) could be used as an indication of where similar data would presumably lie on charts for the present subjects. This approach results in the placement of relaxation characteristics at the right-most extremes of the partial isovolume lines in the individual charts of Figures 5–5 to 5–8. All utterance data lie to the left of these characteristics. Stated otherwise, the rib cage is larger and the abdomen smaller than they would be were the subjects relaxed at the prevailing lung volumes.

Muscular activities that could bring about distortion of this nature are (1) net inspiratory forces operating on the rib cage, (2) expiratory forces operating on the abdomen, (3) a combination of 1 and 2, and (4) a combination of expiratory forces operating on both the rib cage (net) and abdomen, but with the latter predominating. The diaphragm is not included in these alternatives because its action does not cause departure from the relative motion relaxation configuration (see Chapter 4). Therefore, it cannot be determined, on the basis of the present data, whether or not the diaphragm was active during utterances. It seems unlikely that the diaphragm would be active during utterance (see Chapters 3 and 4 and Bouhuys, Proctor, and Mead, 1966; Draper, Ladefoged, and Whitteridge, 1959), except at very high lung volumes for some of the activities for which data are presented in Figures 5–7 and 5–8.

Which alternative is likely to be operating can be surmised on the basis of the presumed sign and magnitude of the muscular pressure required and the relaxation pressure available at the prevailing lung volume (see Chapter

3). The alveolar pressures used by the subjects probably were similar in magnitude to those used by normal-hearing speakers (see Chapter 1). This is because the loudness levels of nearly all the subjects' utterances were comparable to those for normal speakers performing similar tasks under similar instructions. Two of the subjects produced softer-than-normal utterances of a continuous discourse nature. In their cases, it may be that alveolar pressures were slightly lower than those characteristic of normal individuals. The probable relaxation pressure available at each lung volume can be predicted with sufficient accuracy from existing data on healthy, normal subjects (Agostoni and Mead, 1964).

It is assumed that the subjects' utterances of a continuous discourse nature involved the generation of continuous positive muscular pressure and that this pressure increased with decreases in lung volume. Given that utterances generally took place through a lower range of lung volumes than is used by normal individuals, the muscular pressure involved probably averaged somewhat higher than normal. Alternative 4 listed previously seems most likely to account for the observations for runnning speech. Alternatives 1 and 3 probably can be discounted because each includes inspiratory forces that usually are characteristic of only high lung volume segments or very soft speech (see Chapter 3). Alternative 2 seems unlikely because of the predominant rib cage contribution associated with chest wall configuration change. Not only is alternative 4 the most consistent with the observations, it also is consistent with what is known to be the muscular mechanism operating during the same type of speech in normal-hearing individuals (see Chapter 4). The present loud-reading data appear to warrant a similar interpretation as to function but with each part of the chest wall presumably increasing the magnitude of its input relative to that for speech of normal loudness. For certain subjects, the relative volume contribution of the abdomen increased in going to loud reading from normal reading. This suggests that the muscular pressure contribution of the abdomen may have increased more than that of the rib cage.

Continuous discourse utterances of one of the subjects (HV) were characterized by abrupt, extensive, and frequent changes in relative contributions of the rib cage and abdomen. This led to the appearance of relative motion "jogs" in the tracings for his expiratory excursions. The leftward displacement associated with these jogs clearly was synchronous with discrete "individual syllable bursts" in HV's speech. The mechanism associated with these bursts was believed to be one whereby HV was providing abnormally large abdominal wall contractions, muscular pressures, and displacements in syllable-linked gestures. This abnormal abdominal wall activity appears to have been sufficient at times to drive the less active rib cage to a larger size. The jogs appear somewhat in kind to small isovolume maneuvers performed in the presence of a slight air leakage. This interpretation seems even more reasonable when it is considered that much of HV's speech took place at a "background" chest wall configuration involving a generally smaller abdominal size and larger rib cage size than was typical of other subjects (see Fig. 5–6). It would appear that HV's use of his abdominal wall, in a manner far more forcefully than required, drove his less forcefully active rib cage wall upward along the range of sizes it could assume for speech.

It is assumed that sustained vowel and syllable repetition utterances initially involved negative muscular pressure, and then, later, positive muscular pressure (see Chapter 4). The change in muscular pressure sign probably occurred near the uppermost isovolume line in the charts for normal-loudness utterances and at substantially higher lung volumes for loud utterances. Loudness was maintained with each expiratory excursion, so the muscular pressure generated had to become continuously more positive as utterance proceeded (see Chapter 3). More than one of the alternatives mentioned earlier probably accounts for the abdomen being smaller and the rib cage larger than they are presumed to be during relaxation. For the high lung volume range, when muscular pressure is negative, either alternative 1 or 3 is likely to be operating. Each involves inspiratory force that could be used to check excessive relaxation forces characteristic of high lung volumes. Alternative 3 typically is adopted by normal speakers (see Chapter 4) and is the preferred choice to explain the kinematic observations. It seems certain that alternative 3 prevails in cases in which changes involve major inward motion of the abdomen (e.g., see data for MO in Fig. 5–8). Alternative 1 is inconsistent with such an observation. Positive muscular pressure from the chest wall would have to involve either alternative 2 or 4. Alternative 4 seems most likely because both the rib cage and abdomen typically decrease in size simultaneously and because this combination of forces is the same as that used for similar utterances by normals (see Chapter 4). Alternative 2 could not be operating at lung volumes well below FRC because the size of the rib cage is decreased majorly in the face of a concomitant major abdominal drive.

Tracings for loud utterances often were displaced leftward on the motions chart relative to those for normal loudness. This means the abdomen was smaller and the rib cage larger for louder speech. This observation probably reflects a greater increment in abdominal wall activity than in rib cage wall activity as muscular pressure is raised for louder speech. Such a mechanism is consistent with that used by normal individuals for similar utterances (see Chapter 3).

Certain subjects demonstrated abrupt changes in pathway slope on the chart (see Fig. 5–7 and 5–8). These can be accounted for only by rapid muscular pressure adjustments that are superimposed on the major background adjustment of the chest wall. Rapid leftward jogs on the charts probably are the result of greater than normal increases in abdominal drive, whereas rightward jogs probably are attributable to greater than normal increases in rib cage drive. Subject HV's loud repetition of /pɑ/ is particularly informative. At higher lung volumes HV's performance is qualitatively similar to that for his utterances of a continuous discourse nature. That is, he shows leftward motion jogs in association with individual syllables. At just less than 1 L above FRC, however, he shows a change to rightward motion jogs. Thus, he continues to provide discrete chest wall motions for each syllable but with the rib cage predominating instead of the abdomen at lower volumes.

Clinical Implications

USE OF SIMPLIFIED KINEMATIC METHODS. Previous studies on speech breathing kinematics (see Chapter 3 and 4) have involved a demanding set of respiratory maneuvers and sophisticated, trained, subjects to perform them. In this investigation an attempt was made to simplify these methods and to make them clinically applicable to untrained, profoundly hearing-impaired individuals. This simplification involved only the need to perform two isovolume maneuvers. This approach proved highly successful as a means of studying the respiratory kinematics of the present subjects. The outcome is encouraging with regard to further study of hearing-impaired individuals as well as to the clinical study of other groups, such as speakers with neurologically based speech problems.

The present simplified method offers a powerful clinical tool. Its merits include that it is safe, innocuous, precise, rapid, of little inconvenience to the client, unencumbering to natural speech, in a real-time form, and of such a nature as to require little training of either clinician or client. An additional merit is that, from a single oscilloscopic display, changes in lung volume, relative volume contributions of the rib cage and abdomen, and chest wall configuration can be examined.

EVALUATION OF CHEST WALL KINEMATICS IN THE HEARING IMPAIRED. It is important to note that in almost all of the subjects, only the lung volume aspect of kinematic function was abnormal. This suggests that the most relevant kinematic information to be obtained on profoundly hearing-impaired speakers involves a single measurement. A variety of measurement devices could be used to obtain lung volume information. Devices currently more readily available to clinicians than magnetometers include spirometers, respirometers, and flowmeters (volume obtained by integration). Thus, the technological capability for evaluating the abnormal kinematic aspect of the hearing-impaired speaker's respiratory behavior is already at hand for many speech-language pathologists. Measurements need not depend on the sophisticated magnetometer system used here.

Assuming a primary focus on lung volume events, such aspects of speech performance should be evaluated as number of syllables per breath, volume expended per syllable or other suitable segment, length of utterance, linguistic phrasing, nonutterance volume expenditure, and range of lung volumes used.

Although the analysis of lung volume events may warrant emphasis in future clinical endeavors of the nature undertaken here, it is not the intent to suggest that volume analysis alone be conducted. Many individuals, such as the present subject HV, may warrant evaluation on the remaining two aspects of kinematic function.

MANAGEMENT OF CHEST WALL KINEMATICS IN THE HEARING IMPAIRED. The present findings have significant implications for the management of speech problems in profoundly hearing-impaired speakers. The major problem of the subjects was inappropriate lung volume adjustments in association with inefficient valving of the speech airstream. The latter aspect is beyond the scope of the present discussion but is clearly a problem in managing the timing of speech subsystem activities and the precision of laryngeal and upper-airway activities. Such management would be concerned primarily with the modification of articulatory behavior. The former aspect, lung volume adjustments, is of primary interest here. It seems apparent that a major thrust in the management of speakers who exhibit problems of the type manifested by the present subjects should be to attend to the lung volume range through which speech is produced. In many instances it is clear that higher lung volume initiation levels for expiratory limbs should be encouraged. Several benefits accrue from this simple adjustment. These include increased potentials for the following: (1) longer utterance strings between inspiratory refills, (2) an increased number of syllables per expiratory limb, (3) more natural phrasing, and (4) taking advantage of the higher relaxation forces available at higher lung volumes. In the case of subjects who frequently speak at volumes below FRC, a benefit of going to higher volumes is that of eliminating the need to continue expending muscular energy against the inspiratory recoil of the repiratory apparatus.

It is relatively simple to change limb initiation level through verbal instruction and demonstration. This often is not the only lung volume aspect requiring management, however, and verbal instruction and demonstration are often insufficient for changing other aspects. Also requiring management are nonutterance air wastages and inefficient volume expenditures during utterance. The preferred strategy for managing deviant lung volume events is to provide on-line feedback concerning the nature of the subject's performance. A simple and effective means of accomplishing this is to give the subject visual feedback of an analogue of his lung volume change. This can be done via the relative motions chart or it can be done in more conventional time-volume displays involving one of the devices mentioned above for measuring lung volume and a graphic recording. Through use of time-volume displays, the subject can obtain information as to where he is in lung volume and how rapidly he is changing volume.

Volume events have been stressed here because they were found to be deviant in the sample of subjects studied. Management of both the relative contribution of the rib cage and abdomen and the configuration of the chest wall also is possible with biofeedback procedures. In these instances, the most effective means for providing the subject with the needed information is to permit him to monitor the relative motion chart on the screen of the oscilloscope. Figure 5–9 shows the usefulness of this approach for a subject (HV) in the group who exhibited pronounced deviances in chest wall behavior. As discussed previously, HV's speech typically was characterized by frequent and rapid relative volume contribution changes such that, on the motions chart, he exhibited major motion jogs in contrast to the smooth tracings exhibited by normal speakers. It was concluded that the primary reason for these relative motion jogs had to do with HV's belief that each syllable needed to be made with abrupt inward motion of his abdomen. Verbal instruction and speech-language pathologist demonstration were insufficient sources of information for him to be able to modify this respiratory behavior during speech. His behavior was modified successfully, however, through the use of visual biofeedback of chest wall configuration. HV was shown the relative motions chart and instructed as to its meaning.[3] With the display revealing to him the configuration of his chest wall and changes thereof, HV was permitted several minutes of experimentation in which he moved the "dot" (oscilloscope trace) around on the screen and "saw" how its motion corresponded to the maneuvers of his chest wall. He quickly came to an awareness of the correspondence between configuration and position of the dot and could generate any prescribed configuration or changes thereof on command. Convinced that he could control his chest wall through visual biofeedback guidance, he was instructed to do three activites, the data for which are shown in Figure 5–9. First, he performed the standard task of repeating the syllable /pɑ/ throughout most of his vital capacity on a single expiration. Data for this performance are shown in tracing 1 in Figure 5–9. These data are qualitatively similar to those for his previous performances of this activity. Next, he was instructed to do the same task but to "smooth out the tracing." Tracing 2 in Figure 5–9 shows the resulting data. A third performance of the speech task was then accomplished following the instruction of "try it again." Tracing 3 in Figure 5–9 shows the data for this performance.

---

[3]It is useful in instructing a subject to provide him initially with information about the correspondence of motions of the trace along the Y and X axis of the oscilloscope with motions of the rib cage wall and abdominal wall, respectively. A simple way to do this is to alternately ground the two inputs to the oscilloscope so that the subject need only concentrate on the motion of a single part of the chest wall and a single axis of the display. Following his understanding that vertical motions of the trace correspond to rib cage displacements and horizontal motions to abdominal displacements, the subject should then be given experience with the simultaneous relative motions display to enable him to gain an understanding of the chest wall maneuvers required to reach any point on the display. This part of the procedure is facilitated by having the subject displace volume alternately with the rib cage and then the abdomen, solely, and finally with different relative contributions of the two parts.

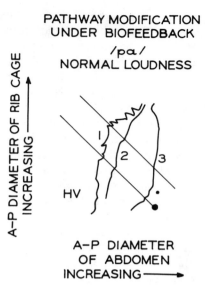

PATHWAY MODIFICATION
UNDER BIOFEEDBACK
/pɑ/
NORMAL LOUDNESS

A–P DIAMETER OF RIB CAGE INCREASING

HV

A–P DIAMETER
OF ABDOMEN
INCREASING

FIGURE 5–9. Relative motion chart showing data obtained for subject HV under conditions of visual feedback of chest wall configuration from a storage oscilloscope display. Tracings are for activities involving syllable repetitions (/pɑ/) in successive trials (denoted in sequence by 1, 2, and 3), the first of which was without feedback and the second and third of which involved feedback. Isovolume lines and tidal breathing extremes are repeated from Figure 5–6.

The data in Figure 5–9 reveal clearly that the subject was able to modify his abnormal chest wall function with remarkable ease. The first attempt at modification (i.e., tracing 2) shows a dramatic reduction in relative motion jogs from HV's typical performance as well as a rightward shifting of the configuration of the chest wall on the relative motions display.[4] The second attempt resulted in an even smoother tracing and one that shifted even further rightward on the display. This tracing is similar to those that would be expected from normal subjects (see Chapter 3). The data in Figure 5–9 are interpreted to indicate that subject HV immediately and appropriately ascribed the abrupt jogs in his first utterance as being caused by the "pulse-like" activities of his chest wall, particularly his abdomen. These activities presumably are decreased in tracings 2 and 3 in terms of their association with individual syllables. It would appear that abdominal wall muscular tone also was rather drastically decreased in this process because the general configuration of the chest wall

---

[4]Although subject HV demonstrated a normal average pitch level in utterances of a continuous discourse nature, he typically performed syllable repetition utterances at an abnormally high pitch. Tracing 1 in Figure 5–9 was accompanied by such an abnormal pitch. Once HV was instructed to remove the motion jogs, his pitch suprisingly dropped to what was judged to be a normal level. Because HV's loudness did not change appreciably, it is assume that this pitch change did not involve a major adjustment in transglottal pressure. Rather, it seems reasonable to speculate that it was accomplished by a laryngeal adjustment. It is possible that this by-product of respiratory behavior change was the result of a generalized decrease in muscular tension throughout the speech apparatus in association with the marked decrease in abdominal tone believed to accompany the tracing's shift rightward on the chart.

shifted rightward on the chart. Whether or not these inferences concerning mechanism are appropriate, the fact remains that under the guidance of visual biofeedback, an ingrained, highly abnormal pattern of chest wall kinematics was subject to modification to normal within less than a minute of utterance. This suggests great potential for the use of such biofeedback procedures in the management of profoundly hearing-impaired speakers who have part of their speech problem based in respiratory dysfunction.

ACKNOWLEDGMENT

The preparation of this manuscript was supported by Research Grant NS-09656 and Research Career Development Award NS-1 K4 41,350 from the National Institute of Neurological and Communicative Disorders and Stroke. The National Technical Institute for the Deaf, especially staff members Joanne Subtelny, Robert Whitehead, and Jean Maki, aided in the work in the course of an agreement with the United States Department of Health, Education, and Welfare.

REFERENCES

Agostoni, E., and Mead, J. (1964). Statics of the respiratory system (pp. 387–409). *In* W. Fenn and H. Rahn (Eds.): *Handbook of physiology. Respiration 1, Sect. 3.* Washington, DC: American Physiological Society.

American National Standards Institute (1969). *Specification for audiometers.* ANSI S3.6-1969. New York: American National Standards Institute.

Bouhuys, A., Proctor, D., and Mead, J. (1966). Kinetic aspects of singing. *Journal of Applied Physiology, 21,* 483–496.

Calvert, D., and Silverman, S. (1975). *Speech and deafness.* Washington, DC: Alexander Graham Bell Association.

Comroe, J., Jr. (1974). *Physiology of respiration.* Chicago: Year Book Medical Publishers.

Connor, L. (1971). *Speech for the deaf child: Knowledge and use.* Washington, DC: Alexander Graham Bell Association.

Draper, M., Ladefoged, P., and Whitteridge, D. (1959). Respiratory muscles in speech. *Journal of Speech and Hearing Research, 2,* 16–27.

Fugl-Meyer, A. (1974). Relative respiratory contribution of the rib cage and the abdomen in males and females with special regard to posture. *Respiration, 31,* 240–251.

Hardy, J. (1961). Intraoral breath pressure in cerebral palsy. *Journal of Speech and Hearing Disorders, 26,* 310–319.

Hudgins, C. (1934). A comparative study of the speech coordinations of deaf and normal subjects. *Journal of Genetic Psychology, 44,* 3–46.

Hudgins, C., and Numbers, F. (1942). An investigation of the intelligibility of the speech of the deaf. *Genetic Psychology Monographs, 25,* 289–392.

Konno, K., and Mead, J. (1967). Measurement of the separate volume changes of rib cage and abdomen during breathing. *Journal of Applied Physiology, 22,* 407–422.

Ling, D. (1976). *Speech and the hearing-impaired child: Theory and practice.* Washington, DC: Alexander Graham Bell Association.

Mead, J., and Agostoni, E. (1964). Dynamics of breathing (pp. 411–427). *In* W. Fenn and H. Rahn (Eds.): *Hand-*

book of physiology. Respiration 1, Sect. 3. Washington, DC: American Physiological Society.

Mead, J., Peterson, N., Grimby, G., and Mead, J. (1967). Pulmonary ventilation measured from body surface movements. Science, 156, 1383–1384.

Moog, J. (1973). Approaches to teaching pre-primary hearing impaired children. Bulletin of the American Organization for Education of the Hearing Impaired, 1, 52–59.

Moore, L., and Mastrotto, L. (1958). Reader's Digest skill builder (pp. 124–125). Pleasantville, NY: Reader's Digest Services.

Pollack, D. (1970). Educational audiology for the limited hearing infant. Springfield, IL: Charles C Thomas.

Rawlings, C. (1935). A comparative study of the movements of the breathing muscles in speech and quiet breathing of deaf and normal subjects, I. American Annals of the Deaf, 80, 147–156.

Rawlings, C. (1936). A comparative study of the movements of the breathing muscles in speech and quiet breathing of deaf and normal subjects, II. American Annals of the Deaf, 81, 136–150.

Simmons-Martin, A. (1974). The oral/aural procedure: Theoretical basis and rationale. Volta Review, 74, 541–551.

Woldring, S. (1968). Breathing patterns during speech in deaf children. Annals of the New York Academy of Science, 155, 206–207.

CHAPTER 6

Speech Breathing Kinematics and Mechanism Inferences

Thomas J. Hixon

M any methods have been used to study speech breathing. None, however, has proved more powerful clinically than kinematic analysis of the chest wall. This chapter discusses this method of analysis and illustrates its use in the study of normal and abnormal function. Discussion is limited to function in adults and to conversational utterances.

THE KINEMATIC METHOD

Figure 6–1 captures the essence of the kinematic method (see Chapter 3). In this method, the chest wall is treated as a two-part system consisting of the rib cage and the abdomen. Each part displaces volume as it moves, whereas together they displace a volume equal to that displaced by the lungs.

Reprinted by permission of the publisher from *Speech motor control*, S. Grillner, B. Lindblom, J. Lubker, and A. Persson (Eds.), pp. 75–93, © 1982, Pergamon Press, Oxford, England.

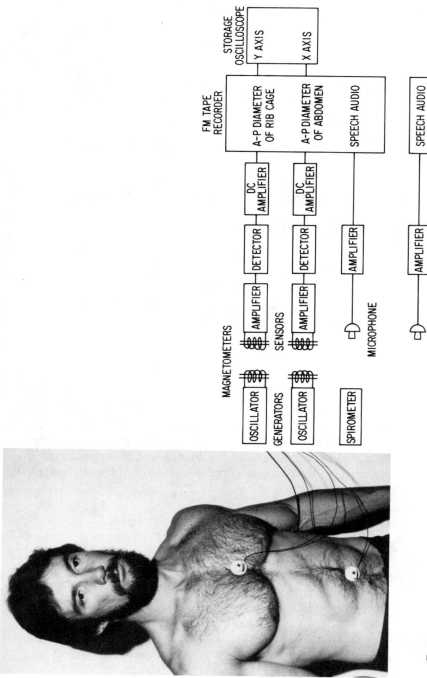

FIGURE 6-1. Coil placements and equipment used.

Changes in the anteroposterior diameters of the rib cage and abdomen are related linearly to their respective volume displacements. Thus, such diameter changes can be used to estimate directly the volumes displaced by the individual parts. This is done most conveniently with magnetometers, electromagnetic coil pairs that provide a voltage analogue of the distance between them. Two such pairs are used, one for the rib cage and one for the abdomen. A generator coil in each pair is fixed to the front of the torso at the midline, that for the rib cage near the nipples and that for the abdomen near the navel. A sensor coil in each pair is fixed to the back of the torso at the midline and at the same axial level as its generator mate. Outputs from the two sensors are processed electronically and are stored on magnetic tape (see Chapter 3).

On tape playback into a storage oscilloscope, a chart in the form shown in Figure 6–2 is generated. In this chart, the anteroposterior diameter of the rib cage is displayed against the anteroposterior diameter of the abdomen, the former increasing upward on the Y axis, and the latter increasing rightward on the X axis. Each point on this chart represents a unique combination of rib cage and abdominal diameters. In addition, each series of points (or pathway) on the chart documents the history of change in the combination of diameters.

Mechanism is inferred from data displayed on a relative diameter chart by considering the forces that could operate to bring about any combination or series of combinations of rib cage and abdominal diameters. The certainty of such inferences is enhanced if a chart is "landmarked" to show the relative

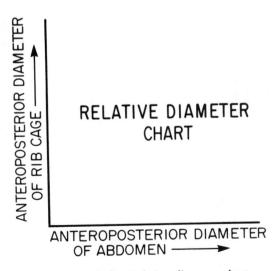

FIGURE 6–2.   Relative diameter chart.

diameter relaxation characteristic of the chest wall. An idealized landmarking is given in Figure 6–3, which shows a line representing an actual characteristic. Circles along this line are at each even 20% of the vital capacity (VC), with the total lung capacity (TLC), functional residual capacity (FRC), and residual volume (RV) designated. The relaxation characteristic can be obtained during tape playback if, during data collection, the subject is required to perform a series of special maneuvers. These involve using the respiratory muscles to adjust lung volume to different levels, whereupon the larynx is closed and the respiratory muscles are relaxed completely. The relative diameter relaxation characteristic is defined by the line formed by interconnecting the data points generated on the chart during the series of relaxations. This line presumably is the same as that which would be obtained were the respiratory muscles flaccidly paralyzed and the lung volume changed passively by a respirator.

Figure 6–4 illustrates the value of relaxation characteristic landmarking. Indicated are the net unbalanced muscular forces that could be operating on the chest wall for data points lying at different locations relative to the characteristic on the chart. RC and AB refer to muscular forces operating on the rib cage and abdomen, respectively. Minus signs and plus signs refer to net inspiratory and net expiratory forces, respectively. Four combinations of forces can prevail for points lying to the left of the characteristic: (1) –RC; (2) +AB; (3) –RC, +AB; and (4) +RC < +AB. Two combinations can prevail for points lying to the right of the characteristic: (1) +RC; and (2) +RC > +AB. Finally, two combinations of forces can prevail for points lying on the relaxation characteristic: (1) relaxation (zero force); and (2) +RC = +AB.

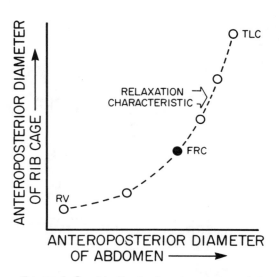

FIGURE 6–3.   Idealized relaxation characteristic.

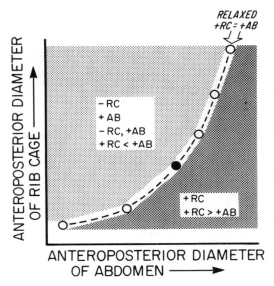

FIGURE 6-4. Muscular force possibilities.

To this juncture, all chart axes have been labeled in anteroposterior diameters. Interpretive convenience is gained if such axes are established in volume displacements. Conversion can be effected during tape playback if, during data collection, the subject is required to perform a special maneuver at FRC. This maneuver is to fix the lung volume by closing the larynx and then slowly displace volume back and forth between the rib cage and the abdomen. The volume exchanged between the two chest wall parts is equal and opposite during such a maneuver. Thus, only the magnitudes of the diameter signals provided by the magnetometers need to be adjusted to be equal and opposite to achieve the desired conversion. Conversion from diameters to displacements is accomplished when, as is shown in Figure 6-5, the pathway followed on the chart during playback of this "isovolume" maneuver forms a line with a slope of −1. Once the axes are converted, it is possible to read the chart directly for the volumes of the rib cage and the abdomen, given by position along the Y and X axes, respectively, and for the relative volume displacements of the two parts, given by the slope of the pathway formed.

Note in Figure 6-5 that, in conjunction with the establishment of the Y and X axes in volume displacements, a third axis has been added to the chart. This axis is for volume displacement of the lungs, which is the sum of the rib cage volume and abdominal volume represented by each point on the chart. On this axis, lung volume is increasing upward and rightward along a 45-degree diagonal. This diagonal can be calibrated graphically if, during data collection,

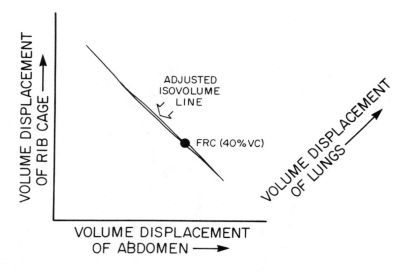

FIGURE 6–5. Adjusted isovolume pathway at FRC.

the subject is required to repeat the isovolume maneuver at different known lung volumes. Figure 6–6 shows the result when this has been done at four lung volume levels, each even 20% VC. Such calibration of the chart makes it possible to read changes in lung volume directly as the distance between any two points perpendicular to adjacent isovolume lines.

Finally, Figures 6–7 is a composite of Figures 6–3 and 6–6, which is the form of backdrop against which the speech data of this chapter are presented.

NORMAL SPEECH BREATHING KINEMATICS

In this section, data are presented from a single subject whose kinematic behavior is representative of normal subjects in general. The upright and supine body positions are considered because of their comparative value in later discussion. The subject studied was a 26-year-old man.

Figures 6–8 and 6–9 present data from upright and supine performances, respectively. The relaxation lines and FRC isovolume lines were generated in the manner described previously. Differences between the two relaxation lines and between the two FRC levels are as would be predicted on mechanical grounds (see Chapter 4). Each tracing represents a single expiratory limb (breath group), and the clusters shown are representative of limbs generated during several minutes of conversation in each body position.

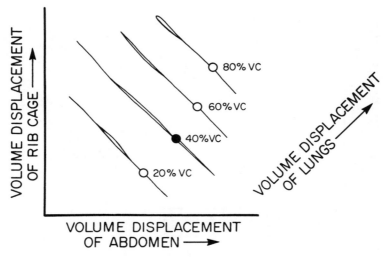

FIGURE 6-6.   Isovolume pathways at each even 20% VC.

Upright Body Position

As is revealed in Figure 6–8, the subject's upright speech was produced through a range of lung volumes that encompassed approximately 60% to 40% VC. This range is typical of normal subjects; most begin utterances from

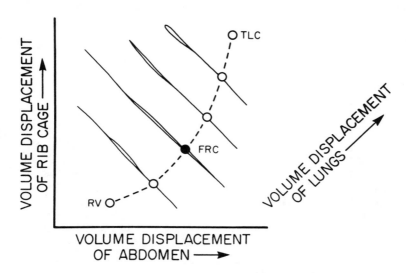

FIGURE 6-7.   Composite of Figures 6–3 and 6–6.

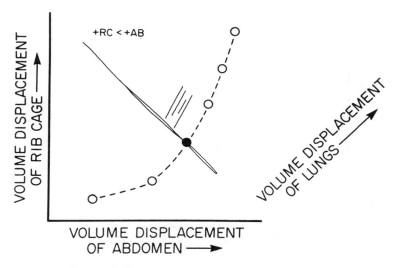

FIGURE 6–8.   Data from an upright normal subject.

about twice resting tidal depth and end utterances above FRC. Limbs in Figure 6–8 show volume excursions of from 10% to 20% VC. Such excursions are characteristic of normal subjects, although variation exists in accordance with linguistic content.

Figure 6–8 shows that the subject's upright speech involved volume displacements of both chest wall parts. As is expressed in the slopes of the tracings, the volume contribution of the subject's rib cage exceeded that of

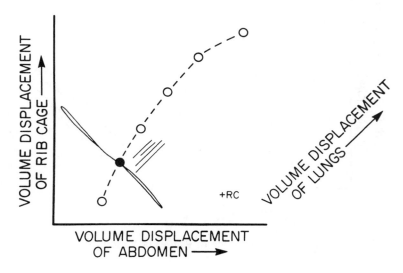

FIGURE 6–9.   Data from a supine normal subject.

his abdomen by a considerable amount. Most normal subjects also displace volumes with both the rib cage and the abdomen during upright speech and show relative volume contributions that favor the rib cage over the abdomen to a substantial degree. A moderate percentage of normal subjects shows a more pronounced rib cage contribution and a lesser abdominal contribution than that shown in Figure 6–8, whereas a small percentage of normal subjects shows roughly equal contributions by the rib cage and the abdomen. All of the tracings in Figure 6–8 are of constant slope. This means that the relative contributions of the rib cage and abdomen were constant throughout each expiratory limb. Most normal subjects also show tracings of constant slope, although a moderate percentage demonstrate gradual changes in slope, either increasing or decreasing, during some expiratory limbs. Most often these changes are associated with breath groups that involve large volume excursions.

As can be seen in Figure 6–8, the data generated lie to the left of the relaxation line on the relative volume chart. This means that, during speech, the subject's abdomen was smaller and his rib cage larger than they were during relaxation at the prevailing lung volume. Normal subjects invariably generate upright conversational data that lie to the left of the relaxation line on their chart. Thus, upright conversational speech must be accounted for through one or more of the four muscular mechanisms listed to the left of the relaxation characteristic in Figure 6–4. Measurement of the actual muscular pressures exerted by each part of the chest wall during upright conversational speech has shown that normal subjects invariably use the last of the mechanisms listed in Figure 6–4 (see Chapter 4). That is, they use expiratory muscle activity by both the rib cage and the abdomen, but with the latter in predominance, +RC < +AB (see Chapter 4).

Supine Body Position

As can be seen in Figure 6–9, the subject's supine speech was generated through a range of lung volumes that encompassed approximately 40% to 20% VC. This range is typical of the conversation of supine normal subjects in general; most begin utterances from about twice resting tidal depth and end them above FRC. Limbs in Figure 6–9 show volume excursions of from 10% to 20% VC. These values are typical of normal subjects, with linguistic content dictating the details.

Figure 6–9 indicates that the subject's supine speech involved volume displacements of both the rib cage and the abdomen. Slopes of the tracings are approximately +1, meaning that the contributions of the two parts were equal. Most other normal subjects also tend toward approximately equal volume contributions from the two chest wall parts under these circumstances. Occasionally, a subject will demonstrate a slight predominance of the rib cage over the abdomen, or vice versa. The limbs depicted in Figure 6–9 are of constant slope. As with upright speech, when changes in slope are observed, they usually are associated with large volume excursions. Slope changes in the supine position invariably result in tracings that are convex toward the Y axis, indicating increases in rib cage contribution and decreases in abdominal contribution as breath groups progress.

All tracings in Figure 6–9 fall to the right of the relaxation line on the chart. This means that the subject's rib cage was smaller and his abdomen larger than they were during relaxation at the prevailing lung volume. Normal subjects invariably present data so positioned on the relative volume chart. Thus, supine conversational speech must be accounted for through one or both of the two muscular mechanisms listed to the right of the relaxation characteristic in Figure 6–4. Measurement of the actual muscular pressures generated by the rib cage and the abdomen during supine speech has revealed that most normal subjects use the first mechanism listed in Figure 6–4 — that of expiratory muscle activity on the part of the rib cage alone, + RC (see Chapter 4).

ABNORMAL SPEECH BREATHING KINEMATICS

Data from four subjects are presented in this section. These subjects demonstrate a variety of speech breathing abnormalities from which insights can be gained with regard to compensatory mechanisms. Included are individuals with congenital deafness, motor neuron disease, Friedreich's ataxia, and acute paralytic poliomyelitis.

Congenital Deafness

A 22-year-old man with a congenital, profound, bilateral sensorineural hearing loss was studied. His unaided better ear average loss for the octave frequencies from 500 to 2000 Hz was 97 dB HL. The subject had worn a hearing aid since childhood and performed expressively in a simultaneous oral-manual mode. His speech was unintelligible and severely disordered; articulation, rhythm, stress, phrasing, rate, and intonation were grossly deviant.

Figure 6–10 presents data from the subject. Recordings were made while he stood erect with his hands at his sides. The relaxation line and FRC isovolume line were generated in the standard manner. The data shown are representative of those generated during the subject's conversational speech. When these data are compared with those from normal subjects, differences are apparent. First, the subject's volume excursions covered 10% VC or less, as compared with normal subjects, whose excursions cover 10% to 20% VC during conversational speech. Second, the subject's speech was produced through a range of lung volumes that encompassed 45% to 25% VC, as compared with normal subjects, who use a lung volume range of approximately 60% to 40% VC for conversation.

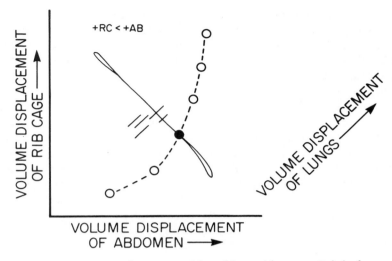

FIGURE 6-10. Data from an upright subject with congenital deafness.

Smaller-than-normal volume excursions can be attributed to the subject's deviant phrasing. Lacking a strategy for producing long stretches of speech, he tended to break his performance into small expiratory chunks of a few syllables each. His producing speech through a range of lung volumes that was about 15% VC lower than normal is explained less certainly, however. The question of importance in this regard is what did the subject gain in exchange for the considerable muscular energy he had to expend to drive his respiratory apparatus through lung volumes that were far lower than those associated with his resting tidal breathing? It seems reasonable to assume that, in the absence of useful auditory sensation, the subject may have been seeking alternative or augmentative sensory information for use in controlling his respiratory apparatus. Perhaps such information is contained in somesthetic sensations attendant to lower lung volumes at which the muscles of the chest wall must work through higher resistive and elastic loads. It may be relevant that the subject produced most of his speech below FRC, whereas subjects with normal hearing produce most of their speech above FRC. Study of the perception of mechanical factors in respiration has shown that the psychophysical relations between various aspects of the respiratory act and the sensory experience of those aspects change in the vicinity of FRC. For example, the exponent of the psychophysical power function involved in the perception of lung volume is known to be different above and below FRC (Salamon, von Euler, and Franzen, 1975).

Subsequent to obtaining the data presented in Figure 6-10, a study was conducted (see Chapter 5) of eight other subjects with profound hearing losses. Several of these subjects were found to produce conversational speech at lower than normal lung volumes, some well below FRC. In a related study done at the National Technical Institute for the Deaf, kinematic observations were made on a group of 15 hearing-impaired subjects, 10 with profound hearing losses and 5 with hearing losses of lesser magnitudes, ranging from moderate to severe (Whitehead, 1980). Those subjects with profound hearing losses frequently produced speech at lower than normal lung volumes. Those subjects with moderate or severe hearing losses produced speech in the normal lung volume range, however. Considering these data, it seems reasonable to conclude that only when the degree of hearing loss is profound might a subject attempt to gain compensatory sensory information from his respiratory apparatus by shifting to low lung volumes. Finally, in attempting to further elucidate the compensatory mechanism that seems to have been identified, it might prove instructive to study lung volume events during the speech of individuals with normal hearing while they are subjected to auditory masking sufficient to disrupt the contribution that the auditory system presumably makes to the control of the respiratory apparatus during speech.

Motor Neuron Disease

The subject studied was a 61-year-old man with a 5-year history of motor neuron disease of the Aran-Duchenne type. That is, he had signs of progressive deterioration of the lower motor neurons of the spinal cord without signs of bulbar or upper motor neuron involvement. He demonstrated mild paresis and atrophy in his limbs and chest wall but was ambulatory and had a vital capacity that was 80% of its predicted value. The subject's speech was judged to be normal.

Figures 6–11 and 6–12 present data obtained from the subject while he was seated erect and lying supine, respectively. The two circles and two lines in each chart designate the relative volumes of the rib cage and the abdomen during standard relaxation maneuvers and isovolume maneuvers, respectively, at FRC and at 1 L above FRC. Straight-line interconnection of the two circles in each chart would describe the subject's relaxation characteristic over the lung volumes delimited. Data tracings in the figures are representative of those obtained. When the subject's upright performance is compared to the upright performances of normal individuals, no significant differences are apparent. When data from the subject's supine performance are compared to analogous data from normal subjects, however, a major difference is apparent. The subject produced speech with repeated, abrupt shifts in the relative volume displacements of the rib cage and abdomen as compared with normal individuals, who produce supine speech with nearly constant relative volume contributions from these two parts. As shown in Figure 6–12, slopes of the subject's expiratory limbs changed erratically and reflected the following: (1) predominance of the rib cage over the abdomen to various degrees, (2) predominance of the abdomen over the rib cage to various degrees, and (3) paradoxing of the rib cage and the abdomen to various degrees, in which one

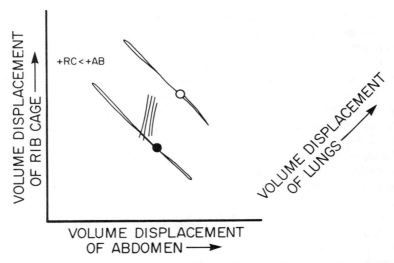

FIGURE 6-11. Data from an upright subject with Aran-Duchenne motor neuron disease.

or the other was displacing volume in the inspiratory direction. The shifts noted suggest a significant departure from the normal mode of controlling supine conversational speech with expiratory rib cage activity alone (+RC). The data are consistent with a changing combination of expiratory forces from both the rib cage and the abdomen, but with the rib cage in predominance (+RC > +AB).

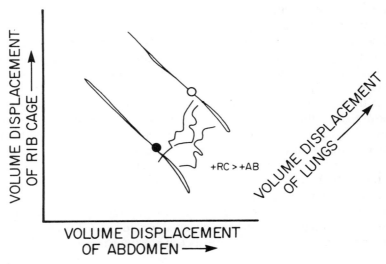

FIGURE 6-12. Data from a supine subject with Aran-Duchenne motor neuron disease.

Why did the subject perform in a normal manner while upright but in an abnormal manner while supine? One possibility relates to his report of orthopnea, the subjective sensation of breathing difficulty while in the supine position. Orthopnea is a frequent symptom in persons with significant neuromuscular involvement of the respiratory apparatus in which the ability of the muscles to perform work is decreased. Examination of the subject's supine tidal breathing tracings revealed a major counterclockwise looping. This suggests a continuous active muscular control of the tidal breathing cycle with the expiratory phase involving significant expiratory activity by the muscles of the rib cage and the abdomen. It seems reasonable to assume that the subject, in response to his subjective sensation of breathing difficulty, engaged his expiratory muscles to achieve a feeling of control over his perceived respiratory embarrassment. Such a mechanism might then be carried over to respiratory cycles involving speech. Given that speech involves prolonged periods of low flows through high resistive loads, it might then cause a heightening of the subject's orthopnea. Faced with an anxious respiratory situation to begin with, the addition of speech to the respiratory load may have been reason enough for the subject to engage in an erratic two-part interplay between the rib cage and the abdomen.

A second possible explanation for the subject's abnormal chest wall behavior while supine relates to the relative novelty of performing speech in that position. Because of the nature of the subject's disease, he was faced with the problem of controlling a respiratory apparatus whose peripheral mechanical properties (e.g., compliance and resistance) were changing in conjunction with changes in its neuromuscular capabilities (e.g., spinal motor neuron deterioration and simultaneous large motor unit reorganization characteristic of the denervation–collateral sprouting–reinnervation process). This means that he had to perform an ongoing reassessment of his status and functionally reprogram his performances to offset these changes. Considering that he routinely practiced speech breathing tasks in the upright position, but not in the supine position, what may have been observed in his erratic supine behavior was poor fine motor control related to the unrehearsed nature of the task.

A third possible explanation for the subject's behavior may be the most controversial of the three offered. Although classical accounts of motor neuron disease emphasize problems of efference, there are potential problems of afference that could be associated with muscle wasting. A remarkable resemblance is noted between the kinematic signs represented in Figure 6–12 and those observed occasionally in individuals with peripheral sensory deficits (Putnam, Hixon, and Stern, 1981). Were important somesthetic or proprioceptive information, or both, lost to the subject, as a result of loss in muscle mass, might he have been engaged in a form of rib cage–abdominal "groping" in his attempts to achieve speech breathing target behaviors? If such were the case, could such "groping" have been a consequence of inadequate afferent information to motor control at unconscious levels, or could it have been done purposefully to gain conscious sensation relative to speech breathing performance?

Whatever the reason for the subject's erratic kinematic behavior during supine conversational speech, it seems clear that his behavior is not idiosyncratic. A related study (Putnam, 1981) has documented similar abnormal chest wall function in the supine body position in a series of other persons with motor neuron disease of various types (see Chapter 8). There is every reason to believe that the body-position effect described is real.

Friedreich's Ataxia

A 17-year-old girl with a 7-year history of Friedreich's ataxia was studied. She had signs of extensive, progressive neuromuscular deterioration that rendered her nonambulatory, with paresis and atrophy in her limbs, chest wall, neck, and head. Her rib cage and diaphragm were moderately to severely paretic and her abdomen was paralyzed. The subject's vital capacity was 30% of its predicted value. Her speech was severely abnormal and only moderately intelligible; problems were apparent with articulation, nasalization, vocal pitch, utterance loudness, rhythm, stress, phrasing, rate, and intonation.

Figure 6–13 presents data from the subject. Recordings were made while she was seated upright. The three circles in the figure designate the relative volumes assumed by the rib cage and the abdomen during relaxation at FRC, 0.5 L above FRC, and 0.8 L above FRC. Straight-line interconnection of these circles would describe the subject's relaxation characteristic over the range of lung volumes considered. The subject was unable to perform standard isovolume maneuvers. Therefore, isovolume data were generated manually by an investigator. This was done by displacing volume into and out of the subject's rib cage and abdomen by alternately and slowly pushing and releasing the rib cage wall and the abdominal wall as she held her breath with a closed larynx at FRC and at 0.5 L above FRC. Two sets of expiratory limbs are shown in Figure 6–13. Those clustered on the right in the chart are representative of data obtained during conversational speech. Those clustered on the left are from an episode of prolonged, spontaneous, seemingly uncontrollable laughter evoked by a comment of an investigator.

When tracings from the subject's conversational speech are compared with those from normal subjects, a striking difference can be seen in where data lie on the chart relative to the relaxation characteristic. Those for the subject lie to the right of the presumed relaxation characteristic on the chart, meaning that her rib cage was smaller and her abdomen was larger than they were during relaxation at the prevailing lung volume. Such data are in sharp contrast to those from upright normal subjects, which invariably lie to the

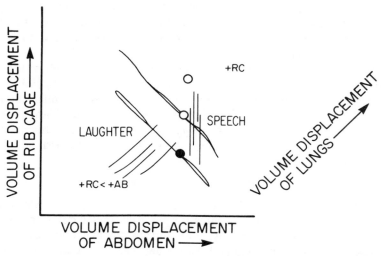

FIGURE 6-13. Data from an upright subject with Friedreich's ataxia.

left of the relaxation characteristic, meaning that the rib cage is larger and the abdomen is smaller than they were during relaxation at the prevailing lung volume. The expiratory limbs in Figure 6–13 suggest a significant departure from the normal mode of controlling upright conversational speech with expiratory activity by both the rib cage and the abdomen, the latter predominating (+RC < +AB). All kinematic signs indicate that the subject's performance involved expiratory activity by the rib cage alone (+RC). Such a conclusion also is consistent with the subject's paralyzed abdomen. It seems reasonable to assume that the general mechanism was one in which the expiratory force generated by the rib cage was spent in part in displacing the paralyzed abdominal wall outward until it offered a relatively firm base against which the rib cage could develop volume compressions.

When expiratory limbs from the subject's spontaneous laughter are compared with those from her conversational speech, the differences are astonishing. First, the range of lung volumes used by the subject during laughter extended from near FRC to near RV, showing no overlap with the range of volumes used during conversational speech. Second, the relative volume contributions of the rib cage and the abdomen during laughter were approximately equal, as compared with the total lung volume change that was contributed by the rib cage during conversational speech. Third, the data for laughter lie to the left of the presumed relaxation characteristic on the chart, meaning that the rib cage was larger and the abdomen smaller than they were during relaxation at the prevailing lung volume, as compared with the data for speech, which are positioned to the right of the relaxation characteristic, indicating that the rib cage was smaller and the abdomen larger than they were during relaxation at the prevailing lung volume. Fourth, and finally, the history of change in the combination of rib cage and abdominal volumes associated with the subject's laughter allows for no other reasonable interpretation of mechanism than that of an expiratory effort by both the rib cage and the abdomen, with the latter predominating (+RC < +AB), as compared with the subject's conversational speech for which expiratory activity by the rib cage alone (+RC) is presumed.

How can the fact be reconciled that for commanded breathing activities and conversational speech the subject had a moderately to severely paretic rib cage and a paralyzed abdomen that enabled her to expire with only moderate force above FRC, whereas for spontaneous laughter she demonstrated extremely forceful expiratory drives from both the rib cage and the abdomen, the latter predominating, that enabled her to expire with great speed to near RV and with extensive motions of the two chest wall parts? What seems a plausible explanation relates to the different natures of the two activities performed. Speech is a highly skilled voluntary act in which a subject must override mechanisms that rhythmically drive the respiratory apparatus. By contrast, laughter, when not contrived but of the all-out, seemingly uncontrollable variety, is an involuntary act that is stimulus dependent and whose program, once triggered, seems to be highly automatic and invariant in form. The vigor of the response from the subject during laughter suggests that the functional capabilities of the spinal lower motor neuron system were relatively intact even though they were not accessed during commanded activities and speech breathing. It is interesting to note that during laughter the predominant muscular activity involved the usually paralyzed abdomen and not the paretic rib cage. Perhaps this relates to a natural predominance of the abdomen over the rib cage for this activity in general. There are several statements commonly heard with regard to a person's outbursts of seemingly uncontrollable laughter that implicate sensations of abdominal predominance. Consider what may be meant in the following four sentences: "I busted a gut laughing," "He just kept us in stitches laughing," "I laughed so hard my sides hurt," "She was doubled over with laughter." It may be possible to explain only feeble muscular action of the respiratory apparatus for speech but vigorous muscular action of the apparatus for uncontrollable laughter by the contribution of the limbic nervous system to motor behaviors with associated emotional components. That is, under commanded breathing activities and speech breathing for the subject, effective voluntary control of the chest wall may have been curtailed severely by the degenerative disease process involved in Friedreich's ataxia. Under conditions calling for an emotional response, however, a contribution from the limbic nervous system may have been invoked that facilitated motor commands to the muscles of the chest wall. Finally, phenomena of this nature may be part of a class of emotionally laden conditions that enhance access to spinal lower motor neurons in other categories of neuromuscular disease. Studies of children with cerebral palsy have shown that although they may be unable to perform major inspiratory or expiratory efforts voluntarily because of chest wall paresis, they may, during the emotional act of crying, engage in deep inspirations followed by expirations that go well below FRC (Hixon, 1976). Once again, the limbic nervous system would appear to allow such actions.

Acute Paralytic Poliomyelitis

The subject was a 48-year-old man who was being studied 18 years after the onset of acute paralytic poliomyelitis. The muscles of his rib cage, diaphragm, and abdomen were flaccidly paralyzed and markedly atrophied. Although dependent on respirators, the subject could free-breathe for short periods by inspiratory efforts of his sternocleidomastoid, scalene, and trapezius muscles and by glossopharyngeal (frog) inspiration. Untrained persons considered the subject's free-breathing conversation to be normal. To the sophisticated listener he showed deviances consistent with the frugal use of his air supply: a strained-strangled voice quality; frequent inspiratory refills; occasional substitutions of glottal stops for fricatives; shortened duration fricatives; and intrusions of glottal stops.

Figure 6–14 presents data from the subject. Recordings were made while he was lying supine. The relaxation line was generated over a 1.25 L range above FRC by applying slow, cyclical pressure variations to the airway opening with a positive-pressure respirator. Isovolume lines were generated manually by an investigator who displaced volume into and out of the subject's rib cage and abdomen by alternately and slowly pushing and releasing the abdominal wall as the subject held his breath with a closed larynx at FRC and at 0.5 L above FRC. Expiratory limbs were nearly invariant and are represented on the chart by an arrow, which is superimposed on the relaxation line and follows it downward over a lung volume range encompassing 0.5 to 0.25 L above FRC. When the subject's data are compared with those from normal subjects, several differences are apparent. First, the subject initiated expiratory limbs at the tidal end-inspiratory level associated with his free-breathing, as compared with normal subjects, who initiate expiratory limbs from about twice resting tidal depth. Second, the subject terminated utterances well above FRC, as compared with normal subjects, who typically end breath groups in the vicinity of FRC. Third, volume excursions associated with the subject's speech were small, covering only about 5% of his predicted vital capacity, as compared with excursions in normal subjects, which cover from 10% to 20% VC. Fourth, and finally, the subject produced speech at rib cage and abdominal volumes identical to those assumed by these two chest wall parts when he was driven through the prevailing lung volume by the respirator, as compared with normal

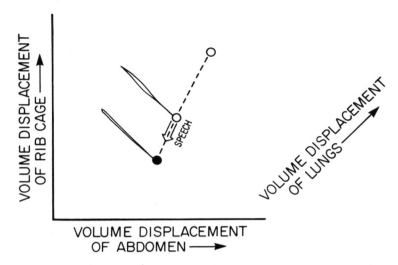

FIGURE 6-14.   Data from a supine subject with acute paralytic poliomyelitis.

subjects, who, when supine, produce speech at a smaller rib cage volume and a larger abdominal volume than those assumed during relaxation at the prevailing lung volume.

It is relevant to consider the manner in which the subject attained the 0.5 L above FRC starting volume for each expiratory limb. Kinematic and surface electromyographic data revealed this to be accomplished through the subject's use of his neck muscles (sternocleidomastoid, scalene, and trapezius) to pull his rib cage axially headward and expand it circumferentially. Once the lung volume had been increased by 0.5 L, the subject closed his larynx, abruptly relaxed his neck muscles, held his breath momentarily against the closed larynx, and then proceeded to produce speech. The importance of the subject's neck effort during each speech breathing cycle was that it served to store potential energy in the respiratory apparatus in the form of expiratory recoil pressure. In more colloquial terms, the subject's neck action "cocked" his respiratory spring in an inspiratory position, where it was held by the larynx until used for speech. During the course of utterance, the return of this spring to its resting length, the FRC level, was governed by intricate metering activities of the larynx and upper airway. The situation was not unlike that involved in limiting the volume decrease of an inflated toy balloon by controlling the flow from its neck.

The limited strength of the subject's neck muscles accounts for his lower-than-normal starting volumes in expiratory limbs. The subject's higher-than-normal termination volumes in expiratory limbs are accounted for by his reaching a level in the lung volume at which the recoil force of the respiratory apparatus was no longer sufficient to drive the larynx and upper airway. That his chest wall followed the relaxation characteristic on the chart is as would be expected because the subject had no muscle capability to depart from the characteristic, save that of his neck muscles, which would be counter-productive to the development of driving pressure. Thus, the subject was, despite his profound neuromuscular impairment, able to produce near-normal speech without respiratory muscle control during the expiratory side of the respiratory cycle. As if all this were not remarkable enough, the subject still had other compensatory mechanisms to help in his speech performance. He was able to recock his respiratory spring in small increments through quick glossopharyngeal inspirations that went unnoticed by casual observers. This mechanism was used at the beginning of expiratory phrases, between words, and even between syllables in multisyllabic words. Once the desired starting lung volume was attained, the subject could, in fact, count continuously for a long period of time by taking repeated glossopharyngeal breaths between numbers. In this way, he could set the general background loudness of his speech by determining the recoil that would be available at the end of a neck inspiration, and then keep the respiratory apparatus at that pressure level by recocking the respiratory spring with a step increase in lung volume that matched the decrease associated with the previous syllable in a string.

There were other compensatory maneuvers performed by the subject that are outside the limited scope of this presentation. The reader interested in more detail should consult Chapter 9, which is devoted exclusively to this one subject.

SUMMARY AND CONCLUSION

This chapter has been an attempt to display the power of kinematic analysis of the chest wall in the study of speech breathing. It should be obvious that this form of analysis has much to offer to investigators and clinicians. Data collected from normal subjects reveal well-defined kinematic patterns for conversational speech breathing that are relatively homogeneous for a given body position. These data provide a useful baseline against which to compare the chest wall data of persons with suspected speech breathing abnormalities. A great deal remains to be done with regard to the kinematic study of abnormal speech breathing. The territory is almost totally unexplored. The four areas considered in this chapter—congenital deafness, motor neuron disease, Friedreich's ataxia, and acute paralytic poliomyelitis—should be viewed as preliminary maps of what lies ahead for the inquisitive investigator and clinician. Definitive answers are not available for some of the questions raised in this chapter. Perhaps those readers who are neurophysiologists have been thinking about how the tools of neurophysiology might be used to gain answers to some of the questions that have been raised in this chapter. Any suggestions the neurophysiologist might have for using kinematic analysis to gain further insights into the control problems of persons with speech breathing abnormalities would be welcomed. For those who are speech scientists and speech-language pathologists, it seems pertinent to mention that kinematic analysis of the chest wall has greatly influenced the approaches now used for the evaluation and management of persons with speech breathing abnormalities. What was recently only a research tool is now an indispensable part of the daily clinical armamentarium.

ACKNOWLEDGMENT

The preparation of this manuscript was supported by Reasearch Grant NS-09656 from the National Institute of Neurological and Communicative Disorders and Stroke. Dr. Anne H. B. Putnam warrants acknowledgment for her conceptual contribution to the section on motor neuron disease.

REFERENCES

Hixon, T. (1976). *The mechanical bases of so-called "reversed breathing" in cerebral palsy.* Progress Report of Research Grant NS-09656 from the National Institute of Neurological and Communicative Disorders and Stroke.

Putnam, A. (1981). *Biomechanics of normal and disordered speech production.* Progress Report of Teacher-Investigator Award NS-00303 from the National Institute of Neurological and Communicative Disorders and Stroke.

Putnam, A., Hixon, T., and Stern, L. (1981). *Speech breathing function in motor neuron disease.* Paper presented at the Eighteenth Annual Meeting of the Federation of Western Societies of Neurological Science, San Francisco.

Salamon, M., von Euler, C., and Franzen, O. (1975). *Perception of mechanical factors in breathing.* Paper presented at the Wenner-Gren International Symposium on Physical Work and Effort, Stockholm, Sweden.

Whitehead, R. (1980). *Some respiratory and aerodynamic characteristics of the speech of the deaf. Clinical implications.* Paper presented at the International Congress of the Deaf, Hamburg, West Germany.

CHAPTER 7

Voice Abnormalities in Relation to Respiratory Kinematics

Thomas J. Hixon
Anne H. B. Putnam

A t one level, voice production is a respiratory phenomenon. Hence, much can be learned about abnormal voice by studying respiratory function. This is true not only with regard to understanding the mechanisms of abnormal voice, but also with regard to evaluating and managing individuals with abnormal voices. This chapter discusses voice abnormalities from a respiratory perspective and illustrates how respiratory data can be used in clinical practice.

Respiratory events can be studied at several levels, each level providing a different type of information. The concern of this chapter is with kinematic observations—those dealing with respiratory events in terms of motions. These observations are chosen for emphasis because of their simplicity and power, and because modern equipment systems for making such observations are

Reprinted by permission of the publisher from *Seminars in Speech and Language*, Volume 5, Number 4, pp. 217-231, © 1983, Thieme-Stratton, New York, NY.

becoming available increasingly in clinical settings. The chapter begins with a discussion of the kinematic method. Next, consideration is given to kinematic data typical of those for conversational utterances of individuals with normal voices. Finally, discussion is directed toward voice abnormalities in relation to respiratory kinematics, illustrated by data from three clients with diverse signs and symptoms.

KINEMATIC METHOD

Figure 7–1 illustrates the kinematic method used. The evolution of this method can be traced through the following sources: Konno and Mead (1967); Mead, Peterson, Grimby, and Mead (1967); and in this volume, Chapters 3, 4, and 6. This method treats the chest wall as a two-part system consisting of the rib cage and abdomen. Each part displaces volume as it moves, and together they displace a volume equal to that displaced by the lungs. Changes in the anteroposterior diameters of the rib cage and abdomen are related linearly to their respective volume displacements. Therefore, diameter changes can be used to estimate directly the volumes displaced by the individual parts. The most convenient way to measure the diameter changes of interest is with magnetometers, electromagnetic coil pairs that provide a voltage analogue of the distance between them. Two such pairs are used routinely, one for the rib cage and one for the abdomen. A generator coil in each pair is attached to the front of the torso at the midline, that for the rib cage near the nipples and that for the abdomen near the navel. A sensor coil in each pair is attached to the back of the torso at the midline at the same axial level as its generator mate. Output signals from the two sensors are processed electronically and stored on FM tape.

On tape playback into a storage oscilloscope, a chart like that shown in Figure 7–2 is produced. In this chart, the anteroposterior diameter of the rib cage, increasing upward on the Y axis, is displayed against the anteroposterior diameter of the abdomen, increasing rightward on the X axis. Each point on the chart represents a unique combination of rib cage and abdominal diameters, and each series of points, or pathway, specifies the history of change in the combination of diameters.

Muscular mechanism can be inferred from the relative diameter chart by considering the forces that could operate to cause any combination or series of combinations of rib cage and abdominal diameters. Inferences are facilitated if the chart is "landmarked" with the relative diameter relaxation characteristic of the chest wall. Figure 7–3 shows a landmarked chart. Circles along the relaxation characteristic are at 20% levels of the vital capacity (VC), with the total lung capacity (TLC), functional residual capacity (FRC), and residual volume (RV) indicated. The relaxation characteristic can be obtained by having

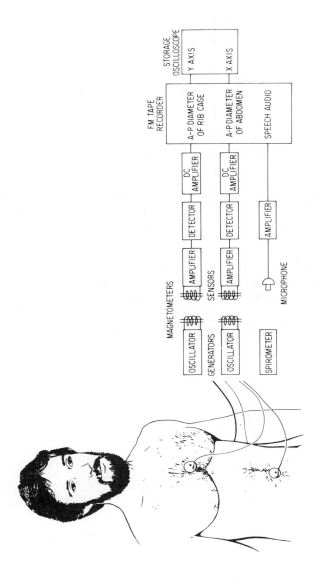

Figure 7-1. Coil placements and equipment.

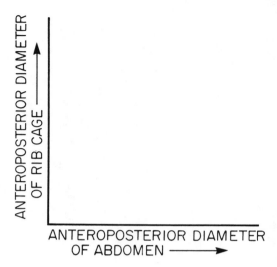

FIGURE 7–2. Relative diameter chart.

the subject perform a series of prescribed maneuvers. These involve using the respiratory muscles to adjust lung volume to different levels, at each of which the larynx is closed and the respiratory apparatus is relaxed. The relative diameter relaxation characteristic is determined by interconnecting the data points generated on the chart during moments of relaxation of the respiratory apparatus.

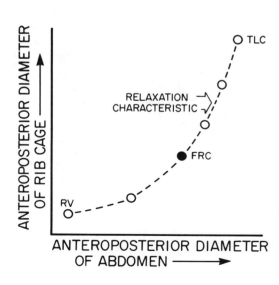

FIGURE 7–3. Relaxation characteristic.

Figure 7-4 designates the net muscular forces that could be operating on the chest wall for data points lying at different locations with respect to the relaxation characteristic on the chart. RC and AB designate muscular forces operating on the rib cage and abdomen, respectively. Minus and plus signs designate net inspiratory and net expiratory forces, respectively. Four force possibilities can prevail for points lying to the left of the characteristic: (1) −RC;   (2) +AB;   (3) −RC, +AB;   and   (4) +RC< +AB. Two force possibilities can exist for points lying to the right of the characteristic: (1) +RC;   and   (2) +RC> +AB. For points lying on the relaxation characteristic, two force possibilities can prevail: (1) relaxation (zero force);   and   (2) +RC = +AB.

Interpretive convenience is gained if chart axes, such as those in Figures 7-1 through 7-4, are converted from diameters to displacements. This can be done following the subject's performance of a prescribed maneuver at FRC. This involves fixing the lung volume by closing the larynx and then slowly displacing volume back and forth between the rib cage and abdomen. The volume exchanged between the two chest wall parts is equal and opposite during such a maneuver. Therefore only the magnitudes of the diameter signals from the magnetometers need to be adjusted to be equal and opposite to effect the axes conversions. When, as is shown in Figure 7-5, the pathway followed on the chart during the prescribed isovolume maneuver forms a line with a slope of −1, conversions are accomplished. It is then possible to read the chart directly for the volumes of the rib cage and abdomen, given by position along

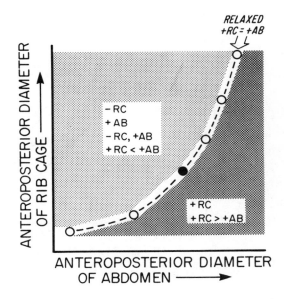

FIGURE 7-4. Muscular force possibilities.

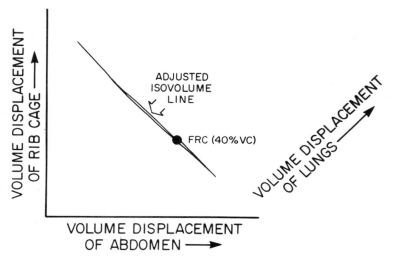

FIGURE 7–5.   Relative volume chart and FRC isovolume line.

their respective axes, and for the relative volume displacements of the two parts, given by the slope of the pathway formed. Notice in Figure 7–5 that, in conjunction with the conversion of the chart axes to volume displacements, a third axis has been added. This axis displays the volume displacement of the lungs, which is the sum of the rib cage volume and abdominal volume

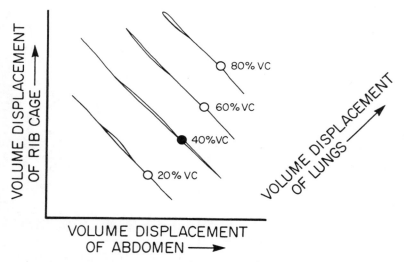

FIGURE 7–6.   Isovolume lines at each even 20% VC.

represented by each point on the chart. On this axis, which runs at a 45-degree diagonal, lung volume increases upward and rightward. This axis can be calibrated by having the subject repeat the isovolume maneuver at different known lung volumes. Figure 7–6 shows the result when this is done at each even 20% VC. Calibration of the chart in such a manner makes it possible to read changes in lung volume directly in terms of the distance between any two points perpendicular to the isovolume lines.

Figure 7–7 is a composite of Figures 7–3 and 7–6. This figure forms the general backdrop against which the voice production data of this chapter are presented.

NORMAL VOICE AND RESPIRATORY KINEMATICS

In this section, data are presented from a 26-year-old male subject whose kinematic behavior during voice production is representative of normal individuals in general. Data from the upright body position are considered because of their comparative value in subsequent discussion of persons with voice abnormalities.

Figure 7–8 presents data from the subject on a relative volume chart. The relaxation characteristic and FRC isovolume line were generated in the standard manner. Each tracing is for a single expiratory limb (breath group), and the cluster of tracings is representative of limbs produced during continuous conversational speech. As is revealed in Figure 7–8, the subject's speech was

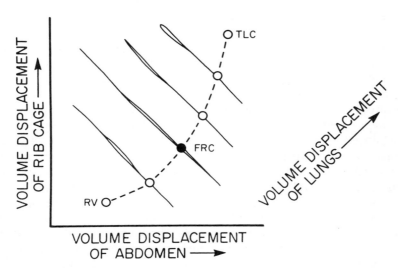

FIGURE 7-7. Composite of Figures 7–3 and 7–6.

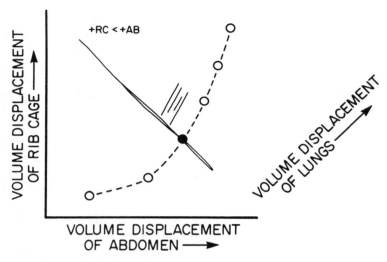

FIGURE 7-8. Data from a representative normal subject.

produced through a range of lung volumes that encompassed approximately 60% to 40% VC. This range is characteristic of normal individuals in that most of them begin utterances from about twice resting tidal breathing depth and end utterances slightly above FRC. As also is revealed in Figure 7–8, the subject's speech was produced with lung volume excursions that covered from 10% to 20% VC. Excursions of this magnitude are typical of normal individuals, although variation occurs, depending on the linguistic content of the speech.

Figure 7–8 shows that the subject's speech involved volume displacements of both parts of his chest wall. More specifically, the slopes of the tracings indicate that the volume contribution of the subject's rib cage exceeded that of his abdomen to a considerable degree. Most normal individuals displace volumes with both the rib cage and abdomen during speech and demonstrate a relative volume partitioning that substantially favors the rib cage over the abdomen. A moderate percentage of normal individuals show a more pronounced rib cage volume displacement and a lesser abdominal volume displacement than that indicated in Figure 7–8, and a small percentage of normal individuals demonstrate approximately equal displacements by the two parts of the chest wall. All of the tracings in Figure 7–8 are of constant slope, which means that the relative contributions of the rib cage and abdomen were constant throughout each breath group. Tracings of constant slope also are characteristic of most normal individuals, although a moderate percentage show gradual changes in slope, either increasing or decreasing, during certain breath groups. Such slope changes most often are associated with breath groups that involve large lung volume excursions.

All of the limbs in Figure 7–8 lie to the left of the relaxation characteristic on the chart, indicating that, during speech production, the subject's abdomen was smaller and his rib cage larger than they were during relaxation at the prevailing lung volume. Normal individuals invariably generate data that lie to the left of the relaxation characteristic on their charts. Deformation of the chest wall in such a fashion must be accounted for through one or more of the four muscular mechanisms listed to the left of the relaxation characteristic in Figure 7–4. Study of the actual muscular pressures exerted by each part of the chest wall during continuous conversational speech in the upright body position has revealed that normal individuals invariably use the last of the mechanisms listed in Figure 7–4 (see Chapter 4). That is, they use expiratory muscle activity by both the rib cage and abdomen, with the latter being of greater magnitude than the former (+RC< +AB).

ABNORMAL VOICE AND RESPIRATORY KINEMATICS

Data from three clients are presented in this section. These clients are selected to demonstrate a variety of voice abnormalities related to a variety of causes. Included are individuals with abnormalities related to functional misuse of the respiratory apparatus, spinal cord injury, and spasmodic dysphonia.

Functional Misuse of the Respiratory Apparatus

The client studied was a 30-year-old woman. She was physically normal and had a normal voice. She was employed as a television weather reporter and was sent to the clinic by her station manager with the complaint that her inspirations during speech were loud and distracting. She reported that the problem was especially prominent during her weather telecasts, that she had become self-conscious about her speech breathing on camera, and that she had been unable to make adjustments in it to her satisfaction. The client's job was relatively fast-paced, particularly during the hour or two preceding each of two daily evening telecasts. She indicated that she felt stressed during these periods and that she smoked many cigarettes at such times in an attempt to relieve tension.

Figure 7–9 presents data from recordings made while the client stood erect with her hands at her sides. The FRC isovolume line was generated in the standard manner. Relaxed TLC and RV configurations are indicated on the chart by open circles. The tracings shown are representative of those generated during continuous conversational speech, the reading of a standard declarative paragraph, and the delivery of a contrived weather telecast. For each of these activities, the client's voice was judged to be normal; however,

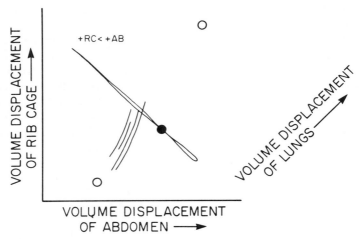

FIGURE 7-9.   Data from a client with functional misuse of the respiratory apparatus.

her inspirations between breath groups were judged to be abnormally loud, both in their own right and in relation to the loudness of her speech.

When the client's tracings are compared with those from normal subjects, two differences are apparent. First, the client's speech was produced through a range of lung volumes that encompassed 45% to 10% VC compared with normal subjects, who use a lung volume range of approximately 60% to 40% VC for similar speech activities. Second, the client's lung volume excursions covered 20% VC or more compared with normal subjects whose excursions cover 10% to 20% VC during speech activities of a similar nature. A third important difference from normal for the client's behavior is not revealed in Figure 7-9. That difference pertains to the durations of her inspirations between breath groups. These averaged approximately 0.4 sec, compared with those for normal subjects, which average about 0.6 sec for similar activities (Horii and Cooke, 1978).

Given the normal physical status of the client, her performance strategy for speech breathing must be considered a matter of choice rather than a matter of compensatory requirement. This makes her behavior puzzling from both mechanical and linguistic perspectives. From an energetics viewpoint, the client's production of speech through a low lung volume range was far more costly of expiratory muscle force than it would have been had she produced speech through the midvolume range used by normal subjects. The reasons for higher cost are twofold: First, higher viscous opposition is encountered in the lower airway as lung volume decreases, and second, higher elastic opposition is encountered in the chest wall as lung volume decreases below FRC. Why did the client use such an uneconomical strategy to produce speech when she could have adopted a more economical strategy? What did she gain in exchange for the considerable muscular energy she chose to expend to drive her respiratory apparatus through lung volumes that were far lower than those associated with her resting tidal breathing? A clue to this low lung volume puzzle may be contained in the client's own statements about her speech. Her reported perception of her voice was that it sounded "more authoritative and business-like" when she spoke in her "usual way" rather than in other ways. On questioning the meaning of her report, it was concluded that she meant her voice was more harsh and less breathy when she spoke in her "usual way." "Usual way," in the present context, means, of course, when she spoke at lower lung volumes rather than at higher lung volumes at which normal speakers usually function. The reader may appreciate this consideration from personal observations of how one's own or another's voice quality changes as the residual volume is approached. Specifically, the voice takes on a slight strained-strangled quality that signals the impending depletion of the available air supply. The client repeatedly contrasted her usual way of speaking with what she described as a "whiney, squeaky tone" to her voice when she produced speech in other manners. Although she demonstrated no conscious awareness of producing speech at low lung volumes, it may be that her method of facilitating the production of a more authoritative and business-like voice, and the avoidance of what she considered to be a whiney, squeaky tone was the perception that led her to adopt a deviant strategy for performance placement within the lung volume range. When an attempt was made to modify the range of lung volumes through which the client produced speech, a change occurred in her voice quality. Specifically, it decreased in harshness and increased in breathiness and took on a "lighter" character. The client expressed a sense of needing less effort to produce voice in a higher lung volume range, although she felt she had "less tight control" over her performance.

The client's larger-than-normal lung volume excursions during speech production can be attributed to her use of a deviant phrasing strategy for performance. Her speech production consistently involved long stretches of utterance without pauses for respiratory refills. Typically she would extend a breath group to cover several phrases or short sentences and rarely did she break her performances into small expiratory chunks of the size used by normal individuals. The client had no awareness that her phrasing strategy was other than normal, and expressed surprise at such a revelation when her abnormal lung volume excursions were brought to her attention in the data chart. Why would the client pass through standard linguistic breaking points for respiratory refills and continue downstream in the flow of her speech? Two explanations seem plausible. First, it is possible that the nature of the client's telecast performances conditioned her to behave in a manner that minimized interruptions in her speech. This possibility seems increased by the fact that she did not work from cue cards or prompts during her telecasts, but rather relied on frequent rehearsals of her telecast performances. With regard to the conditioning of her performances, it should be noted further that her telecasts were characterized by the serial presentation of logical strings of information. This is illustrated by the following example: "It's currently seventy-six degrees in the valley. Skies are partly cloudy and winds are out of the south at six miles an hour. The humidity is thirty-two percent. —(Inspiration)— The expected low for tonight is fifty-one degrees locally, thirty-eight degrees in the White Mountains, Mogollon Rim country, and the skies across the state should be clearing." A desire to deliver her weather information in logical "chunks" may have been a major factor in the client's continuing to speak beyond phrase and sentence boundaries at which other speakers would take an inspiration routinely. In effect, the client may have been functioning as if inspiratory breaks were in competition with her communication goals "on the air."

The second possibility to account for the client's performance in terms of volume excursions is related to her awareness of the consequences of her loud and distracting inspirations. It is possible that she had developed a strategy of avoiding inspirations as much as possible. This would, of course, be the obvious way to do away with the unwanted and distracting noise that detracted from her performance. The specific relationships within such an avoidance paradigm are uncertain. It is possible that the client could have been using the noise from the inspirations as a discriminative stimulus in relation to the concerns of her station manager, or it is possible that her own concern for the noise, per se, was the key factor in avoidance behavior.

Given the client's penchant for producing speech at low lung volumes and for using volume excursions that carried her well into the expiratory reserve volume, she tended to place herself in mechanical situations that were predisposing to the generation of inspirations that were loud in their own right and were perceived in bold relief against the acoustics of her speech performance. It seems likely that her more-rapid-than-normal inspiratory movements and their performance at low lung volumes, at which the resistance of the lower airway is high, would combine to facilitate a relatively intense turbulent noise production on inspiration. The factor of speed alone probably can be accounted for, in part, by the greater inspiratory recoil force available and the more favorable length-tension characteristics of the inspiratory muscles at low lung volumes. Two other factors are potential candidates for contributions to the noisy nature of the client's inspirations. First, her heavy smoking to relieve pretelecast tension could have increased her lower airway resistance and therefore the opportunity for turbulent noise production; and, second, the tension itself could have had some psychogenic influence on airway function.

The client discussed here is the first to be documented with such signs and symptoms. Her rare functional disorder demonstrates clearly how misuse of the respiratory apparatus can be manifested on the inspiratory side of the speech breathing cycle and how acoustic level differences between the two sides of the cycle can become sufficiently contrasting to be perceived as abnormal.

Spinal Cord Injury

A 26-year-old male client had been involved in a motorcycle accident, resulting in spinal cord damage at the C4, C5, and C6 levels. Control of the musculature of his torso and extremities was impaired; his respiratory apparatus showed neurological signs of profound flaccid paresis of the muscles of the abdomen, moderate flaccid paresis of the muscles of the rib cage, and moderate flaccid paresis of the diaphragm. The client's speech signs included inadequate loudness, monoloudness, reduced stress contrasts, short breath groups, and slow inspirations between breath groups. His only speech production symptom was occasional mild dyspnea when he was engaged in prolonged continuous conversational speech.

Figure 7–10 shows data obtained from the client while he was supported upright in a wheelchair by shoulder straps. Two isovolume lines were generated, one at FRC and one at 1 L above FRC. Each was produced with the assistance of a clinician. This was necessary because of the client's muscular weakness and inability to move the rib cage and abdomen through the full ranges of motion required in standard isovolume maneuvers. Assistance amounted to displacing volume into and out of the client's rib cage and abdomen by alternately and slowly pushing and releasing the rib cage and abdomen while the client held his breath with a closed larynx at the two volumes of concern. The tracings shown are representative of expiratory limbs

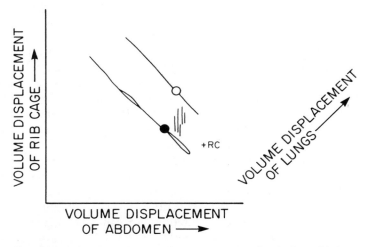

FIGURE 7–10.   Data from a client with cervical spinal cord injury.

generated by the client during continuous conversational speech and the reading of a standard declarative paragraph.

When tracings from the client are compared with those from normal subjects, several differences are apparent. First, the client often initiated breath groups from near the tidal end-inspiratory level (approximately at the 50% VC level for his predicted vital capacity of 5.2 L) compared with normal subjects, who most often initiate breath groups from a depth of about twice that of the tidal end-inspiratory level. Second, the client's volume excursions generally covered about 5% to 10% of his predicted VC compared with normal subjects, whose excursions cover 10% to 20% VC during conversational speech and reading. Third, the client displaced volume with his rib cage only, compared with normal subjects, who show displacement of both the rib cage and abdomen, but with a predominance of the former over the latter. Fourth, data from the client lie to the right of the presumed relaxation characteristic on the chart (a straight line interconnecting the two circles), meaning that his rib cage was smaller and his abdomen larger than they were during relaxation at the prevailing lung volume. Fifth, the tracings suggest a control mechanism dependent on expiratory activity by the rib cage alone, compared with normal subjects, who demonstrate a control strategy that involves expiratory activity by both the rib cage and abdomen, with the latter predominating. Sixth, and not discernible from Figure 7–10 because only the expiratory phases of the client's respiratory cycles are shown, is the fact that the client's inspirations took, on the average, about 1.3 secs to perform, compared with those for normal subjects, who demonstrate average speech breathing inspirations of about 0.6 sec for similar activities (Horii and Cooke, 1978).

It is easiest to appreciate the relationship between the client's speech and voice production and respiratory kinematics by considering the inspiratory and expiratory phases of his speech breathing cycle separately. Several factors appear to have combined on the inspiratory side of the cycle to make the client's performance deviant. His slow and often shallow inspirations in preparation for ensuing breath groups probably are related to two factors: the moderate flaccid paresis of the inspiratory muscles of his rib cage and diaphragm and the profound flaccid paresis of the muscles of his abdomen. Although weakness of the prime inspiratory drivers—the rib cage and diaphragm — logically is related to the client's deviant inspiratory behavior, the role of the abdomen in his performance may be somewhat obscure to many readers and warrants further comment.

The function of the abdomen during inspirations interspersed in normal continuous conversational speech is to displace the abdominal contents inward and the diaphragm headward. This adjustment "tunes" the diaphragm mechanically by increasing its radius of curvature and lengthening its muscle fibers so that on contraction for inspiration they can develop a great deal of force very rapidly. Lacking this important radius-of-curvature adjustment because of a profoundly impaired abdominal musculature, the client's weak diaphragm was placed at a poor mechanical advantage—namely, it was relatively flattened due to the outward distention of the paretic abdominal wall. Accordingly, the client's diaphragm was made to function under conditions in which the delivery of even its available weak drive was hindered further.

The speech signs associated with the expiratory side of the client's speech breathing cycle appear to be consequences of his moderate flaccid paresis of the expiratory muscles of the rib cage and profound flaccid paresis of the muscles of the abdomen. More specifically, the signs of inadequate loudness, monoloudness, and reduced stress contrasts form a cluster of factors influenced by volume compression difficulties related to muscular weakness. Also more specifically, the sign of short breath groups represents a factor that can be related to volume compression difficulties or volume displacement difficulties, or both, caused by muscular weakness. Of course, more shallow than normal inspirations between breath groups, as already discussed, also is a factor in the generation of short breath groups.

The general mechanism involved on the expiratory side of the speech breathing cycle would appear to be as follows. The client's only viable option for providing positive muscular pressure in the lung volume range employed required that he use his rib cage expiratory muscles to drive the respiratory apparatus. This accounts, for the most part, for the fact that the expiratory lung volume changes associated with his utterances involved displacements of the rib cage alone. It also accounts for the general deformation of the chest wall from its relaxed configuration toward one in which the rib cage is smaller and the abdomen larger than they were during relaxation at the prevailing lung volume. It seems reasonable to assume that the process involved was one in which the active expiratory muscles of the rib cage initially spent their force in displacing the essentially paralyzed abdomen outward until the latter offered a sufficiently firm base for the rib cage to work against as an opposing member. By delivering its force against this distended abdominal base, the rib cage then was able to develop the volume compression and volume displacement changes needed for the client's speech production. Although the client's method of compensation obviously was somewhat successful, there were a number of compounding mechanical inefficiencies confronting him because of the necessity for using a solely rib cage control strategy in the face of an essentially paralyzed abdomen.

First, the rib cage, itself impaired, had to move through greater distances to achieve the needed volume compressions for raising alveolar pressure to drive the speech production apparatus. Movement through greater distances was required because the rib cage had an inadequate opposing member against which to pressurize the pulmonary system. Considered colloquially, the bottom was "falling out" of the respiratory apparatus, figuratively and literally, as the flaccid abdomen moved outward in response to the drive being generated by the rib cage. This situation is similar to that involved in squeezing the upper half of a long balloon whereupon the lower half, if not held in position, will expand outward. Not only was the rib cage required to move through greater distances to pressurize the pulmonary system, but it also was required to move through greater excursions to accomplish the volume displacements needed in the client's speech. Considering volume displacements, it is clear that the situation had to be one in which the configurations of the chest wall involved changes in shape that did not necessarily involve changes in lung volume. That is, the movements of the active rib cage were resolved into changes in torso configuration with concomitantly small changes in lung volume. Aside from the rib cage having to assume a greater work load to pressurize the pulmonary system and to displace lung volume during the client's speech, the requirement that it function in the face of a paralyzed abdomen also must be considered. This means that the rib cage was placed in a mechanical situation in which it was operating at lower than normal volumes, that is, rib cage volumes. Accordingly, its expiratory muscles were shortened appreciably from the lengths they would assume normally in generating expiratory force. Thus, like the diaphragm on the inspiratory side of the speech breathing cycle, the expiratory rib cage muscles were placed at a distinct mechanical disadvantage for generating force on the expiratory side of the speech breathing cycle. They were themselves weak and their even weaker partner, the abdomen, had dealt their efficiency a double blow; it had caused them to need to do more work to drive the speech apparatus and had left them in the precarious position of having to make volume compression and displacement compensations under unfavorable performance circumstances.

Finally, the client's only speech production symptom, occasional mild dyspnea during continuous conversational speech, would appear to be related to the muscular weakness manifested by his respiratory apparatus. Such a symptom is common in persons with respiratory muscle weakness despite the fact that their blood-gas composition may contraindicate any departure from normal function. A relatively consistent feature of the perceptions of such individuals with major muscular weakness is that they sense respiratory difficulty for mechanical reasons not yet fully understood, but apparently related to the workloads experienced by their weak musculature.

Spasmodic Dysphonia

The client, a 32-year-old woman, was employed as a travel reservations agent and spent most of her working time engaged in telephone conversations with customers. She came to the clinic through a referral that sought detailed information concerning her respiratory function during speech production.

The client had been diagnosed previously as having adductor spasmodic (or spastic) dysphonia. She had been evaluated both neurologically and laryngologically and showed no clinical signs. Her voice disorder included unpredictable dysphonic and aphonic episodes during conversational speech, reading aloud, and singing. The client's dysphonic episodes ranged in severity from mild to profound and were correspondingly spread across a deviant strained-strangled voice quality continuum to nearly complete voice arrest. Major symptoms during these episodes included the client's feeling that she was choking and that it required a great deal of effort for her to produce speech. The client was observed approximately 6 months following the onset of her problem. She reported that the onset of her problem coincided with the lengthening of her "talking day" by 2 hours through the addition of evening lecture engagements. According to the client, the 6-month course of her problem had been characterized by a great deal of variability in the signs and symptoms of her speech production behavior. An especially unusual feature of the client's history was that several other persons in her work environment also had diagnoses of spasmodic dysphonia.

Figures 7–11, 7–12, and 7–13 present data from recordings made while the client sat upright in a straight-backed chair with her hands in her lap. The isovolume lines in the figures were generated in the standard manner. The lower line in each figure is at FRC; the upper line is at 1 L above FRC.

The tracings in Figure 7–11 are examples of those obtained during the client's performance of running speech activities, as in her usual continuous conversational speech and reading aloud. The dashed pathway depicts the general relative volume course followed on the chart during the client's strained-strangled utterances. The diagonal tracings, which cross this general relative volume course and run parallel to the isovolume lines, portray the courses followed on the chart during various aphonic episodes that interrupted the flow of the client's speech. Each of these diagonal courses was traced rapidly following voice arrest, sometimes by a pair of quick left and right alternating departures from the general relative volume course, but most often by several alternating departures from the general course.

When the client's usual running speech performance is compared with that of normal subjects, two differences emerge. The first difference, and one that is not discernible in Figure 7–11 because time is not designated along the pathways, is that the rate of change in lung volume (i.e., the respiratory flow) associated with those portions of the utterance tracings involving strained-strangled voice averaged about 75 cc/sec compared with the flow for segments generated by normal subjects, which average about 168 cc/sec (Horii and Cooke, 1978). Given that the client's voice was judged to be of normal or greater than normal loudness during strained-strangled segments, and thus that her driving pressure was normal or greater than normal, it seems reasonable to assume that her extremely low respiratory flows were related

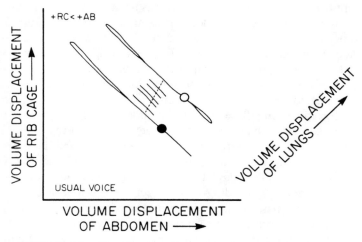

Figure 7-11. Data from a client with spasmodic dysphonia.

to extremely high laryngeal airway resistances. Unfortunately, the nature of the client's abnormal speech production did not allow clinical resistance estimation methods to be applied (Smitheran and Hixon, 1981). The second difference between the client's usual running speech performance and that of normal subjects was her generation of quick left and right alternating departures from the general relative volume course during moments of voice

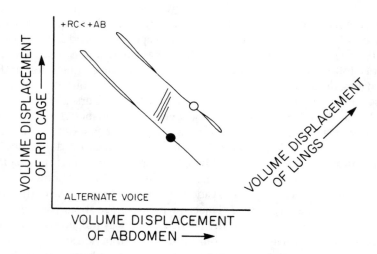

Figure 7-12. Data from a client (same as in Figure 7-11) with spasmodic dysphonia.

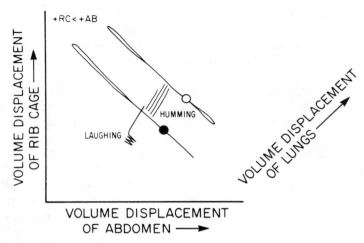

FIGURE 7-13.   Data from a client (same as in Figure 7-11) with spasmodic dysphonia.

arrest. This is in comparison with normal subjects, who maintain the respiratory apparatus in a relatively fixed configuration during pauses in the flow of speech, whether they be brief or involve breath holding of considerable duration while planning further utterance (see Chapter 4).

The physiological mechanism involved in the client's performance during voice arrest appears to be as follows. Presumably the larynx was sealed forcefully and respiratory adjustments were made against an airtight valve. This is inferred from the fact that lung volume did not change during adjustments of the respiratory apparatus and that each aphonic episode was followed by a loud glottal aspiration, indicating that a high pressure had been impounded in the trachea during the period of voice arrest. The alternating shifts in the configuration of the respiratory apparatus during aphonic periods were of a nature akin to the performance of the more extensive isovolume calibration maneuvers the client generated, and they also are akin to maneuvers observed in normal subjects attempting to pant against a fixed resistance at the airway opening (mouth). The exact muscular mechanisms involved in the client's alternating shifts are uncertain. The general background configuration on which the client's quick alternating shifts are imposed (i.e., the dashed course in Figure 7-11) is consistent with the configuration observed in normal subjects and presumably reflects function in which both the rib cage and abdomen are active in the expiratory direction, but the abdomen more forcefully so (+RC < +AB). The alternating shifts themselves could be accounted for by one, or a combination, of the four muscular force possibilities listed to the left of the relaxation characteristic in Figure 7-4. The speed with which the alternations to the left and right of the general background configuration were performed makes it tempting to speculate that the mechanism involved may have been one in which the levels of activity in the already active rib cage and abdomen were varied so as to play one against the other in an expiratory force balance change superimposed on the general configuration. That is, the rib cage and abdomen probably were used as antagonists to and fro while the predominant base was supplied by the generally more forcefully active abdomen. Movements of the rib cage and abdomen in opposite signs in this context would, therefore, reflect the momentary changes in balance between the two opposing force generators.

The client was able to speak conversationally, read aloud, and sing without demonstrating her usual behaviors by using what she called an "alternate voice." This voice was high-pitched, breathy, and harsh, but was accompanied by smoothly flowing utterance events. Figure 7–12 shows data generated during the use of this voice for conversational speech purposes. Compared with data from normal subjects, the tracings in Figure 7–12 are unremarkable and attest to the fact that the client could use her larynx and respiratory apparatus in a manner that permitted fluent oral communication, albeit dysphonic, without episodic interruptions in laryngeal function and abnormal configurational adjustments of the respiratory apparatus.

The client was able to produce a normal-sounding voice under circumstances in which she hummed the suprasegmental features of running speech activities and singing. That is, when she closed her mouth and generated suprasegmental features through her nose, her speech and singing were prosodically normal (e.g., in intonation, rhythm, and stress) and the quality of her voice was normal. Figure 7–13 shows data generated when the client hummed the syllabic and suprasegmental patterns of a standard declarative paragraph. All such data generated in her humming mode fell within the range of respiratory kinematic behaviors typical of normal subjects. Thus, the client was able to use her larynx and respiratory apparatus in a manner that permitted fluent utterances without episodic discontinuities and to do so with a normal sounding voice. Figure 7–13 also shows data obtained from the client as she laughed spontaneously through her nose at the end of the "hummed reading" task. Her laughter was judged to sound normal and kinematic data in Figure 7–13 are of the form observed for the spontaneous laughter of normal subjects.

Several other observations have bearing on the client's utterance capabilities. She was unable to produce fluent and normal suprasegments and voice when asked to do so with her mouth held open and with her oral articulators held in different fixed positions. She also was unable to phonate a sustained vowel throughout her vital capacity without repeated aphonic episodes of the variety discussed with reference to Figure 7–11. She was able to sustain /m/ throughout her vital capacity with a normal-sounding voice, however. The client was unable to sustain /h/ throughout her vital capacity without repeated utterance arrests. She could sustain a glottal fricative through her nose throughout the vital capacity. And, finally, the client was unable to whisper in a normal fashion but could perform whisperlike speech events through her nose.

When considered collectively, the utterance behaviors of the client are clinically perplexing. When sound was generated at the larynx, be it phonation or glottal frication, and passed through the client's nose, her utterances sounded normal and were produced with apparently normal laryngeal-respiratory actions. When the client attempted to generate analogous sound at the larynx but passed it through her mouth, however, her utterances were deviant and in the case of her usual mode of performance were accompanied by aberrant adjustments of the respiratory apparatus. The causal roots of this discrepancy and of the client's inability to generate a normal voice or oral communication are uncertain. Negative neurological and laryngological findings for the client would appear to weigh against a possible neurogenic basis for her abnormal behavior, although such a basis should not be ruled out completely, because in persons with spasmodic dysphonia abnormal neurological signs may be manifested considerably later than the initial occurrence of speech and voice signs and symptoms. In considering a possible psychogenic basis for the client's behavior, the following facts must be weighed: She was able to switch quickly and voluntarily from one form of abnormal voice production to another form of abnormal production; she could use her voice normally under circumstances that were devoid of usual verbal communication; and the gross respiratory adjustments associated with her usual abnormal voice production were bizarre and of such excessive magnitude relative to those that would be expected in struggle behavior against a forcefully closed larynx as to be possibly exhibitionistic. Other observations concerning the client could be viewed from either neurogenic or psychogenic etiologic perspectives. Onset of the client's problem was reported by her to coincide with an increase in the time spent using her probably already overworked voice production apparatus. Further, the unusual feature of her history of several other persons in her work setting also having diagnoses of spasmodic dysphonia indicates a prevalence for the disorder in her environment that is of epidemic magnitude. It is possible, of course, that such a high prevalence could be of neurogenic, psychogenic, or mixed origin.

CONCLUSIONS

This chapter has attempted to demonstrate the clinical relevance of considering voice abnormalities in relation to respiratory kinematics. It has discussed the kinematic method used, documented the relatively well-defined kinematic patterns associated with the speech of normal subjects, and illustrated kinematic patterns associated with dysfunction in three clients. The conviction is that a great deal can be learned about voice abnormalities through the study of respiratory kinematics and that kinematic methods can enhance the practice of speech-language pathology. With regard to the latter, it is believed that kinematic methods increase the precision of evaluation efforts and raise the level of accountability in working with clients with voice abnormalities.

ACKNOWLEDGMENT

The preparation of this manuscript was supported by grants from the National Institute of Neurological and Communicative Disorders and Stroke. Dr. Frances J. Freeman, University of Texas and Callier Center for Communication Disorders, Dallas, Texas, consulted on a portion of the work.

REFERENCES

Horii, Y., and Cooke, P. (1978). Some airflow, volume, and duration characteristics of oral reading. *Journal of Speech and Hearing Research,* 21, 470–481.

Konno, K., and Mead, J. (1967). Measurement of the separate volume changes of rib cage and abdomen during breathing. *Journal of Applied Physiology,* 22, 407–422.

Mead, J., Peterson, N., Grimby, G., and Mead, J. (1967). Pulmonary ventilation measured from body surface movements. *Science,* 156, 1383–1384.

Smitheran, J., and Hixon, T. (1981). A clinical method for estimating laryngeal airway resistance during vowel production. *Journal of Speech and Hearing Disorders,* 46, 138–146.

CHAPTER 8

Respiratory Kinematics in Speakers with Motor Neuron Disease

Anne H. B. Putnam
Thomas J. Hixon

otor neuron disease is a family of degenerative illnesses affecting motor nerve cells in the spinal cord and brain. Its expression in the human neuromuscular system may vary from a so-called "benign" form, which progresses slowly among lower motor neurons, to an acute form, amyotrophic lateral sclerosis (ALS), which progresses rapidly, ravaging upper as well as lower motor neurons (Brooke, 1977). When bulbar motor neurons innervating the laryngeal or upper airway musculature are involved (as in progressive bulbar palsy or in ALS), a dysarthria with flaccid or spastic signs, or both, may result, the perceptual characteristics of which have been well documented (Darley, Aronson, and Brown, 1975; Dworkin, Aronson, and Mulder, 1980). When spinal motor neurons innervating the trunk musculature are involved (as in

Reprinted by permission of the publisher from *The dysarthrias*, M. McNeil, J. Rosenbek, and A. Aronson (Eds.), pp. 37–67, © 1983, College-Hill Press, San Diego, CA.

progressive spinal muscular atrophy or in ALS), wasting and weakness of the chest wall muscles (i.e., those of the rib cage, diaphragm, and abdomen) may result in deterioration of respiratory function. This chapter is concerned with the effects on respiratory function of motor neuron disease in the spinal motor system.

Information about changes in respiratory function associated with motor neuron disease comes primarily from clinical observations of clients with the ALS form of the disease. Their respiratory status often declines rapidly, and they usually succumb to respiratory complications (e.g., atelectasis, aspiration pneumonia, or congestive heart failure) because of reduced ventilatory efficiency (Brooke, 1977; Fallat and Norris, 1980; Keltz, 1965; Kreitzer, Saunders, Tyler, and Ingram, 1978). Some observers of respiratory function in persons with motor neuron disease have described a pattern of anterior horn cell degeneration that may compromise the diaphragm, or the abdomen, earlier or more extensively than the rib cage (Fromm, Wisdom, and Block, 1977; Miller, Mulder, Fowler, and Olsen, 1957; Nakano, Bass, Tyler, and Carmel, 1976; Parhad, Clark, Barron, and Staunton, 1978). This focal pattern of deterioration has implications for respiratory function in general and perhaps also for respiratory function for speech. Heretofore, however, the effects of motor neuron disease on respiratory function for speech have not been studied systematically.

Existing clinical information on the speech breathing capabilities of individuals with motor neuron disease is primarily inferential, deduced from data for nonspeech respiratory tasks and from clients' reports. Unfortunately, respiratory signs of dysarthria characteristic of motor neuron disease rarely are evaluated by the neurologist or the speech-language pathologist. The respiratory apparatus is crucial to sound production in the larynx and upper airway, and apparent abnormalities of voice and articulation in clients with motor neuron disease may be related to abnormal respiratory function. Furthermore, the compensatory tolerance of the respiratory apparatus to the ravages of motor neuron disease may be different from that of the larynx and upper airway with respect to the threshold for overt signs of speech abnormality. Thus, whether or not the respiratory apparatus is involved, and if so, to what extent, constitutes information essential to the accurate evaluation and appropriate management of dysarthria presented by individuals with motor neuron disease.

This chapter summarizes a 3-year investigation of respiratory function in a group of adult subjects with motor neuron disease. It was the purpose of this investigation to document the effects of their disease, if any were discernible, on the behavior of the chest wall, specifically with respect to the demands of speech. Respiratory function during speech was studied in these subjects by means of the kinematic method of Hixon, Goldman, and Mead (see Chapter 3). This method was chosen because of its investigative and clinical utility. It is noninvasive and risk-free, can be applied efficiently and systematically, and requires no performance sophistication on the part of those being studied. Furthermore, there are reliable data on normal chest wall behavior (see Chapter 3), as well as data on chest wall behavior in abnormal populations, including speakers with profound hearing impairment (see Chapter 5), neuromuscular abnormalities (see Chapters 6, 7, and 9), and voice abnormality related to functional misuse of the respiratory apparatus (see Chapter 7).

METHOD

Subjects

Subjects were 10 men with motor neuron disease. Their ages ranged from 34 to 72 years, and their histories of motor neuron disease ranged from 3 to 12 years. Pertinent information on members of the group is presented in Table 8–1, including perceptual judgments of six aspects of their speech. In every case, the neuromuscular disease had been diagnosed on the basis of health history, neurological examination, and electrodiagnostic studies; and, in many cases, a limb muscle biopsy had been performed. All of the subjects had at least spinal motor neuron involvement (MNDsp) with noticeable wasting and weakness in their limb and trunk musculature. All were ambulatory, though some required the assistance of canes or walkers. Most complained of mild to severe orthopnea, the subjective sensation of breathing difficulty when supine. Three of the subjects also had bulbar motor neuron involvement (MNDb) with signs or symptoms of laryngeal (CW), velopharyngeal (FM and FG), labial (FM and FG), or lingual muscle weakness (FM, FG, and CW), and a noticeable dysarthria. Four of the subjects, including the three with bulbar signs, also exhibited upper motor neuron signs and carried the diagnosis of ALS.

Measurement Theory

The theoretical and technical details of the kinematic method can be found elsewhere (see Chapters 3 and 4 and Konno and Mead, 1967; Mead, Peterson, Grimby, and Mead, 1967). Those aspects of the theory that are germane to the present investigation are reviewed briefly here and as the need arises later in the chapter. In theory, the chest wall is considered a two-part system consisting of the rib cage and diaphragm-abdomen[1] arranged in parallel. The

---

[1]The diaphragm-abdomen behaves mechanically as a single structure. Its inner surface is the diaphragm, its outer the abdominal wall, and its incompressible center the abdominal contents (see Chapter 3). Hereinafter, the diaphragm-abdomen will be referred to as "abdomen," although diaphragm-abdomen always is implied.

Table 8-1. *Information on the Subjects of this Investigation Pertinent to their Physical Characteristics, Extents and Histories of Motor Neuron Disease, and the Perceived Abnormalities of their Speech*

Subject	Age (yr)	Height (cm)	Diagnosis (yr)	Voice Quality	Articulation	Nasal Resonance	Breath Group Duration	Utterance Loudness	Utterance Rate
EC	65	183	MNDsp(6)	Normal	Normal	Normal	Normal	Normal	Normal
RF	34	169	MNDsp(3)	Strained-strangled*	Normal	Normal	Short†	Normal	Normal
RR	46	178	MNDsp(5)	Normal	Normal	Normal	Normal	Normal	Normal
KG	41	185	MNDsp(12)	Slightly tremorous	Normal	Normal	Normal	Normal	Normal
VB	61	168	MNDsp(5)	Normal	Normal	Normal	Normal	Normal	Normal
FM	72	165	MNDsp-b(8) (ALS)	Strained-strangled	Imprecise	Hyper-nasal‡	Short	Loud	Slow
LC	66	179	MNDsp(?)	Normal	Normal	Normal	Normal	Normal	Normal
FG	61	173	MNDsp-b(5) (ALS)	Strained-strangled	Imprecise	Hyper-nasal‡	Short	Loud	Slow
KS	49	178	MNDsp(10) (ALS)	Normal	Normal	Normal	Normal	Normal	Normal
CW	68	170	MNDsp-b(3) (ALS)	Strained-strangled*	Normal	Normal	Short	Normal	Normal

*Calculated laryngeal airway resistance was abnormally high (Smitheran and Hixon, 1981).
†This subject exhibited a consistently laconic communication pattern in conversation; breath group duration in reading was normal.
‡Concomitant aeromechanical coupling was verified via nasal air flow recordings (Thompson and Hixon, 1979).

chest wall surrounds the pulmonary system, which consists of the lungs and lower airway. The rib cage and abdomen each displace volume as they move, and their combined displacement equals that of the lungs. Changes in the anteroposterior diameters of the rib cage and abdomen have been shown to be related linearly to the volume each displaces. Therefore, the volume displaced by the rib cage and abdomen can be estimated from their respective diameter changes. An efficient method for measuring these diameter changes uses magnetometer coils attached to surfaces of the rib cage and abdomen (see Chapter 3). Typically, two generator-sensor coil pairs are used. The components of one pair are attached to the midline of the rib cage, front and back, whereas the components of the other pair are placed comparably on the abdomen. Each pair converts a diameter change into a voltage analogue that can be adjusted electronically and interpreted for volume displacement.

The derivation of displacement information from diameter change is predicated on the principle that each part of the chest wall moves with a single degree of freedom. That is, each part can assume only one shape at any given volume of that part. It is necessary to calibrate the relationship between the anteroposterior diameter change of each part and its associated volume displacement. This can be done by means of a chest wall adjustment called an isovolume maneuver, which is performed by the subject with the magnetometers in place. This maneuver reveals the functional relationships between the relative motions of the rib cage and abdomen at particular lung volumes and allows for on-line conversion of the magnetometer signals from diameter change to volume displacement. The use of isovolume maneuvers in this manner is described further in the *Procedure* section.

Equipment

The equipment used for kinematic measurement and analysis is schematized in Figure 8–1. As described earlier, magnetometers were used to sense the anteroposterior diameter changes of the rib cage and abdomen; their signals were displayed on-line oscilloscopically and stored simultaneously on two channels of an FM tape recorder. The speech of the subject and commentary of the investigators were transduced by a microphone and recorded on a third channel of the FM recorder.

Procedure

The magnetometers were attached to the chest wall with double-sided adhesive tape. As shown in Figure 8–1, generating coils were positioned at the midline on the anterior surface of the torso, one for the rib cage near the level of the nipples, and one for abdomen just above the navel. Sensing coils were positioned posteriorly at the midline at the same torso levels as their generator mates.

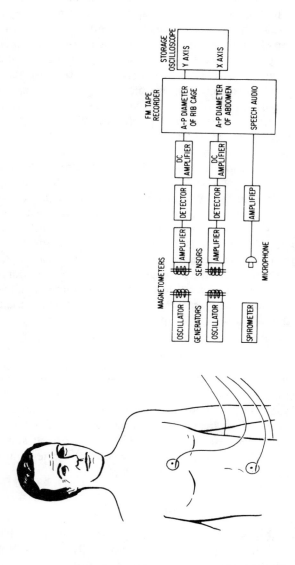

Figure 8–1. Schematic illustration of the equipment used.

The performance demands of the investigation were designed to optimize data collection without overtaxing the subjects' emotional or physical endurance. Accordingly, the protocol included only those nonspeech respiratory tasks necessary to calibrate and otherwise define kinematic landmarks unique to each subject's chest wall, several speech or speechlike tasks that simulated everyday communication demands, and multiple opportunities for resting tidal breathing. As illustrated in Figure 8–2, subjects performed these tasks in two body positions: first while seated upright,[2] and then while lying supine on a foam pad with a small pillow for head support. Five subjects with severe symptoms of orthopnea were not studied in the supine position. Subjects were instructed to avoid raising their arms or shifting their posture during the procedure.

The nonspeech tasks included vital capacity maneuvers, resting tidal breathing, and isovolume maneuvers. Three vital capacity maneuvers were performed by each subject, and an average vital capacity was computed and compared with the subject's predicted vital capacity (using the formula weighted for age and height suggested by Comroe, Forster, Dubois, Briscoe, and Carlsen, 1962). A spirometer was used to obtain the vital capacity data, and each subject wore a nose clip to preclude any loss of volume transnasally. Data for approximately 30 sec of resting tidal breathing were obtained after every task in the protocol. Isovolume maneuvers were performed at lung volume levels corresponding to FRC and approximately 1 L above FRC. For each isovolume maneuver, the subject was instructed to hold his breath and slowly displace volume back and forth between the rib cage and abdomen. A nose clip was worn during these maneuvers to ensure that no volume was lost transnasally. It should be noted that the volume level difference between the two isovolume maneuvers was not always exactly 1 L; the isovolume target above FRC was reached by a measured inspiration from a spirometer, and this volume level was difficult for subjects to achieve precisely in every case. For

---

[2]Note that upright body position data were obtained while subjects were seated, rather than standing, which is the standard reference position (see Chapter 3). The subjects could not tolerate standing and maintaining a stable posture for the one half hour required to complete the procedure in the upright position. Instead, they were seated in a straight-backed chair with their torsos stabilized (but unrestrained) in an upright position they could maintain consistently during the procedure. Shifting from standing to sitting upright may effect a small reduction in the vital capacity (2%) due to changes in the effects of gravity on the chest wall and encroachments on the rib cage volume by headward displacement of the abdominal contents (Campbell, Agostoni, and Newsom Davis, 1970). These changes are small, however, and it would not be predicted that substantially different data patterns would be generated with the subjects seated instead of standing. As a control measure, however, seated data were obtained from a group of 10 neuromuscularly normal men who were matched to the subjects with motor neuron disease on the basis of age and height. On perusal of the control group's data, it was clear that for the respiratory activities of interest, the relative volume patterns of these 10 normal subjects seated upright were consistent with data for normal subjects standing upright (see Chapter 3).

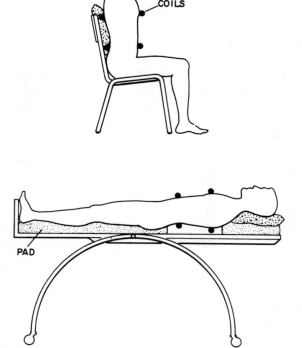

FIGURE 8-2. Schematic illustration of the body positions (seated upright and supine) in which subjects performed the tasks.

this reason, the actual volume differences between each subject's isovolume maneuvers are specified in Tables 8-2 and 8-3.

The speech tasks consisted of several minutes of spontaneous conversation with an investigator and the reading of the Grandfather Passage at normal and twice normal loudness levels. In addition, each subject performed a syllable repetition task that called for intermittent rapid, discrete increments in vocal stress in a pattern repeated several times on a single expiration. The particular instruction for the task was, "Take a deep breath and repeat /ta ta 'ta/ over and over until you run out of breath." The demonstration rate for the repetitions was 3 syllables per sec.

Data Displays: Orientation and Interpretation

Figure 8-3 is a relative volume chart illustrative of those used for data display. Volume displacement of the rib cage increases upward on the Y axis; volume displacement of the abdomen increases rightward on the X axis; and

Table 8–2. *Numerical Data for Respiratory Tasks in the Upright Body Position*

	Vital Capacity		Resting Tidal Breathing				
Subject	Measured (L)	% Predicted	Volume (L)	Frequency (BPM)	Minute Volume (LPM)	% Contribution RC/AB	Isovolume Line Difference (L)
EC	2.40	65*	0.60	25	15.00	57/43	1.20
RF	3.46	87	0.45	19	8.55	71/29	1.15
RR	2.68	67*	0.60	16	9.60	41/59	1.00
KG	4.18	98	1.00	13	13.00	89/11	1.20
VB	3.16	91	0.65	14	9.00	91/9	1.05
FM	2.90	90	0.75	13	9.75	56/44	1.00
LC	3.47	96	0.70	14	9.80	90/10	1.10
FG	1.40	39*	0.25	19	4.75	56/44	1.00
KS	2.30	59*	0.30	22	6.60	33/67	1.00
CW	2.23	66*	0.45	25	11.25	90/10	1.00

*Indicates abnormally reduced from predicted.

Table 8-3. *Numerical Data for Respiratory Tasks in the Supine Body Position*

| | Vital Capacity | | | Resting Tidal Breathing | | | |
Subject	Measured (L)	% Differs from Upright	Volume (L)	Frequency (BPM)	Minute Volume (LPM)	% Contribution RC/AB	Isovolume Line Difference (L)
FM	2.90	0	0.70	17	11.90	30/70	1.15
KS	2.37	3>	0.40	22	8.80	48/52	1.00
KG	3.80	9<	0.90	8	7.20	25/75	1.05
VB	3.22	2>	0.70	13	9.10	39/61	1.05
CW	1.15	52<	0.35	24	8.40	61/39	0.85

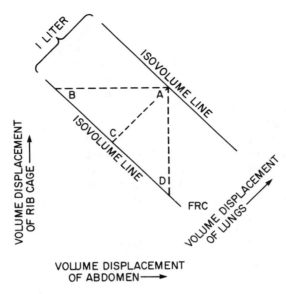

FIGURE 8–3. Relative volume chart (rib cage versus abdomen) illustrative of those used for data display.

their combined volume displacement (i.e., that of the lungs) increases upward on the diagonal axis. The solid diagonal lines in Figure 8–3 are isovolume lines. Each represents the relative volume pathway followed as volume is shifted back and forth between the rib cage and abdomen with the airway closed at a fixed lung volume. The two lines shown represent the FRC level and a level 1 L above FRC. During isovolume maneuvers, the volume exchanged between the two chest wall parts is equal and opposite. The diameter changes of the rib cage and abdomen are not equal during the isovolume maneuver, however. Thus, to make the data on the chart read as if equal diameter changes actually occured, the magnitudes of the coil signals are adjusted electronically so that the line representing the volume shift on the chart has a slope of – 1.

On such a relative volume chart, any series of data points forming a pathway graphs the changing shape of the chest wall during a respiratory behavior. These pathways can be interpreted to reveal lung volume change, relative contributions of the rib cage and abdomen to such volume change, the separate volumes of the rib cage and abdomen, and the configuration of the chest wall. For example, the concomitant change in lung volume along a pathway can be determined by the distance between any two points perpendicular to the isovolume lines (see Chapter 3). Thus, pathways AB, AC, and AD in Figure 8–3 each chart 1 L changes in lung volume. The slopes of these pathways convey how much each part of the chest wall contributed to the associated volume change. That is, the magnitude of the slope may be interpreted as the percentage contribution of the rib cage and the abdomen to the lung volume change. Thus, horizontal pathway AB indicates 100% abdominal contribution to the lung volume change. Vertical pathway AD indicates 100% rib cage contribution to the lung volume change. And pathways with slopes intermediate to those extremes indicate that both the rib cage and abdomen contributed to lung volume change. In Figure 8–3, pathway AC indicates equal rib cage and abdominal contributions (i.e., 50% rib cage, 50% abdomen). Pathways with slopes steeper than AC indicate that the rib cage's contribution was greater than 50%, and pathways with slopes less steep than AC indicate that the contribution of the abdomen to the lung volume change was greater than 50%. Information about the separate volumes of the rib cage and abdomen or the configuration of the chest wall at any point on the relative volume chart may be obtained by reference to the vertical and horizontal axes of the chart.

RESULTS

Vital Capacity Data

Measured vital capacity and predicted vital capacity for all subjects are included in Tables 8–2 and 8–3. In every case, the vital capacity measured in the upright body position was reduced from the predicted value; the measured values ranged from 39% to 98% of predicted. For those five subjects from whom supine position data were obtained, measured vital capacities were slightly larger than, comparable to, or smaller than those obtained from the same subjects upright; the capacity change in the supine position ranged from 3% higher to 52% lower than comparable upright values.

Resting Tidal Breathing—Upright

Resting tidal volumes (in L), frequencies (in BPM), minute volume rates (in liters per minute [LPM]), and percentages of rib cage and abdominal contributions to lung volume change are listed in Table 8–2 for all subjects in the upright body position. Resting tidal volumes ranged from 0.25 to 1 L; frequencies ranged from 13 to 25 BPM, and minute volume rates ranged from 4.75 to 15 LPM. Characteristic resting tidal breathing patterns are illustrated in Figure 8–4 and 8–5. Pathways shown in the figures represent both inspiration and expiration. Slopes of the tidal breathing pathways reflect that both the rib cage and the abdomen contributed to volume displacement, although the contribution of the rib cage tended to predominate in most cases. Note that the pathway slopes are not constant, however. The predominant contribution of the rib cage increased (i.e., the slopes steepen) at the higher volume ends of the quiet breathing cycles for most of the subjects. Estimates of the percentage of rib cage and abdominal contribution to lung volume

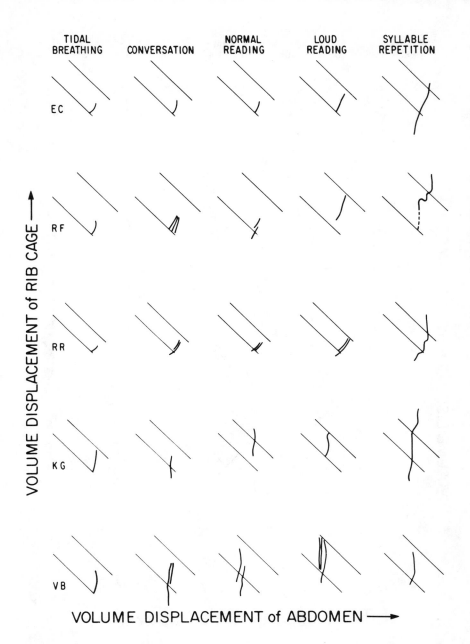

FIGURE 8–4. Relative volume charts for subjects EC, RF, RR, KG, and VB in the upright body position, showing representative data for resting tidal breathing, conversation, normal reading, loud reading, and syllable repetition tasks. The long diagonal lines (−1 slopes) are isovolume pathways, the lower one at FRC and the upper one at approximately 1 L above FRC. See Table 8–2 for precise isovolume line separation in each subject's charts. Data tracings include the remaining solid and dashed lines on the subjects' charts.

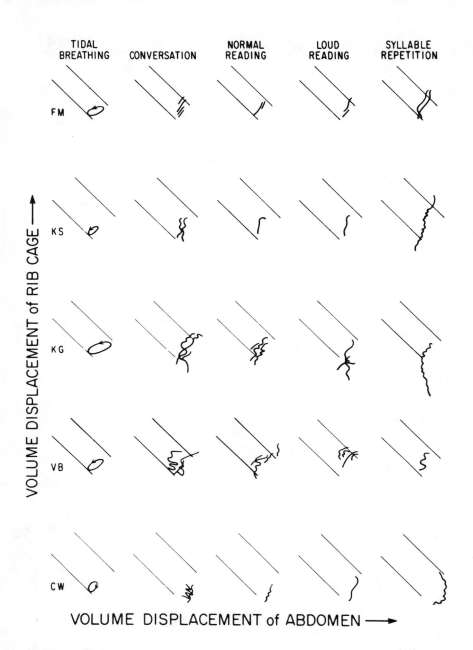

FIGURE 8–5. Relative volume charts for subjects FM, LC, FG, KS, and CW in the upright body position, showing representative data for resting tidal breathing, conversation, normal reading, loud reading, and syllable repetition tasks. The long diagonal lines (–1 slopes) are isovolume pathways, the lower one at FRC and the upper one at approximately 1 L above FRC. See Table 8–2 for precise isovolume line separation in each subject's charts. Data tracings include the remaining solid and dashed lines on the subjects' charts.

change in these data were made from the most extensive portion of each pathway exhibiting a relatively constant slope. On the basis of this measurement scheme, rib cage contribution to lung volume displacement during upright resting tidal breathing was estimated to range from 33% to 91%, and abdominal contribution to range from 9% to 67%. One conspicuous pathway is the looped configuration in the tidal breathing data of subject CW (Fig. 8–5). After a few tidal breaths (dashed pathway), his tidal pathway began to loop clockwise. The left side of the loop represents tidal inspiration, and the right side with the arrowhead represents tidal expiration.

Resting Tidal Breathing—Supine

Supine tidal volumes, frequencies, minute volume rates, and relative contributions of the rib cage and abdomen to lung volume change are listed in Table 8–3 for the five subjects from whom data were collected in this body position. Supine resting tidal volumes ranged from 0.35 to 0.90 L; frequencies ranged from 8 to 24 BPM, and minute volume rates ranged from 7.2 to 11.9 LPM. The volume displacement patterns for supine tidal breathing are displayed in Figure 8–6. Conspicuous in these data are the looped pathways on all the subjects' charts; both inspiratory and expiratory volumes are represented, with arrowheads marking expiration. The loops cycle counterclockwise in four of the subjects, and clockwise in the fifth (CW). Relative volume slopes were estimated roughly as the long axis of each ellipse. On the basis of this measurement scheme, the rib cage contribution to supine resting tidal breathing ranged from 25% to 61%, and the abdominal contribution ranged from 39% to 75%.

Conversation—Upright

Data for the subjects' conversational speech in the upright position are illustrated in Figures 8–4 and 8–5. Each tracing represents a single expiratory limb (i.e., one breath group). Often clusters of such tracings are shown to illustrate breath group pattern variation across a series of consecutive utterances. In other cases, subjects were so consistent in their patterns that a single tracing represents chest wall behavior regardless of linguistic load or length of utterance differences across breath groups. The lung volume levels at which subjects initiated conversation differed. Four subjects (KG, VB, FM, and KS) tended to initiate conversation at or below their resting tidal end-inspiratory levels, four (EC, RF, RR, and CW) tended to begin at levels slightly higher than their tidal end-inspiratory levels, and the remaining two (LC and FG) typically began speaking at twice their resting tidal end-inspiratory levels or higher (although LC's initiation levels were inconsistent). When these breath group initiation levels are considered relative to FRC, all the subjects obviously initiated conversation above that level, and most began speaking at better than

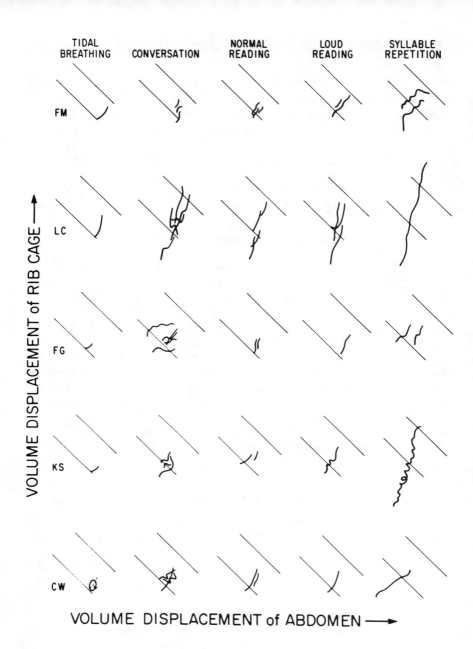

FIGURE 8-6. Relative volume charts for subjects FM, KS, KG, VB, and CW in the supine body position showing representative data for resting tidal breathing, conversation, normal reading, loud reading, and syllable repetition tasks. The long diagonal lines (–1 slopes) are isovolume pathways, the lower one at FRC and the upper one at approximately 1 L above FRC. See Table 8–3 for precise isovolume line separation in each subject's charts. Data tracings include the remaining solid lines on the subjects' charts.

0.50 L above FRC. None, however, with the possible exception of LC, initiated speech at levels 1 L above FRC. In six of the subjects, slopes of the tracings on the charts generally reflect a rib cage predominance in contribution to lung volume change during utterance, ranging for the most part from 65% to 100%. The data of the remaining four subjects (LC, FG, KS, and CW, Figure 8–5) exhibit marked changes in slope across a cluster of connected utterance tracings, or abrupt shifts in the slopes of individual tracings. For example, note the cluster of conversational speech data for subject FG; he uttered some breath groups with a predominant rib cage contribution, whereas for others he used primarily an abdominal contribution to effect lung volume change. Subject CW's data cluster indicates that his expiratory limbs were characterized frequently by tracings whose slopes changed abruptly from predominantly rib cage to predominantly abdominal contributions. Furthermore, in the unusual slope data of these four subjects and perhaps even a fifth (FM), the tracings often indicate paradoxical displacements of the rib cage and the abdomen.[3]

Conversation—Supine

The data for conversation in the supine body position are illustrated in Figure 8–6. The lung volume levels at which subjects initiated conversation differed. Starting levels ranged from approximately the tidal end-inspiratory level to approximately twice the tidal volume depth. Relative to the FRC of each subject, the supine conversation initiation levels of three (KG, VB, and FM) were often 1 L or more above FRC, although VB began at that level only rarely, and FM showed a noticeable decrease in starting level over time. The remaining two subjects (KS and CW) never initiated supine conversation 1 L above FRC. The slopes of the data tracings changed abruptly in all but one of the supine subjects (FM), in whom the rib cage contribution to lung volume change was 60%. Among the other four supine subjects, the abruptly changing slopes, with some evidence of rib cage and abdominal paradoxing, had been noted already in the upright conversational data of two (KS and CW), but were novel for KG and VB.

Reading—Upright

The displacement data for the subjects' readings of the Grandfather Passage in the upright body position at normal and twice-normal loudness levels are illustrated in Figures 8–4 and 8–5. Six of the subjects (EC, RF, RR, VB, FM, and LC) tended to initiate normal reading near or below their resting

---

[3]Paradoxical displacements of the rib cage or abdomen are ones in which the displacement of the part is opposite in sign to lung volume displacement.

tidal end-inspiratory levels, three (FG, KS, and CW) began at levels somewhat higher than their tidal end-inspiratory levels, and one (KG) initiated his reading considerably higher than his tidal end-inspiratory volume. Considering these initiation levels relative to FRC, nine subjects typically initiated normally loud upright reading at volumes less than 1 L above FRC. Only KG initiated his reading 1 L or more above that level. When instructed to read the passage at twice normal loudness, seven of the subjects initiated utterances at lung volume levels higher than their normal reading starting levels. Two subjects (CW and LC) exhibited essentially no change in lung volume initiation levels between the two reading conditions, and one subject (KG) initiated loud reading at lower lung volume levels than those at which he had read the passage normally. The slopes of the tracings in all cases indicate that both chest wall parts contributed to lung volume displacement during the reading tasks, although, in general, the rib cage tended to predominate more or less. There are examples, however, of tracings for which equal contributions of rib cage and abdomen are apparent (e.g., see RR or FM), or for which the contribution is exclusively that of the rib cage (see VB). Subject KS exhibited some abrupt changes in the slopes of his expiratory limbs during the loud reading performance with chest wall paradoxing similar to that which characterized his conversational data.

Reading—Supine

The data generated by the supine subjects for reading are illustrated in Figure 8–6. Lung volume initiation levels for normally loud reading were roughly comparable to or below resting tidal end-inspiratory levels in one subject (KG) and somewhat higher in the other four (FM, KS, VB, and CW). Among the latter, however, only VB initiated his reading 1 L or more above FRC, although inconsistently so. Four subjects' attempts at loud reading usually were initiated higher than the lung volume levels at which they had begun reading normally; subject KG, however, tended to initiate the loud reading at or below his normal reading initiation level. Slopes of the tracings for reading supine in three subjects (KG, VB, and CW) exhibited a number of abrupt shifts in relative contributions to lung volume change with evidence of rib cage and abdominal paradoxing within single expiratory limbs, although CW was inconsistent with respect to this characteristic between the two reading conditions. Subjects FM and KS exhibited data slopes without numerous abrupt shifts in either reading condition, although their data in the loud reading performance do exhibit several gradual changes in slope.

Syllable Stress Task—Upright

Data generated by the subjects on the syllable repetition stress task in the upright body position are illustrated in Figures 8–4 and 8–5. In six cases (EC, RF, RR, KG, LC, and KS) subjects initiated this task at lung volume levels at least 1 L or more above FRC (in response to the instruction, "Take a deep breath"). Five of these six also continued the task below FRC (as per instructions to continue "until you run out of breath"). The sixth subject (RF) always stopped performing the task well above FRC, however, and expired quietly to FRC as indicated by the dashed portion of his relative volume tracing for this activity (Fig. 8–4). The remaining four subjects generated data that were initiated at much lower levels. Two of these (VB and FG) also produced data that were curtailed at end-task level, stopping at or just below FRC; the other two (FM and CW), although they started at low lung volumes, were able to continue the task well below FRC. The slopes of the tracings generated by the subjects on this task exhibit several patterns. Four subjects (EC, KG, VB, and LC) generated data in which a rib cage contribution to lung volume change prevailed. Other subjects (RF, RR, FM, FG, and KS) exhibited slopes in which the predominance of rib cage and abdomen alternated abruptly in contribution to lung volume change. In the cases of FM and KS, the abrupt shifts in the tracings consistently were related to the occurrence of stressed syllables during utterance of the task; in the other cases, such shifts in relative contributions apparently were unrelated to the occurrence of stressed syllables. There are numerous signs of rib cage or abdominal paradoxing in the data; the signs are subtle in subjects RR, KG, and VB, and obvious in RF, KS, and CW. CW's tracing reflects noticeable abdominal paradoxing as he began the task and then equal contributions of rib cage and abdomen to lung volume change as he continued. There also are indications of rib cage paradoxing among the abrupt slope changes in the data of RF and FM.

Syllable Stress Task—Supine

The data generated by the supine subjects for this task are illustrated in Figure 8–6. Lung volume initiation levels were more than 1 L above FRC in two subjects (FM and KS), and less than 1 L above FRC in the other three. At the termination level of the task, FM, VB, and CW ended at FRC; KS and KG continued below FRC. The slopes of the tracings for four subjects (KS, KG, VB, and CW) exhibit abrupt shifts in relative contributions to lung volume change consistently related to the occurrence of stressed syllables in the task. In addition, there is evidence of paradoxical motion of the abdomen among the abrupt slope changes for those four subjects and an occasional sign of rib cage paradoxing. The data for FM show slight changes in slope, which apparently were unrelated to the occurrence of stressed syllables during utterance, with evidence of abdominal paradoxing near the end of one performance.

DISCUSSION

It is of interest first to discuss the data for vital capacity maneuvers and resting tidal breathing. These provide insight into the basic respiratory capabilities of the subjects on which demands for speech were superimposed. Measured vital capacities for all subjects in the upright body position were reduced from predicted values. A measured vital capacity is not considered abnormally low, however, unless it is reduced by more than 20% of the predicted value (Comroe et al., 1962). Applying this criterion to the measured upright vital capacity data of the present subjects, the values of five were within normal limits. The values of the remaining five (asterisked in Table 8–2) were reduced markedly, ranging from 39% to 67% of predicted. When body position is shifted from upright to supine, a small change in the measured vital capacity, usually a reduction, is not unexpected (Comroe et al., 1962). Hence, for four of the subjects, supine vital capacity values varied slightly from upright in unremarkable amounts. Subject CW, however, exhibited a 52% reduction in vital capacity when shifted from upright to supine. What information do such remarkable differences convey with respect to the effect of motor neuron disease on the respiratory apparatus?

Reduction in the measured upright vital capacity from expected values has been cited often as a consequence of neuromuscular disease when the chest wall musculature is involved (Comroe et al., 1962; Gibson, Pride, Newsom Davis, and Loh, 1977; Kreitzer et al., 1978; McCredie, Lovejoy, and Kaltreider, 1962; Nakano et al., 1976; Newsom Davis, Stagg, Loh, and Casson, 1976; Stone and Keltz, 1963). The discrepancy between measured and predicted vital capacity may be attributed to fatigue, weakness, or both, in any one or all of the chest wall components. A large discrepancy between the vital capacity measured in the upright and supine positions, with the latter remarkably reduced, has been associated with diaphragmatic weakness. In the supine position, gravitational forces normally effect an inward displacement of the abdominal wall and a headward displacement of the diaphragm, which, when relaxed, may encroach on the expiratory reserve volume and alter the mechanical constraints on the chest wall. Such constraints as well as an increase in pulmonary blood volume in this position (Comroe et al., 1962) may render the supine measured vital capacity reduced slightly from upright values. If the diaphragm is weak or paralyzed, it also may be displaced headward passively during inspiration in the supine position, thus reducing the efficiency of the remaining inspiratory muscles. This imposes a limitation on the inspiratory capacity and may greatly exaggerate a normal tendency toward a reduced vital capacity when supine. This phenomenon may explain the 52% reduction in measured vital capacity for subject CW when he was shifted from upright to supine. His data resemble those reported by McCredie and colleagues (1962) and Newsom Davis, Goldman, Loh, and Casson (1976) on patients with documented diaphragm paresis or paralysis, who tended to exhibit supine vital capacities reduced by 50% or more from their upright values.

Compared to the normal resting tidal volume excursion of 0.45 to 0.60 L (Comroe et al., 1962), four of the subjects had upright resting volumes within normal limits, two fell below, and four fell above the normal range. In the supine position, one subject fell below, one within, and three above the normal range. Compared to the normal resting tidal frequency range of 11 to 14 BPM (Comroe et al., 1962), four of the upright subjects fell within the normal range, and six had abnormally high resting tidal frequencies. In the supine position, one subject fell below, one within, and three above the normal frequency range. When the resting tidal depths and frequencies are considered in terms of minute volume rates, the normal reference is 5.2 to 8.8 LPM, using normative data of Comroe and colleagues (1962), applied to the nomogram of Radford, Ferris, and Kriete (1954), and corrected for altitude. Relative to these figures, in the upright position one of the subjects fell below that range, two fell within it, and seven exceeded it. In the supine position, three of the subjects fell within the normal range, and two exceeded it.

Alterations in the depth and frequency of resting tidal breathing and changes in minute volume rate have a well-documented association with weakness of the respiratory muscles. Small resting tidal volumes and rapid tidal frequencies, such as those seen in six of the subjects upright and three supine, have been cited as characteristic of chest wall weakness, especially diaphragmatic, and accompanied by evidence of hypoventilation (Fromm et al., 1977; Gibson et al., 1977; Newsom Davis, Goldman, Loh, and Casson, 1976; Newsom Davis, Stagg, Loh, and Casson, 1976; Parhad et al., 1978) and decreased diffusing capacity (Nakano et al., 1976). High resting minute volume rates, such as those seen in seven of the subjects upright and two supine, have been associated with alveolar hyperventilation in patients with restricted chest wall excursion due to respiratory muscle weakness in motor neuron disease (Kreitzer et al., 1978) or secondary to spinal cord injury (Stone and Keltz, 1963) and resemble respiratory behavior induced experimentally by chest wall strapping in normal subjects (Gibson et al., 1977). In this context it also is appropriate to comment on the implications of orthopnea that was reported as a more or less troublesome symptom by most of the subjects. Orthopnea is the subjective sensation of breathing difficulty when supine, with or without accompanying evidence of ventilation-perfusion abnormality. It is acknowledged as a symptom in many patients with neuromuscular disease of the chest wall and may be suggestive of weakness or fatigue in any or all of the chest wall components. Because the symptom characterizes supine respiratory function, however, flaccid paresis or paralysis of the diaphragm or spastic paresis or paralysis of the abdominal wall, or both, are most often implicated owing to an exaggeration of the normal effects of the supine position on the mechanical behaviors of these two chest wall components when they are disabled by neuromuscular disease (Comroe et al., 1962; McCredie et al., 1962; Miller et al., 1957; Newsom Davis, Goldman, Loh, and Casson, 1976; Parhad et al., 1978; Stone and Keltz, 1963).

Thus far, given their tendency toward reduced vital capacities and systematic alterations in the temporal and volumetric characteristics of resting tidal breathing, accompanied by frequent reports of orthopnea, the subjects' data are consistent with a picture of chest wall muscle weakness—particularly inspiratory—presented in the literature on abnormal respiratory function in neuromuscular disease. With the preceding information in mind, consider the relative volume data for resting tidal breathing. In general, the slopes of the pathways reflect normal patterns of rib cage and abdominal contributions to volume change, the contribution of the rib cage predominating in most of the subjects upright, and the contribution of the abdomen predominating in most of the subjects supine (see Chapter 3). These normal tendencies notwithstanding, there are two unusual details in the specific configuration of the tidal breathing pathways that deserve discussion. Normal relative displacement patterns for quiet breathing usually form a single, relatively straight pathway for both inspiration and expiration (Chapter 3). Many of the quiet breathing data on the present subjects, however, exhibited unusual hooked or looped configurations. For example, most of the upright resting tidal pathways are noticeably hooked toward the Y axis at their higher volume ends where the slopes of the pathways become markedly steeper. This unusual configuration change denotes a shift to a greater rib cage contribution near the end of inspiration, with evidence of abdominal paradoxing in RF and VB, perhaps reflecting fatigue of the diaphragm's contribution to the inspiratory gesture.

The other configuration among the data for resting tidal breathing that is unusual is a looped pathway that appears on the chart of subject CW in the upright position and on the charts of all the subjects supine. CW, after his first few resting tidal breaths upright (which exhibited a hooked configuration; note the dashed line in Figure 8–5), produced a pathway that looped in a clockwise direction. The inspiratory pathway that forms the left side of the loop denotes motion of the rib cage in the inspiratory direction but motion of the abdomen in the expiratory direction. Furthermore, it should be noted that CW's neck muscles bulged visibly during each inspiration. The expiratory path of his loop denotes rib cage displacement in the expiratory direction but abdominal displacement in the inspiratory direction. This relative volume pattern and associated neck muscle activity on inspiration also were characteristic of his resting tidal breathing when supine. If these kinematic data are coupled with his vital capacity and numerical tidal breathing statistics, the picture is consistent with signs of diaphragm weakness. Specifically, his abnormally reduced upright measured vital capacity (66% of predicted); the abnormally large reduction in his supine measured vital capacity compared with his upright value (down 52%); his low resting tidal volume, high tidal frequency, and high minute volume rate; kinematic pathways that imply paradoxing of the abdominal wall during portions of both inspiration and expiration (Newsom Davis, Goldman, Loh, and Casson, 1976); and a habitual tendency to assist inspiration with neck muscle effort all suggest that his diaphragm, normally a major muscle of inspiration, was not normally active during his resting tidal inspiration in either body position.

The other looped pathways in the resting tidal breathing data were characteristic of the supine data of four subjects and followed a counterclockwise course. The inspiratory sides of the loops follow the expected pattern for this body position (see Chapter 3) but uncharacteristic of normal subjects, the expiratory pathways are displaced to the left of the inspiratory data on the charts. This leftward departure implies that the subjects used expiratory muscular forces of the rib cage and the abdomen, and perhaps more predominantly the latter, to facilitate lung volume decrease for the duration of resting tidal expiration, which is normally a predominantly passive phenomenon involving relaxation forces during its last two-thirds (see Chapter 1). Several explanations may be offered for this behavior. Because all four subjects complained of mild to moderate orthopnea, their tidal expiratory muscle efforts may represent a strategy to take active control over a usually passive process and offset the emotional discomfort of orthopneic symptoms (McCredie et al., 1962). It also is conceivable that these tidal expiratory data may reflect strategies to facilitate subsequent inspiration when the diaphragm is mildly weak and easily fatigued (Newsom Davis, Goldman, Loh, and Casson, 1976). That is, abdominal muscle efforts during tidal expiration may ensure headward displacement of the diaphragm to a position that is mechanically advantageous for its next inspiratory contraction; and relaxation of the abdominal muscles at the end of a tidal expiration may be helpful in initiating footward motion of the diaphragm during the subsequent inspiration (although this latter strategy would be more effective with the torso upright, the position for which it was reported by Newsom Davis, Goldman, Loh, and Casson (1976) and Gibson (1977).

The placement of kinematic data for conversation and reading on the relative volume charts provides information about the background torso configuration prevailing during the chest wall displacement charted. The reference point for placement was the intersection of a subject's resting tidal expiratory pathway with his FRC isovolume line.[4] In Figures 8–4 and 8–5, note that the data for conversation and reading upright tend to cluster on the charts slightly to the left of where each tidal expiration pathway intersected the FRC line. This is consistent with the normal torso configuration for speech upright, in which the rib cage tends to be larger and the abdomen smaller than their presumed relaxed configurations at the prevailing lung volume. In Figure 8–6, the data for conversation and reading supine tend to cluster on the charts slightly to the right of the tidal end-expiration points. This, too,

---

[4]The reference points for assessing appropriate placement for kinematic data on relative volume charts traditionally have been the *relaxed* configurations of the chest wall at the prevailing lung volumes (see Chapters 3 and 4). The relaxation maneuvers required to establish such reference points are tedious, however, and were not included in the protocol. Instead, it was decided to use the tidal end-expiratory level as a reference: It usually corresponds to the resting level (FRC) of the respiratory apparatus, and the point at which the tidal expiratory pathway intersects the FRC isovolume line most nearly approaches the relaxed configuration of the chest wall at that level.

is consistent with the normal torso configuration for speech supine, in which the rib cage is smaller and the abdomen larger than their presumed relaxed configurations at the prevailing lung volume. These data placements imply that the subjects had sufficient strength in their chest walls to assume a normal torso configuration for these speech activities.

Abnormalities in the data for conversation and reading include low lung volume initiation levels and abrupt changes in rib cage and abdominal contributions to lung volume change during utterance. Consider the lung volume initiation level discrepancy first. Normal speakers typically begin normally loud utterance at about twice their resting tidal depths and, depending on the linguistic load and individual phrasing styles, typically end utterance at or just above FRC (see Chapter 3). The majority of the present 10 subjects, however, failed to initiate conversation or normally loud reading at the expected lung volume level in either body position, and many initiated utterance no higher than their resting tidal end-inspiratory levels. For the loud reading, most of the subjects demonstrated that they were able to initiate speech at higher lung volumes than those at which they had read normally, as normal speakers are wont to do for loud utterance (Chapter 3). That they did so only when compelled, however, and often lapsed in their efforts before the reading passage ended, suggests that the more forceful inspirations necessary for the loud reading were effortful maneuvers that they could not perform repetitively without fatigue or discomfort. These data are consistent with the suggestion of inspiratory muscle weakness noted in other respiratory performances of these subjects.

Low lung volume levels of speech initiation can be a liability to utterance length and to the expiratory recoil they provide for utterance loudness. Furthermore, when inspiratory muscle weakness is coupled with significant expiratory muscle weakness, low levels of initiation may compromise both volume displacement and volume compression in the expiratory direction. The weak expiratory muscles of the rib cage are not stretched to an optimal mechanical advantage, and the abdomen may be a weak opposing partner to rib cage compression. This may translate to inadequate loudness for sound generation and stress contrasts as well as short breath groups in speech, not to mention ineffectual power for more strenuous chest wall activities like coughing and clearing secretions (Brooke, 1977; Fallat and Norris, 1980; Kreitzer et al., 1978). Among these possible consequences of low lung volume initiation levels in speech, only short breath groups were a noticeable sign in three of the subjects (CW, FM, and FG) at the time of this investigation. Among these three, only CW's short phrases could be attributed exclusively to chest wall weakness. (He had high laryngeal airway resistances [Smitheran and Hixon, 1981] and no perceptible signs of upper airway valving incompetence.) Subjects FM and FG, however, in addition to exhibiting signs of respiratory weakness, also demonstrated pervasive velopharyngeal incompetence during speech, forfeiting much of their expiratory flow transnasally. In their cases, both respiratory and upper airway inadequacies probably combined to reduce the pressure and flow available for speech production on any one expiration.

Before leaving this issue of the implications and liabilities of low lung volume initiation levels in speech, one other aspect deserves consideration in the interest of client management and counseling. When the kinematic data reveal signs of inspiratory muscle weakness, it would be helpful to know the extent to which the weakness is partitioned between the rib cage and diaphragm. In this investigation, only the data of CW provide enough nonspeech and speech information to support specific implication of the diaphragm as the weak inspiratory component. The apparently reduced inspiratory capabilities of many of the other subjects, although suggestive, are not so readily attributable to either inspiratory rib cage or diaphragm weakness without further information. To resolve this ambiguity, and a similar one that could arise for expiration between the rib cage and abdomen, investigators and clinicians would do well to assess the inspiratory and expiratory reserve volumes in subjects with motor neuron disease and to monitor the behavior their chest walls during tasks which compel their use of these extremes of the vital capacity.

The other abnormality of interest in the data for conversation and reading among the subjects was the appearance of unusual changes in slope along the volume displacement pathways. Comparable data for the normal chest wall manifest slope changes during utterance, although such changes tend to be gradual. Furthermore, when normal slopes change in steepness during utterance, their direction is still more or less downward and leftward on the relative volume chart indicating in-phase motion of the rib cage and abdomen in the expiratory direction (see Chapter 3). The slope data of some of the subjects were aberrant for both these characteristics. First, the slope changes were noticeably abrupt and frequent within a single breath group, indicating numerous seemingly erratic changes in rib cage and abdominal contributions to lung volume change. And second, the direction of some of the pathways after an abrupt change in slope often coursed upward and leftward on the charts, indicating paradoxical motion of the rib cage, or downward and rightward, indicating paradoxical motion of the abdomen. Four subjects exhibited these erratic pathways during conversational speech in the upright position. None of these subjects, however, or any others, exhibited such aberrations when reading at normal loudness levels upright. In the supine position, all but one of the five subjects demonstrated the unusual pathway changes in conversation, and three of the five also demonstrated them in reading at both loudness levels. Considering the performance contexts in which the aberrant slope data were observed, note that they were more or less apparent depending on the constraints of the material uttered and the body position in which the speech behavior was elicited. Yet they were not associated with any perceptible changes in utterance quality or loudness. What, then, could be the significance of these unusual but acoustically unobtrusive behaviors of the chest wall?

Pertinent to the interpretation of these data is the fact that the chest wall affected by motor neuron disease undergoes considerable neuromuscular reorganization (Brooke, 1977). Hence, the speaker with motor neuron disease must adjust his or her respiratory pump for speech with a neuromuscular system whose control properties are altered and perhaps even deficient as a result of motor neuron death, chest wall muscle atrophy, and susceptibility to fatigue. Under these circumstances, the kinematic evidence of abrupt exchanges between chest wall parts for predominance in lung volume displacement during utterance may represent rib cage-abdominal "groping" as a consequence of reduced afferent feedback for fine motor control of rib cage and abdominal coordination due to loss of proprioceptors in atrophied muscle. It also is conceivable that the trade-off between efforts of the rib cage and abdomen during utterance may be a strategy to counteract fatigue in their respective muscle groups, which has been well-documented as a troublesome symptom and noticeable sign in muscles affected by motor neuron disease (Norris, Denys, and Ü, 1980).

That the unusual slope data were more or less apparent depending on tasks and body position also may be interpreted in terms of abnormal chest wall control capabilities. In the upright body position, unusual slopes characterized the kinematic data of some subjects' conversation but not their reading. The utterance constraints imposed by the reading task may have given the subjects finite expiratory phrasing boundaries within which to organize speech breathing support strategies. Consecutive conversational utterances, on the other hand, were spontaneous and had to be grouped into expiratory gestures extemporaneously by the subjects. Of these two speech tasks, then, reading and spontaneous conversation, the unrehearsed or unmarked nature of the latter might be more likely to challenge fine motor control of the chest wall for on-line adjustments. In the supine position, the aberrant slopes were apparent not only in the conversational speech data of four of the five subjects but also in the reading data of three of the five. Furthermore, for two of these, the unusual pathway shifts during utterance were novel characteristics that did not exist in their upright data. That these unusual slope changes were more prevalent in the supine position may imply that the relatively unrehearsed nature of speech supine challenges fine motor control of the abnormal chest wall even more than speech produced upright. It also is conceivable that the respiratory load of speaking while lying supine might exaggerate a subject's orthopnea and anxiety (McCredie et al., 1962), and that speaking under such conditions might be reflected in erratic interplays between the rib cage and abdomen. Whatever their explanation, these unusual slope data and the variation in their prevalence with speech mode and body position may have important implications for the identification and management of a respiratory disorder in motor neuron disease and deserve further investigation.

Finally, this discussion would not be complete without some consideration of the tasks involving syllable repetition with alternating stress. These showed variation across subjects with respect to lung volume initiation and termination levels and unusual patterns of rib cage and abdominal contributions to lung volume change, including evidence of rib cage and abdominal paradoxing. Nevertheless, all the subjects met the task demands of the stress pattern /tɑ tɑ 'tɑ/. Hence, to the extent that a talker uses the chest wall as a major contributor to the loudness increase associated with heavy stress on every third syllable of the utterance pattern, all the subjects were able to muster the muscle forces necessary to imitate the stress pattern requested.[5] It is difficult to interpret the kinematic data for this task in relation to chest wall weakness. For example, the number of times a subject could repeat a triad on one breath varied from one to as many as 15 times and appeared to be associated with the depth of inspiration that preceded the task as well as the lung volume at which the subject chose to terminate the task. But, such level differences could be attributed to things other than neuromuscular weakness. Subjects differed in their interpretations of the instructions as well as in their abilities to follow them, even with a model to imitate. Some admittedly were inhibited about performing such a nonsense task in the presence of their spouse and strangers. Others appeared to be unwilling to push their respiratory apparatuses to inspiratory or expiratory extremes to comply with the instructions. "Unwilling" is used here not in a pejorative way but simply to convey that the weakness and fatigability that characterize muscular systems affected by motor neuron disease exert emotional as well as physical limitations on subjects' abilities to use these systems, regardless of their intentions to cooperate.

CONCLUSIONS

The numerical vital capacity and tidal breathing data obtained from the subjects of this investigation were aberrant in ways suggestive of chest wall muscle weakness, particularly in the inspiratory direction, and consistent with pulmonary function data on similar groups of subjects in the literature. The chest wall kinematic data complemented the numerical data with information about chest wall displacement during tidal breathing and speech, which also

---

[5]It was noted that the subjects also tended to make the stressed syllables higher in frequency and longer in duration, which are two other parameters that can be manipulated to create the perceptual impression of heavy stress.

suggests inspiratory muscle weakness and possibly abnormal chest wall function during utterance. It is important to consider these data in practical relation to the respiratory demands of everyday speech and the expected destruction pattern of motor neuron disease. Normal speakers in the upright body position produce conversation between 60% and 40% of the vital capacity (40% and 20% supine); this amounts to approximately 20% of the average adult male 5 L vital capacity (see Chapter 3). Thus, conversational speech normally demands and consumes only a moderate portion of the midrange lung volume. An extensive literature on respiratory function for nonspeech tasks in subjects with motor neuron disease, some of which was cited here, reports that chest wall muscle weakness and wasting, whether generalized or focal, tend first to curtail the inspiratory and expiratory extremes of the lung volume range. Thus, it might reasonably be expected that such weakness would have to be extensive in all parts of the chest wall, or selectively and profoundly destructive to one of the chest wall components, to encroach noticeably on the midvolume range of the vital capacity and compromise breathing for conversational speech. Based on the study of these 10 subjects, who differed extensively in age, history, and distribution of signs and symptoms of motor neuron disease, that expectation appears to be a valid one. To be sure, some subjects exhibited unusual patterns of rib cage and abdominal contribution to lung volume change during speech, and most subjects initiated speech tasks at low lung volumes. All, however, were still able to muster adequate volume displacement and, apparently, volume compression for the demands of conversation, in spite of signs of chest wall muscle weakness or abnormal control. Unfortunately, such signs, although subtle in most of the subjects at the time of this investigation, proved to be liabilities to their pulmonary health and harbingers of further neuromuscular deterioration.

ACKNOWLEDGMENT

The preparation of this manuscript was supported by grants from the National Institute of Neurological and Communicative Disorders and Stroke. For their interest in and cooperation with the research, Dr. Lawrence Z. Stern, neurologist, and the Muscular Dystrophy Association of Tucson, Arizona, are gratefully acknowledged.

REFERENCES

Brooke, M. (1977). *A clinician's view of neuromuscular diseases*. Baltimore: Williams & Wilkins.

Campbell, E., Agostoni, E., and Newsom Davis, J. (1970). *The respiratory muscles: Mechanics and neural control*. Philadelphia: Saunders.

Comroe, J., Jr., Forster, R., II, Dubois, A., Briscoe, W., and Carlsen, E. (1962). *The lung: Clinical physiology and pulmonary function tests*, (2nd ed.). Chicago: Year Book Medical Publishers.

Darley, F., Aronson, A., and Brown, J. (1975). *Motor speech disorders*. Philadelphia: Saunders.

Dworkin, J., Aronson, A., and Mulder, D. (1980). Tongue force in normals and dysarthic patients with amyotrophic lateral sclerosis. *Journal of Speech and Hearing Research*, 23, 828–837.

Fallat, R., and Norris, F. (1980). Respiratory problems. *In* D. Mulder (Ed.): *The diagnosis and treatment of amyotrophic lateral sclerosis*. Boston: Houghton-Mifflin.

Fromm, G., Wisdom, P., and Block, A. (1977). Amyotrophic lateral sclerosis presenting with respiratory failure. *Chest*, 71, 612–614.

Gibson, G., Pride, N., Newsom Davis, J., and Loh, L. (1977). Pulmonary mechanics in patients with respiratory muscle weakness. *American Review of Respiratory Disease*, 115, 389–395.

Keltz, H. (1965). The effect of respiratory muscle dysfunction on pulmonary function. *American Review of Respiratory Disease*, 91, 934–938.

Konno, K., and Mead, J. (1967). Measurement of the separate volume changes of rib cage and abdomen during breathing. *Journal of Applied Physiology*, 22, 407–422.

Kreitzer, S., Saunders, N., Tyler, H., and Ingram, R. (1978). Respiratory muscle function in amyotrophic lateral sclerosis. *American Review of Respiratory Disease*, 117, 437–447.

McCredie, M., Lovejoy, F., and Kaltreider, N. (1962). Pulmonary function in diaphragmatic paralysis. *Thorax*, 17, 213–217.

Mead, J., Peterson, N. Grimby, G., and Mead, J. (1967). Pulmonary ventilation measured from body surface movements. *Science*, 156, 1383–1384.

Miller, R., Mulder, D., Fowler, W., and Olsen, A. (1957). Exertional dyspnea: A primary complaint in unusual cases of progressive muscular atrophy and amyotrophic lateral sclerosis. *Annals of Internal Medicine*, 46, 119–125.

Nakano, K., Bass, H., Tyler, H., and Carmel, R. (1976). Amyotrophic lateral sclerosis: A study of pulmonary function. *Disorders of the Nervous System*, 37, 32–35.

Newsom Davis, J., Goldman, M., Loh, L., and Casson, M. (1976). Diaphragm function and alveolar hypoventilation. *Quarterly Journal of Medicine*, 45, 87–100.

Newsom Davis, J., Stagg, D., Loh, L., and Casson, M. (1976). The effects of respiratory muscle weakness on some features of the breathing pattern. *Clinical Science and Molecular Medicine*, 50, 10p–11p.

Norris, F., Denys, E., and Ü, K. (1980). Differential diagnosis of adult motor neuron diseases. *In* D. Mulder (Ed.): *The diagnosis and treatment of amyotrophic lateral sclerosis*. Boston: Houghton-Mifflin.

Parhad, I., Clark, A., Barron, K., and Staunton, S. (1978). Diaphragmatic paralysis in motor neuron disease. *Neurology*, 28, 18–22.

Radford, E., Ferris, B., and Kriete, B. (1954). Clinical use of a nomogram to estimate proper ventilation during artificial respiration. *New England Journal of Medicine*, 251, 877–884.

Smitheran, J., and Hixon, T. (1981). A clinical method for estimating laryngeal airway resistance during vowel production. *Journal of Speech and Hearing Disorders*, 46, 138–146.

Stone, D., and Keltz, H. (1963). The effect of respiratory muscle dysfunction on pulmonary function. *American Review of Respiratory Disease*, 88, 621–629.

Thompson, A., and Hixon, T. (1979). Nasal air flow during normal speech production. *Cleft Palate Journal*, 16, 412–420.

CHAPTER 9

Speech Production with Flaccid Paralysis of the Rib Cage, Diaphragm, and Abdomen

Thomas J. Hixon
Anne H. B. Putnam
John T. Sharp

T his chapter considers the breathing behavior of an adult subject with total expiratory paralysis and nearly total inspiratory paralysis as sequelae to acute paralytic poliomyelitis. Despite these deficits, this subject was able to maintain his speech skills at socially useful levels. Study of this subject is important because it provides (1) insight with regard to the human potential for restoration of a damaged system, and (2) information of use in evaluating and managing persons with abnormal speech related to poliomyelitis or other problems, such as spinal cord injury, myasthenia gravis, spinal muscular

Reprinted by permission of the publisher from the *Journal of Speech and Hearing Disorders,* *48*, pp. 315–327, © 1983, American Speech-Language-Hearing Association, Rockville, MD.

atrophy, peripheral neuropathy, and muscular dystrophy. Although new cases of poliomyelitis are rare, a wave of postpoliomyelitic motor neuron disease now is occurring among persons with a history of polio (Campbell, Williams, and Pearce, 1969; Mulder, Rosenbaum, and Layton, 1972). Hence, speech-language pathologists may be called on to serve a population with whom they rarely have been concerned during the past two decades.

THE SUBJECT

The subject, a 48-year-old man, was studied 18 years following the onset of acute paralytic poliomyelitis. His clinical signs included flaccid paralysis of the extremities and most of the torso. Physical examination and electrodiagnostic testing revealed that the muscles of his rib cage, diaphragm, and abdomen were paralyzed and markedly atrophied. He was continuously at ventilatory risk and was maintained most of the time on one of three devices—a positive-pressure respirator, a rocking bed, or a torso pneumobelt.

The subject was able to spend brief periods "free breathing." This he accomplished through two compensatory modes of breathing. One of these was based on his retention of some secondary inspiratory capability via the operation of the sternocleidomastoid, scalenus, and trapezius muscles. Using these muscles, he was able to bring about to-and-fro displacement of the rib cage in a manner that met his resting ventilation needs. Hereinafter, this mode of breathing will be referred to as neck breathing, and the muscles that effected it will be referred to as neck muscles. The subject's other compensatory mode of breathing was a form of self-generated positive-pressure breathing in which he used structures of the larynx and upper airway to pump small volumes of air into his lungs. A series of these pumping gestures inflated his lungs in a stepwise fashion above the functional residual capacity (FRC). Referred to technically as glossopharyngeal breathing, this form of breathing is colloquially termed "frog breathing" because it resembles the breathing of frogs and other amphibia that inflate their lungs by "pushing" air into them.

Of interest here are the subject's speech skills during free breathing. Untrained persons who conversed with the subject during such periods judged his speech to be normal. Three clinicians evaluated the subject's conversational speech, and five other clinicians evaluated a tape recording of the same utterances. The live speech and tape recorded samples received identical reactions—the subject's speech was judged to be fully intelligible and marked by only a few deviances. Voice quality was mildly to moderately "strained-strangled." Linguistic phrasing was moderately deviant with inspirations sometimes occurring at inappropriate points. Articulatory deviances included occasional substitutions of glottal stops for oral fricatives, shortened durations of fricatives, and intrusions of glottal stops. The subject's language and hearing were normal, and he had no abnormalities of the larynx or upper airway.

METHOD

The measurement technique was the kinematic procedure described in Chapter 3. This procedure treats the chest wall as a system composed of the rib cage and abdomen, wherein the volume displaced by each part is related linearly to anteroposterior diameter change of that part. By means of magnetometers attached to the surfaces of the rib cage and abdomen, the anteroposterior diameter changes of these parts are measured during prescribed breathing maneuvers and free-breathing activities. Data are combined in relative volume charts (rib cage versus abdomen), from which inferences are drawn concerning the muscular mechanism that prevailed during the activities studied (see Chapter 3).

Magnetometers were attached with adhesive tape. Generating coils were positioned at the midline on the anterior surface of the chest wall, one for the rib cage near the level of the nipples and one for the abdomen near the level of the navel. Sensing coils were positioned posteriorly at the midline at the same axial levels as their generator mates. Signals from the magnetometers were fed to two channels of an FM tape recorder for subsequent playback into a storage oscilloscope.

All tasks were performed as the subject lay supine with his head slightly elevated by a pillow. Tasks were of two types: breathing activities and utterances.

Breathing Activities

Four breathing activities were performed—two by an investigator and the subject jointly and two by the subject alone. Activities involving the investigator substituted for the prescribed breathing maneuvers called for in the procedure described in Chapter 3 that this subject could not perform on his own.

To obtain data on the subject's relative volume relaxation characteristic, an investigator applied slow, cyclical pressure changes to the subject's airway opening (mouth) with a positive-pressure respirator. The subject sealed his lips around a mouthpiece coupled to the respirator (he wore a noseclip) and otherwise relaxed while the respirator pumped him "up and down" in the manner of a toy balloon being inflated and deflated by internal pressure changes. The respirator was adjusted to pump the subject between FRC and 1.25 L above FRC; numerous cyclings were performed, each taking 10 sec.

To obtain data on the volume-motion relationship for each part of the subject's chest wall, an investigator shifted volume manually between the subject's abdomen and rib cage. This was done at FRC and 0.5 L above FRC. For each measurement, the subject closed his larynx while the investigator slowly pushed and released the subject's abdominal wall.

The breathing activities performed by the subject alone were his two compensatory modes of breathing—neck breathing and glossopharyngeal breathing. For the former, the subject was instructed to breathe quietly "by neck," whereas for the latter, he was instructed to inspire to various lung volume levels well above FRC, using his glossopharyngeal method.

Utterances

Utterances included two groups of activities. The first group involved four tasks of a connected speech nature wherein the subject was given the following instructions:

1. Engage in 2 min of spontaneous conversation
2. Count in a long continuous string at typical loudness
3. Read a declarative paragraph at typical loudness—the first paragraph of "The Rainbow Passage" by Fairbanks (1960)
4. Read the first few sentences of the same paragraph as in 3 above at twice normal loudness.

The second group of utterance activities included sustained vowel and syllable repetition tasks. For each task, the subject was instructed to inspire deeply, using glossopharyngeal inspiration, and then do the task on a single expiration until it could no longer be performed. Tasks included the following:

1. Sustained production of /ɑ/ at the subject's typical quality, pitch, and loudness
2. Sustained production of /ɑ/ at the subject's typical quality, pitch, and twice normal loudness
3. Sustained production of /ɑ/ at the subject's typical quality, pitch, and loudness, with intermittent abrupt emphatic stressing
4. Repetition of /hɑ/ at a rate of 2 per sec, at the subject's typical quality, pitch, and loudness.

RESULTS AND DISCUSSION

Relative Volume Charts and Their Interpretation

Figure 9–1 is an idealized relative volume chart (see Chapter 6). Volume of the rib cage is shown on the vertical axis, volume of the abdomen on the horizontal axis, and volume of the lungs on the diagonal axis. Solid lines in the figure portray pathways traced during the shifting of volume back and forth between the rib cage and abdomen at fixed lung volumes, FRC and 0.5 L above FRC. Slopes of these isovolume pathways are adjusted to show equal volume changes for equal diameter changes of the rib cage and abdomen. The dashed line in the figure portrays the relative volume relaxation characteristic traced during the cycling imposed by the respirator. Circles on this line correspond to points at FRC, 0.5 L above FRC, and 1.25 L above FRC.

As configured, the chart enables direct reading of (1) changes in lung volume—given by the distance perpendicular to the isovolume lines, (2) changes in the volumes of the rib cage and abdomen—given by the slope of any line, and (3) separate volumes of the rib cage and abdomen (i.e., chest wall configuration)—given by position along the chart axes.

The relative volume chart also can be used to infer muscular mechanism. Such inferences depend on comparisons of chest wall configuration during relaxation and free-breathing activities with departures from the relaxation characteristic on the chart reflecting some form of muscular activity. Listed below the chart in Figure 9–1 are the only options that could prevail for the present subject. The designations *left, on,* and *right* refer to positions on the chart relative to the relaxation line. Use of the chart to make inferences concerning mechanism for the present subject involves only two possibilities— data for self-generated activities must fall either to the left of the relaxation line or on it, implying that the neck muscles are either active or relaxed, respectively. When the neck muscles are active, the extent of departure to the left of the relaxation line can be taken as a first approximation of the magnitude of the inspiratory force involved.

Breathing Activities

Representative data from breathing activities are shown in Figure 9–2.

RELAXATION CHARACTERISTIC. The upper left chart in Figure 9–2 shows the relative volume relaxation characteristic obtained when the subject's breathing apparatus was driven by the respirator. Inflation and deflation pathways were superimposed. The data reveal that both the rib cage and abdomen changed volume in the same sign as did the lungs, the volume change of the rib cage exceeding that of the abdomen.

ISOVOLUME LINES. The upper right chart in Figure 9–2 repeats the subject's relaxation characteristic together with the relative volume lines obtained when his breathing apparatus was subjected to the manual shifting of volume back and forth between the rib cage and abdomen at fixed lung volumes. The pathways followed were essentially independent of the direction of volume shift and are represented by nearly closed loops, each being approximately linear. Lower and upper isopleths are at FRC and 0.5 L above FRC, respectively. The single-valued nature of the isopleths, their linearity, and their parallelism all are consistent with relative volume data obtained for normal subjects (see Chapter 3), and bear witness to the success of manually imposed isovolume maneuvers.

TIDAL BREATHING. The lower left chart in Figure 9–2 repeats the upper right chart (shown hereinafter for reference in all displays) together with the

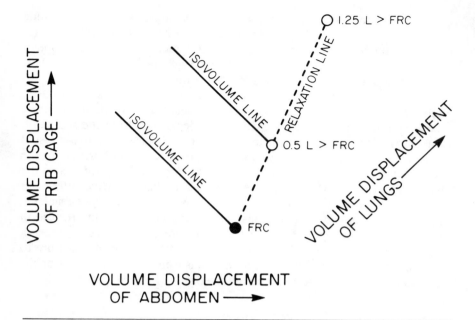

FIGURE 9-1. Idealized relative volume chart (rib cage versus abdomen) of the form used to display the data, and capsulizations of the different muscular actions that could account for positions on the chart relative to the relaxation characteristic for the subject.

relative volume data obtained during the subject's tidal breathing by neck. Inspiratory and expiratory pathways were identical. The data reveal volume excursions during tidal breathing of 0.5 L, with both the rib cage and abdomen contributing, the former substantially more than the latter. The data further reveal that the volume contributions of the abdomen were paradoxical during both inspiration and expiration, such that when the volume of the lungs

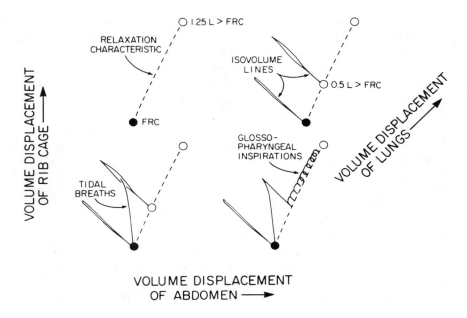

FIGURE 9-2. Relative volume charts showing representative data for breathing activities.

increased, that of the abdomen decreased, and vice versa. Specifically, each 0.5 L excursion was the result of a rib cage volume change of 0.58 L and an abdominal volume change of 0.08 L in the opposite direction [$V_{RC} + V_{AB} = V_L$; 0.58 L + (−0.08 L) = 0.5 L]. Data positioning on the chart indicates that the volume of the rib cage always was larger and the volume of the abdomen always was smaller during inspiration and expiration than were their volumes during apnea at FRC or during relaxation at the prevailing lung volume. Deformation of the chest wall to such larger rib cage volumes and smaller abdominal volumes increased with increases in lung volume and decreased with decreases in lung volume. Tidal breathing took place at a cycling rate of 12.5 BPM, temporally patterned by cycle to include an inspiratory time of 1.2 sec, an expiratory time of 1.0 sec, and an apneic time of 2.6 sec. The minute volume rate was 6.25 LPM.

The subject's effectiveness at neck breathing is shown by the values for tidal volume, breathing rate, and minute volume rate, which are essentially identical to those for average normal subjects while rest breathing (Comroe, 1965). This effectiveness was gained through temporal patterning and control mechanisms that presumably are unique to the subject.

Temporal patterning for tidal breathing was characterized by relatively short inspiration and expiration and relatively long apnea. This contrasts with tidal breathing in normal subjects, which is characterized by relatively long inspiration and expiration, and brief apnea (Comroe, 1965). On a percentage basis, inspiratory time, expiratory time, and apneic time occupied 25%, 21%, and 54% of each breathing cycle of the subject, respectively. Experimentally inexperienced normal subjects (Mead and Agostoni, 1964), those most appropriate to compare with the present subject, show proportional values for inspiratory time, expiratory time, and apneic time of 41%, 55%, and 4%, respectively. Unlike normal subjects, the present subject accomplished his inspiratory and expiratory volume excursions rapidly and then engaged in a long pause before proceeding with the next cycle. While free breathing by neck, the subject actually moved air only 46% of the time, whereas when normal subjects engage in tidal free breathing, they spend 96% of their time moving air (Mead and Agostoni, 1964).

The control mechanism for the subject's tidal breathing by neck seems relatively straightforward. During inspiration, muscles of his neck were activated to provide a continuously increasing pull on the rib cage from FRC to the tidal end-inspiratory level. This is evidenced by the increasing leftward departure of the tidal breathing line from the relaxation characteristic on the chart as inspiration deepens. This pull resulted in axial elevation and circumferential expansion of the rib cage, a decrease in pleural pressure, and circumferential expansion of the lungs. Given the paralyzed state of the diaphragm, the subject's breathing apparatus functioned as a single container in which the lowered pleural pressure was accompanied by a corresponding decrease in abdominal pressure. This latter decrease caused a hydraulic pull on the inner surface of the abdominal wall, such that it was dragged in the expiratory direction. This is indicated on the relative volume chart by the paradoxical inward displacement of the abdominal wall in association with the outward displacement of the rib cage during inspiration. During expiration, the subject gradually decreased his neck pull. This is revealed by the decrease in leftward departure of the tidal breathing line from the relaxation characteristic as expiration proceeds. Accompanying this subsiding neck pull was an axial lowering and circumferential reduction in the size of the rib cage, an increase in pleural pressure, and a circumferential decrease in the size of the lungs. Along with the pleural pressure increase involved, an equivalent increase in abdominal pressure resulted across the paralyzed diaphragm, causing the abdominal wall to move outward as the rib cage moved inward during expiration. During apnea at the end-expiratory level, the subject relaxed his neck muscles completely. This is documented on the relative volume chart in that the end-expiratory level lies on the relaxation characteristic at the exact chest wall configuration that prevailed during relaxation at FRC.

GLOSSOPHARYNGEAL BREATHING. The lower right chart in Figure 9–2 shows data obtained while the subject used glossopharyngeal breathing to inflate his breathing apparatus. For the maneuver shown, the subject inspired to 1.2 L above FRC. (He was able to inspire substantially in excess of this level and would boast facetiously that he could "bust a lung while frog breathing.") When instructed to breath glossopharyngeally, the subject invariably first inspired to 0.5 L above FRC using his neck muscles (in the manner he did for tidal breathing), closed his larynx and relaxed his neck muscles (indicated by a return to the relaxation characteristic on the chart on a course parallel to the isovolume lines), and proceeded to produce a series of stepwise increments in lung volume. For the activity charted in Figure 9–2, nine such steps were generated. On the average, individual steps involved a volume change of 75 cc and took 0.75 sec to complete. The pathway followed on the chart reveals that each step had three features—a leftward departure of the tracing from the relaxation characteristic generally parallel to the isovolume lines, an upward coursing generally parallel to the relaxation characteristic, and a rightward return of the tracing to the relaxation characteristic generally parallel to the isovolume lines.

The mechanism involved in the subject's glossopharyngeal breathing appears to be as follows. Each stepwise adjustment began with the subject's activating his neck muscles slightly. This is revealed on the chart by the small leftward departure of the tracing from the relaxation characteristic. The purpose of this neck activation probably was axial fixation of the chest wall to prevent its footward displacement in response to the positive pressure applied during the ensuing glossopharyngeal compression. (Axial fixation is analogous to holding the barrel of a syringe while plunging air into it or gripping the neck of a balloon while blowing it up.) The next event was a positive-pressure stroke, by which a mouthful of air was forced into the lungs, in a manner akin to working a small plunger. The result of such action is the lung volume increase shown by the upward coursing of the tracing. That the tracing stays to the left of the relaxation characteristic during the glossopharyngeal stroke is evidence that the neck maintained its fixation of the chest wall throughout the compressive pumping phase. The final event in each stepwise adjustment was the subject's relaxation of his neck muscles. This is revealed by the rightward return of the tracing to the relaxation characteristic.

The subject was very skilled in his use of glossopharyngeal breathing. His intact larynx and upper airway enabled him to develop a vigorous and efficient form of glossopharyngeal compensation, the success of which was apparent by the depth of inspiration he could achieve. The first documentation of glossopharyngeal breathing in an individual with profound breathing muscle impairment subsequent to acute paralytic poliomyelitis was by Dail in 1951. Since then, many occurrences have been reported, although none has been studied using the kinematic procedure employed with the present subject. Some individuals with acute paralytic poliomyelitis have learned glossopharyngeal breathing spontaneously, some have learned it by imitating other persons with whom they have been hospitalized, and some have learned it as a result of formal instruction from professional workers (Affeldt, 1964; Dail, Affeldt, and Collier, 1955; Dail, Zumwalt, and Adkins, 1955; Kelleher and Parida, 1957). Whatever the origins of the skill, investigative study (Ardran, Kelleher, and Kemp, 1959; Collier, Dail, and Affeldt, 1956; Lawes and Harries, 1957) has characterized it as having four stages: first, with the larynx closed and the mouth open, the cycle is begun by taking a mouthful and throatful of air by depressing the tongue, mandible, and larynx and widening the pharynx; second, with the larynx still closed, the mouth is closed and the velum is raised to form an airtight cavity consisting of the oral and pharyngeal segments of the upper airway; third, in conjunction with an opening of the larynx, the mandible and tongue are raised, the tongue is moved backward, and the pharynx is constricted—actions that collectively compress the air within the upper airway and force it into the trachea; and fourth, the larynx is again closed to trap the air contained within the pulmonary system—thus, the larynx functions as a one-way flow valve. The mechanism reported for the present subject, wherein his neck muscles fixed the chest wall to prevent its footward displacement during the compressive stroke, may well be a functional characteristic in other glossopharyngeal breathers. Previous investigators have not reported observations that would elucidate such neck action were it a part of the general mechanism involved.

Finally, both the temporal and volumetric aspects of the subject's glossopharyngeal breathing compare favorably with those for the 100 subjects studied by Dail, Affeldt, and Collier (1955). On the average, the subject took a glossopharyngeal breath of 75 cc every 0.75 sec, whereas the subjects studied by Dail, Affeldt, and Collier demonstrated average step magnitudes of 59 cc and average stroke durations of 0.6 sec.

Connected Speech Activities

Representative data for connected speech activities are presented in Figure 9–3. Charts show tracings typical of those for breathing cycles involving conversational speech, counting, normal reading, and loud reading. (The subject's attempt at loud reading was judged to be no different in level from his reading performance at normal loudness. Separate considerations of the two activities are maintained here, however, because the two involved different mechanisms.) Pathways followed for the different activities were essentially identical. Closed loops formed clockwise, starting and ending at the resting FRC position on the chart. Three major features characterized the pathways—first, a relatively straight line that traced the same course as that considered earlier for tidal inspiration by neck; second, a straight line that

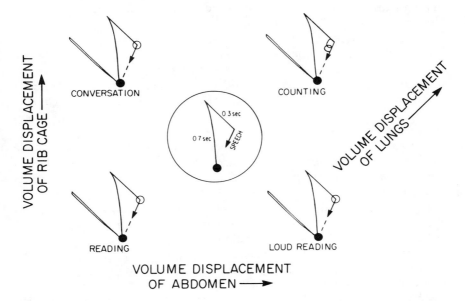

FIGURE 9-3. Relative volume charts showing representative data for connected speech activities.

traced a pathway to the relaxation characteristic on a course parallel with the isovolume lines; and, third, a relatively straight line that followed the relaxation characteristic downward on the chart back to the resting FRC position. Inspiratory segments of the tracings were executed in approximately 0.7 sec, whereas segments paralleling the isovolume lines were performed in approximately 0.3 sec. Segments that followed the relaxation characteristic varied in duration. Most of these segments involved utterance in the first one half to two thirds of their course (to the tip of each arrowhead), followed by nonspeech expiration during the latter one half to one third of their course (from the tip of each arrowhead to the FRC level). Utterance portions of the segments proceeded irregularly, sometimes beginning after a pause immediately following neck relaxation at the start of an expiratory breath group, and sometimes being interrupted by pauses once utterance had begun. Pauses were of two types, one in which progression of the segment stopped and the tracing stayed in a fixed position on the relaxation characteristic, and one in which one or more small clockwise loops were formed to the left of the relaxation characteristic on the chart. These loops were of the general form of those discussed earlier in association with glossopharyngeal inspirations. The chart for counting contains two such loops. Loops also occurred during certain pauses in conversation and normal reading, although they are not shown to avoid cluttering the charts.

When all utterance portions of the segments were considered for conversational speech, counting, reading, and loud reading, respectively, the average number of syllables generated per breath group (syllables/breath group) was 8.9, 10.8, 6.5, and 7.0; the average volume of air expended per syllable (cc/syllable) was 19.6, 20.9, 33.4, and 39.3; and the average flow (cc/sec)—determined from average volume expenditure and average breath group duration—was 98.9, 102.0, 95.6, and 153.0.

Recall that the speech of the subject was judged to be fully intelligible and marked by only a few deviances. These observations point to the subject's having compensated effectively in the face of profound biomechanical deficits in the breathing apparatus. The control mechanism involved appears to be elucidated by the data, is unique, and includes compensatory adjustments in the breathing apparatus, and in the larynx and upper airway, in joint biomechanical and linguistic adaptations.

Each breathing cycle for connected speech was begun with a neck inspiration to the subject's usual (postmorbid) tidal end-inspiratory level. This is revealed on the relative volume charts by the straight-line segments that trace pathways identical to those generated for tidal inspiration by neck (compare data in Fig. 9–2 and Fig. 9–3). Once the end-inspiratory level was attained, the subject closed his larynx and relaxed his neck muscles completely. Evidence of this on the charts is the rightward return of the data tracings to the relaxation characteristic along a course that parallels the isovolume lines. In the course of inspiring with his neck, the subject stretched his breathing apparatus and stored energy in it, as a coil spring might be stretched, which, when deformed further and further from its resting position, generates greater and greater recoil force. Having "cocked" his "breathing spring" with his neck muscles, the subject made himself capable of generating speech on the ensuing expiration, during which he could release the expiratory energy he had stored.

It is relevant that the duration of inspiration was quite different for the subject's tidal free breathing and connected speech breathing. The former took 1.2 sec to perform, while the latter took only 0.7 sec. A shorter inspiration for speech breathing than for tidal breathing is consistent with data for normal subjects (see Chapter 3 and Horii and Cooke, 1978). In Chapter 4 it is suggested that running conversational speech constitutes a circumstance in which the speaker desires to transmit information in as continuous a fashion as possible. The inspiratory refills required in running speech are undesirable and in a linguistic sense represent inherent performance constraints. It is reasonable, therefore, that speakers would design their chest wall control strategies to minimize the durations of such interruptions and thereby facilitate the continued transmission of information. Clearly, such a strategy was adopted by the present subject, even within the confines of his breathing impairment.

His success in this endeavor is reflected in the abruptness of his neck inspirations, which, being 0.7 sec, come remarkably close to the average 0.6 sec value for inspirations in the connected speech of normal adult subjects (Horii and Cooke, 1978).

During the expiratory side of the subject's speech breathing cycle, control was vested almost entirely in laryngeal and upper airway metering of the air stream provided by the release of stored expiratory energy. This is documented on the relative volume charts by the fact that, during speech performance, data tracings follow the relaxation characteristic downward, meaning that no muscular force (i.e., no neck muscle force) was operating. Restriction of speech during only the first one half to two thirds of the course of each expiratory excursion presumably was dictated by the reduction in recoil force to a magnitude insufficient to drive the larynx and upper airway (Hixon and Abbs, 1980). At this point, the subject opened his larynx and allowed the expiratory excursion to be completed passively. This was revealed by a quick return to the resting FRC position on the chart along a course that followed the relaxation characteristic downward. Some stoppages immediately before and during utterance segments were related to fixation of the breathing apparatus by breath holding at the larynx. Such an interpretation is consistent with the maintenance of the prevailing lung volume without departure of the tracing from the relaxation characteristic on the chart. Other stoppages immediately before and during utterance segments were related to the generation of quick glossopharyngeal inspirations (the small clockwise loops mentioned earlier) and represent the only moments during which the larynx and upper airway were not solely in control. These quick inspirations served unobtrusively to "cock" the breathing apparatus further before initiation of the breath group or to recock it slightly at times during the course of the breath group. Mechanically, these miniature inspirations achieved two things: first, they stretched or restretched the apparatus (increased lung volume) and, therefore, increased the expiratory recoil force; and second, they extended the potential for utterance continuation without having to pause for a breathing refill via neck drive. Thus, during connected speech activities, the subject used both negative- and positive-pressure breathing forms—external neck pull to inflate his breathing apparatus during the inspiratory phase of the breathing cycle and internal glossopharyngeal pumping to inflate the apparatus during the expiratory phase of the cycle.

The manner in which neck breathing and glossopharyngeal breathing were combined in the subject's connected speech is illustrated in Table 9–1. There transcripts are shown for performances of the four activities studied: conversation, counting, reading, and loud reading. Each line in the transcripts was performed on a separate neck breath, whereas the circles above each line indicate when glossopharyngeal inspirations were employed. Ellipses designate noticeable pauses. Table 9–1 reveals that glossopharyngeal inspirations

Table 9-1. *Transcriptions for the Running Speech Activities Studied: Conversation, Counting, Reading, and Loud Reading*

Conversation

°°Well, I ... uh ... °like to talk about my fam'lies.
°I have a wonderful family.
°I have two children and a wife.
My boy just got married this summer ...
June third.
°An ... uh ... °both him and his wife°moved in this area.
So he'll be a tremendous help to me.
Be able to get home on weekends an ...
°Fact, I was invited out
°To dinner last night°to his house ...
For a spaghetti dinner which I enjoyed very much.
    (Are you froggy breathing at all now?)
°No, just with my neck muscles.

Counting

One, two, three, four
°Five, six, °seven, °eight, °nine, °ten
°Eleven, °twelve, °thirteen, °fourteen, fifteen, °sixteen, °seventeen, °eighteen
Nineteen, °twenty, °twenty-one, °twenty-two, °twenty-three, °twenty-four.

Reading

°When
°The sunlight strikes°°°rain°drops in the air, °they act like a
°Prism and
°Form a rainbow.
°The rainbow is a
°Division
Of white light into many beautiful colors.
°These take the shape
Of a long round,
Arch,
°With it°path high°above
°And it°two ends apparently°beyond the°°horizon?
    (I don't know where these glasses are.)
There is,
According to the legend,
°A boiling pot of gold
At the end ... °People look, but°°no one ever finds it.
°When a man looks°for°something beyond his reach,
His friends say°be ...
He is looking
°For a pot of gold at the end of the rainbow.

(continued)

Table 9-1. *(continued)*

Loud Reading (Paragraph read only partially)

When the sunlight strikes raindrops in the air, they act like a pri . . .
Prism and form
A rainbow.
The rainbow
Is a division of white light
Into many beautiful colors.

Each line was produced on a separate neck breath. Circles above the lines indicate moments when glossopharyngeal inspiration was used. Ellipses designate noticeable pauses.

occurred both between words and within them (e.g., "strikes°°°rain°drops"). Note that during conversation an investigator asked the subject, "Are you froggy breathing at all now?" and the subject replied, "°No, just with my neck muscles." Not only had the subject been using glossopharyngeal inspiration frequently, although he denied it, but he even used it during his negative response to the inquiry about its use. Note in the transcript for the counting activity that the subject breathed glossopharyngeally before most of the numbers spoken. This strategy enabled him to remain at a relatively constant lung volume during the task by quickly recocking the expiratory spring to resupply the volume expended during utterance of the preceding number. Accordingly, the subject was able to produce relatively long strings of numbers of relatively equal loudness on single neck breaths. Note finally in Table 9-1 that glossopharyngeal inspirations were not used during the subject's attempt to read at twice normal loudness. Rapid depletion of the air supply may have been more than could be offset economically through glossopharyngeal inspirations.

The control of expiratory function by laryngeal and upper airway adjustments downstream of the breathing apparatus is analogous to controlling the expenditure of potential energy in an inflated toy balloon by regulating the flow of air from its neck. The manner in which this was accomplished is an important feature of the compensatory mechanism adopted for connected speech performance by the subject. Specifically, the subject demonstrated behaviors that were biomechanically and linguistically frugal with his air supply. Biomechanical frugality is revealed in data on the average number of syllables per breath group, average volume expended per syllable, and average flow per breath group. The subject's average syllables/breath group values of 8.9, 10.8, 6.5, and 7.0, although less than the dozen or more syllables/breath group typical of normal subjects (see Chapter 5), are viewed as relatively high. At the same time, the average volume expended per syllable by the subject involved cc/syllable values of 19.6, 20.9, 33.4, and 39.3, which, when compared with the 42.0 cc/syllable value reported for normal subjects by Horii and Cooke (1978), is considered relatively low. Further, the subject's cc/sec values of 98.9, 102.0, 95.6, and 153.0 are well on the low side of average flow per breath group values characteristic of connected speech activities produced by normal subjects, a suitable comparison being the 167.9 cc/sec value obtained for normal subjects reading at normal loudness by Horii and Cooke (1978). When syllables per breath group, volume per syllable, and flow per breath group values are considered collectively, the functional interpretation is that the subject valved the airstream more efficiently than usually is the case for normal individuals. This picture is consistent with the strained-strangled voice quality noted for the subject and may be a reflection of his attempt to meter the airstream in a more-efficient-than-normal manner by "tightening down" the laryngeal valve.

Frugality at the linguistic level is inferred from the nature of the articulatory adjustments made by the subject in his connected speech activities. These included programming adjustments in the larynx and upper airway that used less of the available air supply than would be consumed by normal subjects during similar types of utterances. For example, the subject's use of glottal stops as substitutes for oral fricatives, his shortening of fricative durations, and his intrusive use of glottal stops can be interpreted as linguistic program modifications to conserve air. Collectively, these adjustments decreased the influence of high flow activities by using lower flow alternatives in their place.

Finally, the subject was unsuccessful in his attempt to produce speech at twice normal loudness. That he attempted to make adjustments to do so is indicated by the fact that he generated substantially different average volumes per syllable (33.4 cc/syllable and 39.3 cc/syllable) and average flows per breath group (95.6 cc/sec and 153.0 cc/sec) when normal and loud efforts were involved. The subject's attempt to produce speech at twice normal loudness was carried out through exactly the same lung volume range as normal loudness utterance. Because identical expiratory recoil forces were available to him at corresponding lung volumes, the volume expenditure and flow differences noted had to be related to differences in the metering function of his downstream subsystems, presumably the larynx being the most important. Increased air expenditure per syllable and increased average flow per breath group in the face of identical driving pressures indicate that the average resistance to expiratory drive was lower for the subject's attempt to produce speech of twice normal loudness than for his generation of speech of normal loudness. It is somewhat surprising that he did not prepare for attempts to produce loud speech by inspiring to a deeper level with his neck muscles. (He was able to inspire to 0.75 L above FRC by neck.) This would have afforded him the opportunity of taking advantage of the greater expiratory recoil forces available at higher lung volumes. It may have been, however, that the increased recoil pressure gained between his usual tidal end-inspiratory level of 0.5 L and his inspiratory capacity level of 0.75 L was not enough to make a significant difference in loudness and thus warrant the additional major expenditure in neck effort that would have been required to cock the breathing apparatus more extensively.

Sustained Vowel and Syllable Repetition Activities

Representative data for sustained vowel and syllable repetition activities are presented in Figure 9–4. Only the expiratory segments of the breathing cycles are displayed. Each activity was initiated from 1 L or more above FRC and traced the relaxation characteristic downward on the chart. Activities terminated at lung volumes near 0.25 L above FRC. The subject's attempts to perform the activities were successful only for the sustained production of /ɑ/ at normal loudness. Attempts to produce /ɑ/ at twice normal loudness did not result in a loudness greater than that for the vowels sustained at the subject's normal level. The subject's attempts to produce /ɑ/ so as to simulate emphatic stressing yielded no stress changes. Rather, he closed the larynx during stress attempts and generated the series [ɑːʔ|ɑːʔ|ɑːʔ| . . . .]. Attempts

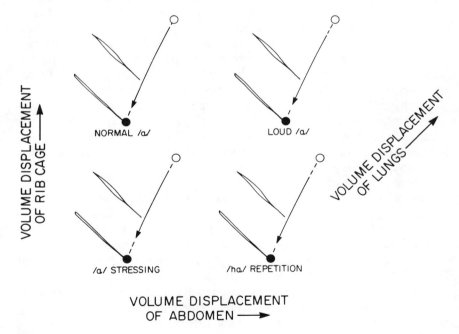

FIGURE 9–4. Relative volume charts showing representative data for sustained vowel and syllable repetition activities.

to repeat /hɑ/ were unsuccessful in that the subject could not produce the glottal fricative /h/ without losing large quantities of air. His sole means of preventing this devastating loss, laryngeal closure, was at odds with the open larynx required for /h/ generation. In his attempt at the task, the subject produced a glottal stop in place of the glottal fricative and terminated each syllable with a glottal stop. The result was the series [ʔɑʔ|ʔɑʔ|ʔɑʔ| . . . .].

Average flow for each activity was determined by dividing the volume excursion involved by the time elapsed during the excursion. Values for normal /ɑ/, loud /ɑ/, /ɑ/ stressing, and /hɑ/ repetition were 78.6 cc/sec, 112.5 cc/sec, 71.4 cc/sec, and 40.9 cc/sec, respectively. All activities were performed with a strained-strangled voice quality.

The general mechanism involved for the sustained vowel and syllable repetition activities appears to be as follows. After attainment of the pre-utterance end-inspiratory level, the subject closed his larynx and relaxed his neck muscles completely. This was revealed on the relative volume chart by a rightward return of the tracing to the relaxation characteristic and a brief maintenance of the prevailing lung volume. Thereafter, the airtight laryngeal seal was broken and utterance ensued under sole control of the larynx, drive being provided by expiratory energy that had been stored during the earlier inspiratory effort. Evidence of solely laryngeal control, in the absence of neck muscle activity, is contained in the fact that, during the course of utterances, the data tracings followed the relaxation characteristic downward on the chart. Utterances were terminated somewhat above the FRC level, presumably because the expiratory recoil force had reduced to a magnitude insufficient to drive the larynx. Thereupon, the subject opened his larynx and expired passively to FRC, evidenced by a rapid return to that level along the relaxation characteristic. That laryngeal valving varied from one activity to another is revealed in the different average flows manifested for the activities, there being a threefold difference, for example, between the average flow for the attempted loud production of /ɑ/ and the attempted serial repetition of /hɑ/. For the single activity the subject was able to perform as prescribed—the sustained utterance of /ɑ/ at normal loudness—the average flow from the breathing apparatus was 78.6 cc/sec. This value is well below the 100 cc/sec or more that would be expected for the performance of this activity by normal subjects (see Chapter 3). A relatively low flow coupled with the subject's strained-strangled voice quality suggests a compensatory attempt on his part to valve the airstream frugally with the larynx. Although the subject was unable to compensate successfully under three of the four utterance activities involved, it should be realized that the activities on which he failed are among the most taxing that might be imposed on the breathing apparatus.

Finally, the subject's unsuccessful attempt to produce a sustained vowel at greater than normal loudness warrants comment. It is clear that the subject attempted to adjust his performances between the normal /ɑ/ and loud /ɑ/

activities. This is shown by the substantial difference in average flow between the two (78.6 cc/sec versus 112.5 cc/sec). Because the two activities were performed through the same lung volume range, the expiratory recoil force available during their generation was identical. Accordingly, differences between the two flows must be attributed to differences in downstream valving of the breathing output. There seems no plausible explanation other than that the larynx adjusted its metering action differently for the two vowel utterances, airway resistance being substantially lower for the attempt at loud utterance than for the normal-loudness utterance. Resistance offered by the larynx generally increases with loudness increases in normal subjects (Isshiki, 1964; Kunze, 1962) in contrast to the decrease in resistance noted for attempted loudness increase for the present subject.

CONCLUSIONS

The present data appear to have implications for (1) understanding the human potential for developing restorative mechanism in the face of profound functional disability, and (2) improving the clinical evaluation and management of other individuals with neuromuscular dysfunction of the breathing apparatus.

The Human Potential for Functional Restoration

The subject's disease left him confronted with a muscularly powerless and functionally inert breathing apparatus. From this predicament, he was able to develop two new functional systems—neck breathing and glossopharyngeal breathing—for use in free breathing, and he was able to combine features of these two with other biomechanical and linguistic adaptations into still another functional system for speech production. By any measure, the subject's compensatory behaviors for neck breathing, glossopharyngeal breathing, and speech breathing must be considered remarkable. These accomplishments bear strong witness to the human restorative potential in response to damage to the breathing apparatus in both its ventilatory and speech communication functions. It seems appropriate to view the subject's breathing behaviors from a perspective that encompasses the concepts of Pavlov-Luria-Anokhin concerning the potential behaviors of functional systems (Hatfield, 1981). Briefly, such a conceptualization considers a functional system to comprise a group of interconnected acts that are united dynamically in the performance of a given task. Such systems are highly plastic to the extent that the initial and final links of a system—for example, the intention of its acts and the realization of that intention—remain intact, whereas the intermediate steps required to achieve a given function can be changed within very wide limits.

Implicit in such a conceptualization is the possibility of recreating a functional system when components have been impaired or destroyed. As such, the conditions of compensation displayed by the present subject demonstrate attempts to recreate functional systems for the breathing apparatus in its ventilatory functions and for use of the apparatus in speech breathing.

The subject improvised relatively well with very little that even remotely resembled his premorbid capabilities. Rather than surrender to inertness, he used intricate and resourceful compensations to perform familiar tasks by new methods. A colloquial analogue to these compensatory functions may be the adaptive control that occurs when the "proficient violinist breaks a string during a recital but continues without interruption by reprogramming the usual fingering, playing the required notes on different strings" (Wolff, 1981). In this case, the motor idea controlling the performance does not dictate a fixed relation between notes and finger movements. Rather, it enables the generation of functionally equivalent finger sequences that preserve the musical intent.

The time course of adaptive control can provide insight with regard to inbuilt aspects of restorative function. On this point, it seems relevant to document some results of interviews with approximately three dozen individuals with severe to profound breathing impairment resulting from flaccid paresis related to spinal cord injury. Nearly all of those interviewed had recollections of behaviors that occurred at the time of injury or shortly thereafter that might be interpreted as signs or symptoms of spontaneous adaptive reorganization. Common reports were that noticeable changes occurred in the depth of breathing or in its patterning in torso motions—all of which seemed to be automatic. Other common reports were that speech was readily produced immediately following injury, even though certain individuals were profoundly impaired. For some individuals, expiratory muscles that had been used routinely for speech were functionally inert, and the spontaneous development of novel compensatory muscular activities appeared to be the only explanation that could account for continuing abilities to produce acceptable speech. Spontaneous adaptive control in the normal speech apparatus is well documented (see Chapter 3 and Hughes and Abbs, 1976; MacNeilage, 1970; Netsell, Kent, and Abbs, 1980). That normal speakers do not have to "learn" to make adaptations for mechanical intrusions to their speech apparatus appears to argue that the correction processes involved are a normal and inbuilt aspect of speech control. Furthermore, that such correction processes would extend to the damaged functional system seems reasonable. Although the centers of origin and the processes involved in compensation remain largely unknown, it seems clear that the human breathing apparatus has an astounding flexibility to accommodate automatically to a broad spectrum of conditions that would otherwise significantly impair function.

Clinical Evaluation and Management Concerns

The subject's compensatory behaviors suggest several considerations with regard to clinical evaluation and management of other individuals with neuromuscularly based speech breathing abnormalities.

It is obvious from the present data that neck breathing is a viable compensatory mechanism. The extent to which such a mechanism might be used in other individuals with breathing dysfunction related to paresis or paralysis of the muscles of the chest wall and with adequate neck muscle function seems promising. For example, individuals with progressive spinal motor neuron deterioration and its consequence of chest wall muscle paresis (see Chapter 8) might well be encouraged to develop compensatory neck breathing in anticipation of advanced stages of their disease. This, in fact, has been done to foster the gradual development of such a compensatory mechanism in an individual with amyotrophic lateral sclerosis. During the course of the weakening of the inspiratory muscles of the chest wall, a gradual increase in inspiratory neck muscle drive became apparent visually in increased axial elevation of the upper rib cage and prominent neck muscle activity. Experience with this individual suggests that it probably is most advantageous to begin training programs for neck breathing once the signs of chest wall muscle paresis suggest moderate levels of dysfunction. This encourages a gradual transfer of prime mover function to the neck muscles from the inspiratory muscles of the chest wall as the latter decline in force-generating potential with disease.

It also is obvious from the present data that glossopharyngeal breathing is an effective compensatory mechanism. There may be other individuals with chest wall muscle paresis or paralysis who could benefit greatly from learning to inspire glossopharyngeally during connected speech. Given the ease and the unobtrusiveness with which the present subject used glossopharyngeal inspirations in his speech, it would not be surprising to find that other individuals who have learned glossopharyngeal breathing for other purposes are incorporating it advantageously in their motor programs for speech. Since studying the present subject, two other individuals have been identified who use glossopharyngeal inspirations in their connected speech production. It may well be that such inspirations, because of their quickness and subtleness, go undetected by all but the most astute observers of speech in persons with chest wall muscle dysfunction, and their detection may only be ensured when suitable physiological monitoring is accomplished on the breathing apparatus. Whatever the case may be, it seems clear that glossopharyngeal inspiration is a powerful mechanism for the facilitation of connected speech production in persons with severe or profound chest wall muscle dysfunction. Encouraging aspects of the mechanism are that it is simple to teach and relatively inconspicuous visually and acoustically in the speech product that ensues.

Although proven programs of instruction for glossopharyngeal breathing are available (Dail, Zumwalt, and Adkins, 1955), success cannot be expected for all individuals. Those with impairment of bulbar musculature (i.e., the musculature of the larynx and upper airway) may be unable to muster the strength or coordination needed to inflate the breathing apparatus by positive pressure. There also are medical concerns, because glossopharyngeal breathing may have undesirable effects on certain individuals. The prolonged inspiratory phase of multistepped glossopharyngeal breathing represents intermittent positive-pressure breathing in its worst form (Collier et al., 1956). The heightened intrathoracic pressure associated with such breathing decreases the gradient of venous return to the chest, and cardiac output may decrease significantly. Collier and colleagues (1956) have suggested that glossopharyngeal breathing is "contraindicated in individuals without normal vasomotor reflexes and . . . the mean tracheal pressure should be kept as low as possible" (p. 583). The general medical wisdom seems to be that the breathing method is safe for most individuals if the tidal volume is kept below 1 L and the breathing time is kept to short intervals. Thus, in the case of the incorporation of glossopharyngeal breathing into connected speech in the manner of the present subject, medical concerns are nil. If the desire might be to increase an inspiratory capacity to levels that would enable an individual to extend the length of breath groups by starting at high lung volumes, however, medical concerns may become relevant. The best advice to the speech-language pathologist who envisions potential gains for a client through the use of glossopharyngeal breathing is to consult a physician well versed in pulmonary function and obtain medical clearance before initiating a program of training.

The downstream metering strategies adopted by the present subject centered on air conservation by the larynx and upper airway and were an important part of his utterance compensations. Given their success, it would seem that the management of aeromechanical valving efficiency should be considered a high priority concern for persons with breathing impairment related to significant muscular paresis or paralysis. Successful management along such lines has the advantages of prolonging breath groups, reducing the number of breaks for inspiratory refills, and maintaining the breathing apparatus at lung volume levels at which the expiratory recoil force is adequate for conversational speech purposes. Experience in attempting to teach such compensations to other individuals with a wide variety of neuromuscular impairments of the breathing apparatus is that they are best accomplished through programs involving a mixture of standard behavioral methods and flow biofeedback instrumentation arranged to enable the individual to gain an awareness of air expenditure during utterance and during pauses between utterances (see Chapters 2 and 5).

The potential for making significant compensatory adjustments at the laryngeal level is great because of the structure's strategic location as the initial outlet valve of the pulmonary system. It is not surprising, therefore, that the present subject found it profitable to modify his laryngeal behavior to (1) accommodate breath holding without chest wall muscle participation, and (2) reduce air consumption during voicing. It is relevant, with regard to the latter, to consider the significance of the mildly to moderately strained-strangled voice quality the subject demonstrated. It would appear that this quality was related directly to his efforts to reduce the rate at which air left his lungs during voicing. That is, this quality was associated with the subject's presumably "greater-than-normal" laryngeal opposition to expiratory driving pressure in his effort to use efficiently his limited air supply. Relevant to this apparent physiological-perceptual linkage may be other experiences in studying individuals with flaccid paresis of the breathing apparatus subsequent to spinal cord injury. Many of these individuals likewise present a strained-strangled voice quality that is more severe than would be expected in the absence of neurogenic laryngeal signs. Based on this experience, it seems reasonable to consider the perceptual sign of strained-strangled voice quality in the presence of major breathing impairment for speech to be a reflection of the attempts of some disabled individuals to compensate physiologically with "tighter-than-normal" valving efforts by the larynx. The main task for the clinician attempting to treat a strained-strangled voice in a person with significant chest wall muscle involvement is to determine whether the basis for the sign is functional-compensatory or neurogenic. That is, the question must be answered as to whether the voice quality is a manifestation of a functionally intended laryngeal adjustment that is a by-product of aeromechanical compensation or whether it is a laryngeal manifestation of a disease process that is co-affecting both the breathing apparatus and the laryngeal apparatus. If the former, it would not need clinical attention, unless it was judged that laryngeal misuse and its consequences for the potential development of laryngeal pathology was of concern. Without such consequences, the clinician should simply view the quality of the client's voice as something to accept in exchange for longer breath groups and more fluent speech production. To attempt to normalize voice quality in a client using such a compensatory mechanism would be counter productive, because normalization would lead to an increase in the rate of expenditure of the available air supply.

The potential for compensatory adjustments at the upper airway level carries with it a wider range of possibilities than does the potential at the larynx, because the upper airway incorporates multiple valving sites and is involved more importantly in the execution of the phonetic program. It is reasonable, therefore, that the present subject took advantage of modifications in upper airway valving efficiency and in selected aspects of his phonetic program. It seems relevant to note that the subject's modifications tended to concentrate on valving and program changes for phone types that are heavy consumers of aeromechanical energy. For example, fricative durations were shortened, stops were substituted for fricatives, and stops were used intrusively at times when flow might normally prevail. Upper airway valving adjustments and adjustments in phonetic program have been observed in other individuals with paresis of the breathing apparatus, but never to such a major extent as in the present subject. Such extensive adjustments on his part can be appreciated within the articulatory compensation framework suggested by Hardy (1961) for persons with neuromuscular involvement of the upper airway. It is Hardy's contention that a reduced vital capacity alone will not result in a speech abnormality if downstream valving is made to be more efficient than normal to compensate for the smaller than normal air supply. The present subject's vital capacity was reduced by 86% of its predicted value (0.75 L for 5.3 L), and he performed connected speech over a volume range of only 0.25 L (one half of his tidal free-breathing volume by neck). Despite the fact that he used only about 5% of his predicted vital capacity for speech, he was still able to perform remarkably well. Hardy's belief that a reduced vital capacity can be compensated for by efficient downstream valving with the articulatory apparatus would appear to be substantiated by the present data, which also illustrate the extent to which such compensations can pervade the speech act. Embedded within this conclusion is the important notion of interdependence of function among various speech apparatus subsystems. In both this example of upper airway adjustment and the previous one of laryngeal adjustment, it is clear that other subsystems figuratively came to the rescue of the impaired breathing subsystem.

Finally, there is a powerful clinical implication in the manner in which the present subject gained restorative function for speech purposes. His neck breathing developed spontaneously following the onset of his disease, and sometime later (several months by the subject's account) he was taught glossopharyngeal breathing. It seems important to note that the subject was never instructed to combine glossopharyngeal breathing and neck breathing for speech activities. Therefore, it must be presumed that sometime after he learned to breathe glossopharyngeally, he began to incorporate this skill into the breathing strategy he had acquired spontaneously. The subject denied any original conscious intent to include glossopharyngeal breathing in his connected speech performances. His report, plus the observation that he seemingly was unaware that he used glossopharyngeal breathing during speech, point to the inclusion of a breathing form in an activity without conscious awareness of that form by the subject. This may be an example of how an act that has been learned purposefully can be included unconsciously within the performance of another, more elaborate goal-directed act. This observation for speech breathing may be similar to those made for other motor systems by Grillner (1982), in which already learned behaviors are incorporated into functional groupings that form new, more elaborate behaviors. The clinician should be aware that some already-learned behaviors might be combined with others to benefit the client. An obvious goal would be to work toward automating appropriate behavioral combinations. The notions just considered may be extended to more than just the teaching of new or better breathing control strategies when compensations are called for following debilitating disease. Both laryngeal and upper airway functions should be viewed from a similar perspective when it comes to rehabilitation processes and procedures.

ACKNOWLEDGMENT

The preparation of this manuscript was supported by grants from the National Institute of Neurological and Communicative Disorders and Stroke. At the time of data collection, the first author was Visiting Researcher in Pulmonary Medicine, Veterans Administration Medical Center, Hines, Illinois.

REFERENCES

Affeldt, J. (1964). Neuromotor paralysis. *In* W. Fenn and H. Rahn (Eds.): *Handbook of physiology. Respiration II, Sect. 3.* Washington, DC: American Physiological Society.

Ardran, G., Kelleher, W., and Kemp, F. (1959). Cineradiographic studies of glossopharyngeal breathing. *British Journal of Radiology, 32,* 322–328.

Campbell, A., Williams, E., and Pearce, J. (1969). Late motor neuron degeneration following poliomyelitis. *Neurology, 19,* 1101–1106.

Collier, C., Dail, C., and Affeldt, J. (1956). Mechanics of glossopharyngeal breathing. *Journal of Applied Physiology, 8,* 580–585.

Comroe, J., Jr. (1965). *Physiology of respiration.* Chicago: Year Book Medical Publishers.

Dail, C. (1951). Glossopharyngeal breathing by paralyzed patients: Preliminary report. *California Medicine, 75,* 217–218.

Dail, C., Affeldt, J., and Collier, C. (1955). Clinical aspects of glossopharyngeal breathing: Report of use by one hundred postpoliomyelitic patients. *Jour-nal of the American Medical Association, 158,* 445–449.

Dail, C., Zumwalt, M., and Adkins, H. (1955). *A manual of instruction for glossopharyngeal breathing.* New York: National Foundation for Infantile Paralysis.

Fairbanks, G. (1956). *Voice and articulation drillbook* (2nd ed.). New York: Harper and Row.

Grillner, S. (1982). Possible analogies in the control of innate motor acts and the production of sound in speech. *In* S. Grillner, B. Lindblom, J. Lubker, and A. Perrson (Eds.): *Speech motor control.* Oxford: Pergamon Press.

Hardy, J. (1961). *A study of pulmonary function in children with cerebral palsy.* Doctoral Dissertation, University of Iowa.

Hatfield, F. (1981). Analysis and remediation of aphasia in the USSR: The contribution of A. R. Luria. *Journal of Speech and Hearing Disorders, 46,* 338–347.

Hixon, T., and Abbs, J. (1980). Normal speech production. *In* T. Hixon, L. Shriberg, and J. Saxman (Eds.):

Introduction to communication disorders. Englewood Cliffs, NJ: Prentice-Hall.

Horii, Y., and Cooke, P. (1978). Some airflow, volume, and duration characteristics of oral reading. *Journal of Speech and Hearing Research*, 21, 470–481.

Hughes, O., and Abbs, J. (1976). Labial-mandibular coordination in the production of speech. Implications for the operation of motor equivalence. *Phonetica*, 33, 199–221.

Isshiki, N. (1964). Regulatory mechanism of voice intensity variation. *Journal of Speech and Hearing Research*, 7, 17–29.

Kelleher, W., and Parida, R. (1957). Glossopharyngeal breathing: Its value in respiratory muscle paralysis of poliomyelitis. *British Medical Journal*, 5047, 740–743.

Kunze, L. (1962). *An investigation of the changes in subglottal air pressure and rate of air flow accompanying changes in fundamental frequency, intensity, vowels, and voice registers in adult male speakers*. Doctoral Dissertation, University of Iowa.

Lawes, W., and Harries, J. (1957). Spirographic studies in glossopharyngeal breathing. *British Medical Journal*, 5055, 1205–1206.

MacNeilage, P. (1970). Motor control of serial ordering of speech. *Psychological Review*, 77, 182–196.

Mead, J., and Agostoni, E. (1964). Dynamics of breathing. *In* W. Fenn and H. Rahn (Eds.): *Handbook of physiology. Respiration 1, Sect. 3*. Washington, DC: American Physiological Society.

Mulder, D., Rosenbaum, R., and Layton, D. (1972). Late progression of poliomyelitis or forme fruste amyotrophic lateral sclerosis? *Mayo Clinic Proceedings*, 47, 756–761.

Netsell, R., Kent, R., and Abbs, J. (1980). *The organization and reorganization of speech movements*. Paper presented at the Society for Neuroscience, Cincinnati.

Wolff, P. (1981). Theoretical issues in the development of motor skills. *Developmental disabilities in preschool children*. Chicago: Spectrum Publications.

CHAPTER 10

Respiratory Kinematics in Classical (Opera) Singers

Peter J. Watson
Thomas J. Hixon

S inging is a complex biomechanical process. This process is unitary, but often it is conceptualized as involving respiratory, laryngeal, velopharyn-geal-nasal, and oral components of function. A rich folklore surrounds singing, and there are many opinions about the process among teachers of singing and singers. Unfortunately, there have been few investigations of the biomechanical bases of singing.

The investigation reported in this chapter applied modern techniques to the study of respiratory function for speaking and singing in a group of highly trained singers. Classical singers, those trained to perform operatic, song, and oratoric literatures, were chosen for study. Such singers receive more formal training than other types of singers, and it is around their art that the most passionate and expanded controversies have developed concerning the use

Reprinted by permission of the publisher from the *Journal of Speech and Hearing Research*, *28*, pp. 104–122, © 1985, American Speech-Language-Hearing Association, Rockville, MD.

of the respiratory apparatus. Furthermore, classical singing is, perhaps, the most physically demanding of singing styles. It is performed without amplification, goes on for prolonged periods, and taxes essentially the entire gamut of vocal ability. Finally, most would agree that classical singers are at the top of the technical hierarchy of singing.

The method chosen for this investigation was the kinematic procedure described in Chapter 3. This procedure is noninvasive and requires little experimental sophistication on the part of those being studied. Previous investigations have demonstrated that comprehensive accounts of respiratory function can be developed using this approach, both for normal individuals (see Chapters 3 and 4) and for individuals with various abnormalities (see Chapters 5 through 9). These same investigations also have demonstrated that accurate determinations can be made of the inherent and volitional forces involved in the respiratory activities studied.

METHOD

Subjects

Six normal men served as subjects. Data on certain of their physical characteristics are given in Table 10–1. Subjects were chosen who had extensive classical singing training and performance experience and were of a single gender and voice classification. Extensive training was defined as encompassing those who had studied classical singing for at least 5 years beyond high school and had completed graduate training, or were in graduate training, in vocal performance or choral conducting. Extensive performance experience was defined as encompassing those who had performed widely in opera, oratorio, concert, graduate recital, or any combination of these. All the subjects were baritones. Years of singing training, performance experience, and competition awards of the subjects are summarized in Appendix A.

Observation Conditions

Observations were made under conditions resembling a vocal recital. The performance site was a church auditorium that was similar to a music hall. The auditorium had a high wooden ceiling and plaster walls. It was furnished with padded seats and carpeting and had a seating capacity of approximately 900. At the front of the auditorium was a well-lighted stage raised 4 ft (1.2 m) off the main floor and having dimensions of approximately 40 ft (12 m) across and 10 ft (3 m) deep. A baby grand piano, used to accompany the subjects during singing, was positioned toward the front in the center of the stage.

Table 10-1. *Selected Data on Physical Characteristics of the Subjects Studied*

Subject (ID)	Age (yr)	Height (cm)	Weight (kg)	Vital capacity (L)
TA	38	188.0	88.6	4.7
DM	31	175.3	81.8	4.4
PW	31	182.9	81.8	4.6
WL	30	195.6	87.3	4.6
JD	26	182.9	72.7	5.1
SF	23	188.0	100.0	5.6

Subjects stood on stage in the crook of the piano. They faced out toward the auditorium with a music stand positioned in front of them (Fig. 10–1). Subjects were permitted to place their hand(s) on either the piano or the music stand before they began each activity; however, having done so, they were not to change their placement during that activity. Each subject wore a loose-fitting hospital gown over his torso.

Six individuals served as the audience. These included two investigators, an accompanist, a page turner who assisted the accompanist, a video equipment operator, and an audio equipment operator. In an attempt to put a live performance "edge" on the subjects, they were told—and truthfully so—that their singing performances would be audio and audio-video tape-recorded for later listening and viewing by highly experienced and nationally known singing teachers.

Procedure

Two weeks before the observations each subject was given a form to complete and musical scores of the songs he was to perform in common with the other subjects. The form instructed the subject to write separate descriptions of how he believed he inspired and expired during classical singing. Subjects were told to familiarize themselves with the musical scores and to practice their performances extensively. Each subject also was asked to be prepared to sing an aria of his choice during the investigation, one with which he was thoroughly familiar, which he had practiced extensively, which was demanding but within his perceived technical ability, and which favorably displayed his singing skill.

For the investigation proper, three types of observations were made: audio recordings, audio-video recordings, and recordings of the kinematic behavior of the respiratory apparatus. Figure 10–1 includes a diagram of the equipment.

Audio and audio-video recordings were made with high-quality recording systems. For audio recordings, the acoustic signal was sensed with an air microphone, amplified, and recorded on a reel-to-reel tape recorder. For audio-video recordings, the acoustic signal was sensed with a second air microphone

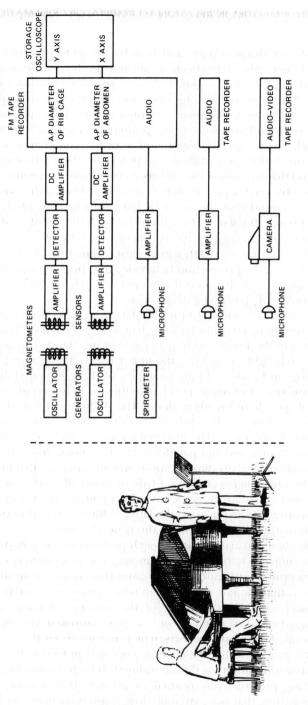

FIGURE 10–1. Subject positioning and diagram of equipment.

and amplified, while the video signal was sensed with a color video camera. The audio-video combination was recorded on an audio-video cassette recorder. To allow synchronization of the audio and audio-video recordings with recordings of the kinematic behavior of the respiratory apparatus, a third air microphone was used to sense the acoustic signal. Its output was amplified and fed to a direct record channel of an FM tape recorder whose other channels (see subsequent discussion) recorded kinematic data.

Respiratory data were obtained using a streamlined form of the kinematic procedure described in Chapter 3. This procedure treats the chest wall as a two-part system consisting of the rib cage and abdomen. Each part displaces volume as it moves, and together they displace a volume equal to that displaced by the lungs. Volume changes of the rib cage and abdomen are related linearly to changes in their respective anteroposterior diameters. Therefore, only diameter changes need to be determined to obtain measures of the volumes displaced by these individual parts and the lungs. In this investigation, such diameter changes were sensed with magnetometers, electromagnetic coil pairs that provide a voltage analogue of the distance between them. Two such pairs were used, one for the rib cage and one for the abdomen. A generator coil in each pair was attached to the front of the torso at the midline, that for the rib cage between the nipples and that for the abdomen just above the navel. A sensor coil in each pair was attached to the back of the torso at the midline and at the same axial level as its generator mate. Output signals from the two sensors were processed electronically and recorded on FM tape.

The streamlined procedure required that subjects perform several respiratory activities. These included vital capacity maneuvers, muscular relaxations of the respiratory apparatus at different lung volumes, and isovolume shape changes of the respiratory apparatus at a single lung volume. Three vital capacity maneuvers were performed. For each, the subject (wearing a noseclip) inspired fully, placed his lips around a mouthpiece attached to a spirometer, and expired fully. The largest of the three measured expiratory excursions was designated the subject's vital capacity (VC). Muscular relaxations were performed several times at the total lung capacity (TLC), the functional residual capacity (FRC), and the residual volume (RV). For these, each subject used his respiratory muscles to adjust lung volume to the appropriate level, at which he closed his larynx and relaxed his respiratory apparatus completely. Isovolume shape changes were performed several times at FRC. For these, the subject fixed his lung volume, closed his larynx, and slowly displaced volume back and forth between his rib cage and abdomen by alternately moving his abdominal wall inward and outward.

Each subject performed four speaking activities. For the first, the subject engaged in approximately 2 min of spontaneous conversation with the investigators. The second speaking activity involved reading aloud a declarative passage, in what the subject judged to be a typical manner. The third activity repeated the second, except that the passage was read at what each subject judged to be twice his normal loudness. For the last speaking activity, the subject read, from a musical score, the words to the first verse of the American national anthem (*The Star Spangled Banner*).

Four singing activities also were performed by each subject. These included *The Star Spangled Banner*, two Italian songs (*Amarilli mia Bella* by Caccini and *Che Fiero Costume* by Legrenzi), and an aria of the subject's choice. *The Star Spangled Banner* was sung in A^b major and covered the range A_2^b–E_4^b. It is characterized musically as vigorous and fortissimo. The two Italian songs chosen, *Amarilli mia Bella* and *Che Fiero Costume*, are from the same musical period, were performed in F minor, and encompassed approximately the same ranges (C_3–D_4 and C_3–F_4, respectively). These two songs are contrasting in that the former is slow and sustained, whereas the latter is fast and declarative and involves vigorous facile pronunciation. *Amarilli mia Bella* was performed at a tempo of 60 beats/min and at an utterance rate of 0.63 syllable/sec. *Che Fiero Costume* was performed at a tempo of 76 beats/min and at an utterance rate of 2.6 syllables/sec. Appendix B provides information on the arias sung by the subjects. These encompassed a wide variety of musical characteristics and were performed in four languages (two in French, two in Italian, one in German, and one in English).

Data Charts

Data charts were formed in which the anteroposterior diameter of the rib cage, increasing upward on the Y axis, was displayed against the anteroposterior diameter of the abdomen, increasing rightward on the X axis. To facilitate direct reading of the charts, their axes were converted from diameters to volume displacements. This was done by adjusting the amplifier gains on the Y and X channels of a display oscilloscope during playback of each subject's performance of isovolume shape changes at FRC until the resulting isovolume line on the screen had a slope of -1 (Fig. 10–2). In conjunction with the conversion of the Y and X axes of the charts, a third axis also was added. This axis displayed the volume displacement of the lungs, the sum of the rib cage volume and abdominal volume represented by each point on the chart. On this axis, running at a 45-degree diagonal, lung volume increases upward and rightward. With data charts so formed, it was possible to read them directly for (1) the volumes of the rib cage and the abdomen, given by position along their respective axes; (2) the relative volume displacement of the two parts, given by the slope of any pathway formed; and (3) the volume displacement of the lungs, given by the distance between any two points parallel to the third axis on the charts.

RESULTS

Figures 10–3 to 10–8 contain kinematic data from the subjects.

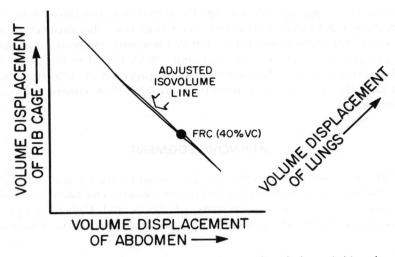

FIGURE 10-2. Relative volume chart and FRC (functional residual capacity) isovolume line.

Respiratory Activities

Data for respiratory maneuvers are shown in the upper left-most panels of the figures and are reproduced selectively in other panels. The upper and lower unfilled circles in each panel designate the relative volumes obtained during relaxation against a closed larynx at TLC and RV, respectively. The filled circle in each panel specifies the relative volume obtained during analogous relaxation at FRC. FRC was found to be approximately 40% VC for each subject. The curved dashed line in each panel estimates the relative volumes that would have been measured had the subject relaxed against a closed larynx at all lung volumes. Estimations are based on relaxation characteristics of other normal male adults (see Chapters 3 and 4). The solid diagonal line in each panel represents the adjusted (to − 1 slope) FRC isovolume line. Actual isovolume tracings were flat loops or single lines, each being linear or approximately so. The three dashed diagonal lines in each respiratory maneuvers panel are estimations of isovolume tracings that would have been measured had the subjects performed isovolume shape changes at 20%, 60%, and 80% VC. Estimations are based on isovolume line data generated by other normal male adults (see Chapters 3 and 4).

Speaking Activities

Speaking activities data are shown in the right-most four upper panels of Figures 10-3 to 10-8. Three representative data tracings are portrayed in each panel. Each tracing is for one respiratory cycle. Dotted ends of the tracings specify inspiratory starting positions.

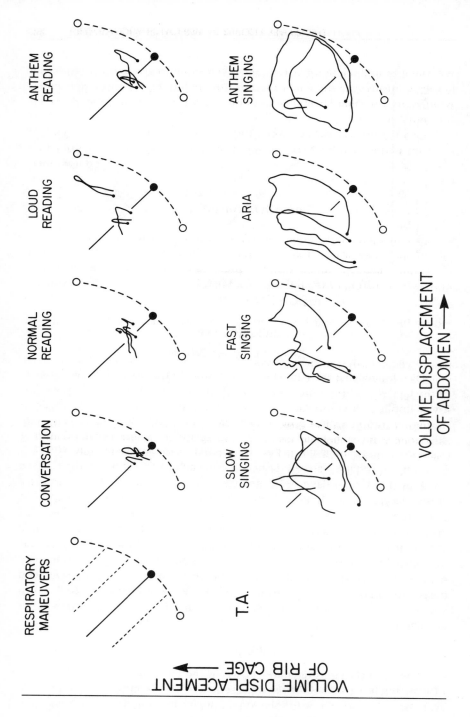

FIGURE 10-3. Kinematic data for subject TA. (See text for explanation.)

344

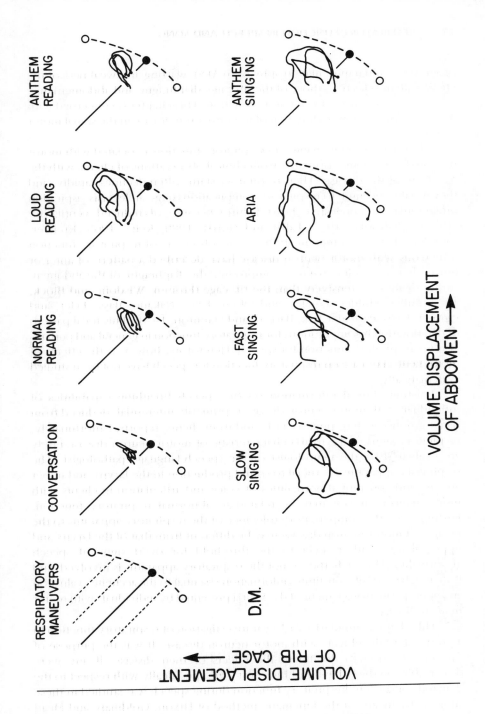

FIGURE 10-4. Kinematic data for subject DM.

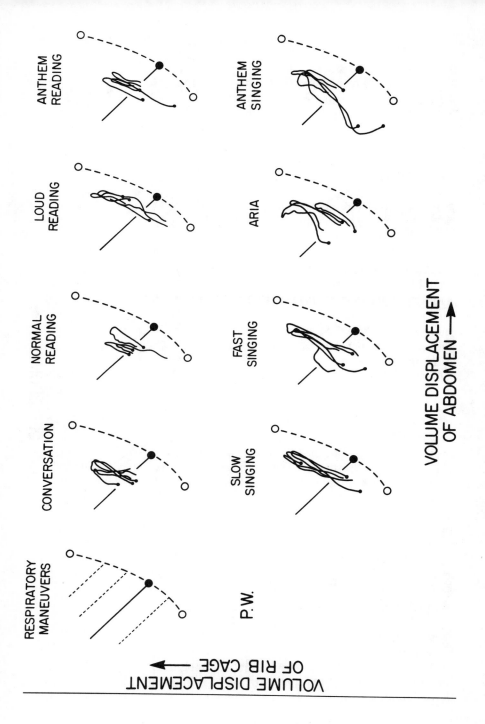

FIGURE 10-5. Kinematic data for subject PW.

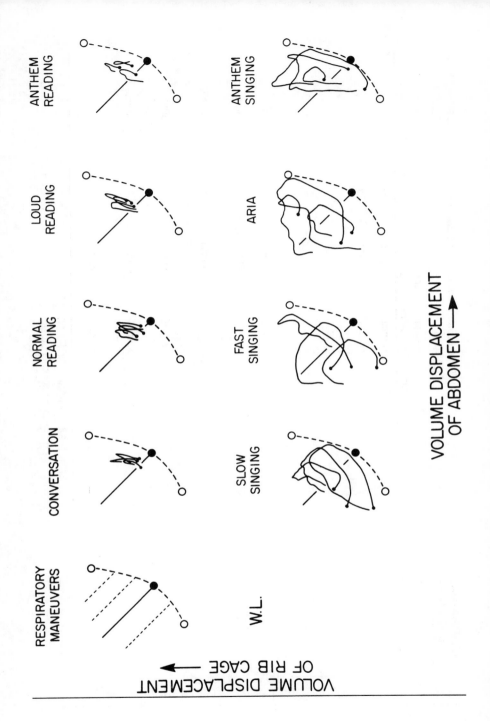

FIGURE 10-6. Kinematic data for subject WL.

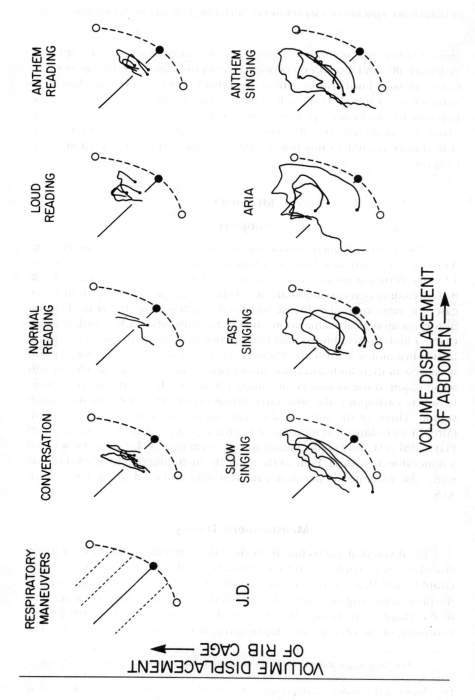

FIGURE 10-7. Kinematic data for subject JD.

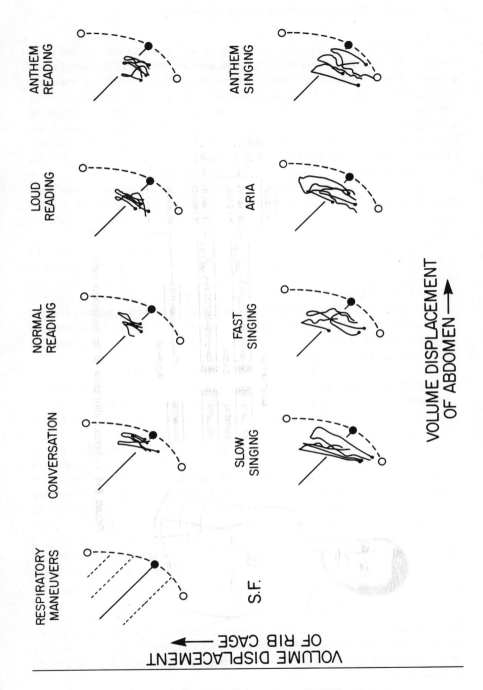

FIGURE 10-8. Kinematic data for subject SF.

LUNG VOLUME. Lung volume almost always was restricted to the middle 50% VC. For conversation, normal reading, and anthem reading, most breath groups (expiratory phases) were begun from within a range of volumes encompassing 70% to 50% VC. Findings were mixed with regard to initiation levels for loud reading. Subjects TA, DM, and PW often started loud reading from higher lung volumes (usually about 10% to 25% VC higher) than those from which they started other speaking activities, whereas the remaining subjects started breath groups for loud reading from about the same lung volume levels they used for other speaking activities.

Breath groups for speaking activities usually were terminated near FRC (typically between 50% and 30% VC). Exceptions were certain breath groups for subject PW, which encroached significantly on the expiratory reserve volume (ERV).

Most subjects typically displaced 10% to 25% VC during the inspiratory and expiratory excursions associated with conversation, normal reading, and anthem reading. Subject PW, an exception, frequently displaced volumes in excess of 25% VC for these activities. For loud reading, findings were mixed with regard to typical excursions. Subjects DM and PW demonstrated volume changes that routinely exceeded those for other speaking activities, whereas the remaining subjects showed only an occasional larger volume change for loud reading (see data for subject TA).

RELATIVE VOLUME DISPLACEMENTS OF THE RIB CAGE AND ABDOMEN. A wide variety of relative displacements of the rib cage and abdomen were responsible for the lung volume changes associated with speaking.

For the inspiratory phase of the respiratory cycle, data tracings revealed that, for most subjects (TA, PW, WL, JD, and SF), the volume contribution of the rib cage typically exceeded that of the abdomen. In some instances for these subjects, a predominant rib cage displacement characterized the first part of the lung volume increase, followed by equal rib cage and abdominal displacements (see data for subjects TA and PW). In other instances for the same subjects, the converse was true (see data for subject WL). Only subject DM showed inspirations in which the relative contribution of the abdomen typically exceeded that of the rib cage. In his case, abdominal displacement predominated for much of the inspiration, followed by equal rib cage and abdominal contributions, and followed, in turn, in some instances, by a predominant rib cage contribution. For some inspirations, subject DM demonstrated paradoxical movement of the rib cage. That is, although the volume displacement of the lungs was in the inspiratory direction, the displacement of the rib cage was in the expiratory direction (see DM's loud-reading data).

For the expiratory (or breath group) phase of the respiratory cycle, data tracings revealed relative volume displacements ranging from a marked predominance of the rib cage to a marked predominance of the abdomen.

Such extremes were manifested by subjects PW and DM, respectively. Other subjects demonstrated relative contributions that fell between these extremes (see TA's data), there being a tendency for the remainder of the subject group to show predominant rib cage displacement of varying degrees.

No group trends in relative displacements were discernible across the different speaking activities. Subjects who demonstrated differences among activities did so idiosyncratically (see normal versus loud reading for subject TA versus subject JD).

Relative volume contributions often changed markedly within individual breath groups. These changes differed in kind, with some relative displacements going from essentially all rib cage contribution to all abdominal contribution, or vice versa (see data for subjects TA and DM). Involved in certain of these changes were paradoxical movements of either the rib cage or the abdomen, particularly the latter, in which one or the other of the parts moved in the inspiratory direction during some segment of the breath group. An example of rib cage paradoxing can be seen in the middle loud-reading tracing for subject DM, whereas examples of abdominal paradoxing can be seen in the anthem reading tracings for subject SF.

SEPARATE VOLUMES OF THE RIB CAGE AND ABDOMEN. Nearly all speaking activities were performed within the range of rib cage and abdominal volumes associated with relaxation between TLC and RV. For most subjects, the volume of the rib cage almost always was in excess of that associated with relaxation at FRC. Subject PW departed from this group trend most often when, at times, he encroached significantly on his ERV (see his reading data). For conversation, normal reading, and anthem reading, most breath groups were initiated from within the range of rib cage volumes associated with relaxation between 80% and 60% VC. Subjects PW and JD initiated some breath groups from appreciably higher rib cage volumes (see PW's data for conversation). Breath groups associated with loud reading were initiated at higher rib cage volumes than for normal-loudness activities in some subjects (see data for subjects TA and DM), whereas for others, breath groups were initiated at similar rib cage volumes regardless of loudness.

Speaking breath groups usually were terminated at rib cage volumes encompassing the range of rib cage sizes associated with relaxation between 60% and 40% VC. Exceptions at the lower end of this range were confined almost exclusively to subject PW, whereas exceptions at the higher end involved mainly the loud reading of subjects TA and DM.

Typical rib cage excursions for conversation, normal reading, and anthem reading were the equivalent of 10% to 20% VC changes in relaxed rib cage volume through the vital capacity midrange. Subject PW was an exception, in that he routinely used larger rib cage excursions. For loud reading, half of the subjects (TA, DM, and PW) showed a tendency to use rib cage excursions that were greater than those associated with the other speaking activities.

It can be seen in Figures 10–3 to 10–8 that during speaking activities the volume of the abdomen usually was maintained at or below the volume it assumed during relaxation at FRC. For conversation, normal reading, and anthem reading, most breath groups were initiated within the range of abdominal volumes associated with relaxation between 40% and 20% VC. Subject DM was an exception on the high side of this range at times (see his data for normal reading and anthem reading), whereas subject SF was an exception on the low side for anthem reading. For loud reading, several subjects initiated breath groups at abdominal volumes that were larger than those associated with relaxed FRC (see data for TA, DM, PW, and JD). The most striking effect was demonstrated by subject DM, who, at times, started breath groups at abdominal volumes approximating the volume his abdomen was estimated to assume during relaxation at 80% VC.

Breath groups for speaking activities were terminated over a wide range of abdominal volumes, but most often from within the range of abdominal volumes associated with relaxation between 35% VC and RV. On occasion, subjects TA, DM, and PW decreased the volume of the abdomen to magnitudes less than that at relaxed RV (see DM's loud-reading data).

Abdominal excursions varied widely among breath groups. Most were of magnitudes ranging between comparable 10% to 30% VC changes upon relaxation. In some cases, however, excursions ranged in excess of 75% of the abdominal volumes associated with relaxation between TLC and RV (see loud-reading data for DM).

Considering the separate volume data for speaking activities relative to those for the subjects' presumed relaxation characteristics, it is found that speaking took place to the left of the relaxation configurations of the chest wall in each panel in Figures 10–3 to 10–8. Thus, the rib cage was relatively more and the abdomen was relatively less expanded than they were in the relaxed state at corresponding lung volumes.

Singing Activities

Singing activities data are shown in the lower four panels of Figures 10–3 to 10–8. Each panel contains three representative data tracings. Complete respiratory cycles are portrayed, with the dotted end of each tracing specifying the start of the inspiratory phase.

LUNG VOLUME. Lung volume for singing activities encompassed essentially the full range of the vital capacity. For all four activities, the majority of breath groups started from within the 90% to 60% VC range. Exceptions above the high end of this range most often involved aria singing (see data for subjects DM, WL, and JD), whereas exceptions below the low end of the range occurred for all activities but slow singing. Subject SF typically began breath groups at lower than 60% VC for anthem singing. Findings were mixed with regard to the initiation levels used by different subjects. Some subjects were relatively consistent in lung volume initiation levels across activities (see data for PW), whereas others demonstrated idiosyncratic variations in starting levels across activities (see data for subjects DM and WL). Variation in initiation level within activities often was considerable (see fast singing for subjects TA, WL, and JD), with the smallest variation observed for slow singing (see data for subjects DM, PW, WL, and SF).

Most singing breath groups were terminated within ERV, with the bulk of the utterances ending between 35% and 15% VC. Exceptions above the high end of this range were most frequent for anthem singing (see data for subject PW), whereas exceptions below the low end of the range were most frequent for the aria activity (see subjects TA, WL, and JD).

A wide range of volume changes occurred during the inspiratory and expiratory excursions associated with singing. These encompassed as much as nearly 100% VC and as little as 15% VC, although most excursions involved displacements of between 65% and 30% VC. Exceptions above the high end of the 65% to 30% VC range were confined mainly to aria singing and anthem singing (see data for subject JD). A trend also was observed for slow singing to involve larger volume excursions than the other singing activities (see tracings for subject SF).

RELATIVE VOLUME DISPLACEMENTS OF THE RIB CAGE AND ABDOMEN. Lung volume changes during singing resulted from a wide range of relative volume displacements by the two chest wall parts.

For the inspiratory phase of the cycle, data tracings revealed two principal patterns. In one, the volume contribution of the rib cage typically exceeded that of the abdomen (see data for Subjects PW and SF). In the other, the contribution of the abdomen typically exceeded that of rib cage during the first part of inspiration, followed by equal rib cage and abdominal displacements, and followed, in turn, by a predominant rib cage contribution during the latter part of inspiration (see data for fast singing by DM, WL, and JD). Four of the subjects used one or the other of these displacement patterns almost exclusively (see PW and SF versus WL and JD), whereas two subjects, TA and DM, used both patterns. Paradoxical movement of the rib cage or abdomen or both was manifested during many inspirations. Paradoxing of the rib cage, in which it moved in the expiratory direction while lung volume was increasing, often occurred during the first part of inspiration (see tracings for fast singing for subject JD, aria singing for subject DM, and slow singing for subject WL). Abdominal paradoxing, in which the abdomen moved in the expiratory direction (inward) while lung volume was increasing, often took place during the first and last parts of inspiratory excursions. Examples of such paradoxing during the first part of inspiration can be seen in the fast-singing and anthem-singing data for subject PW, whereas examples for the last part of inspiration are apparent in the fast-singing data of subjects TA and DM.

For the expiratory, or singing breath group, phase of the cycle, two general relative volume patterns prevailed. For one of these, the volume contribution of the rib cage typically was greater than that of the abdomen throughout most, or all, of the expiratory excursion. For the other, the contribution of the abdomen typically exceeded that of the rib cage during the first part of the excursion, followed by equal rib cage and abdominal displacements, and followed, in turn, by a sole or predominant rib cage contribution during the last part of expiration. The first of these patterns can be seen in the slow-singing data for subjects PW and SF, whereas the second can be seen in subject DM's slow-singing data and subject JD's fast-singing data. The use of both patterns within an activity is revealed in subject TA's data for slow singing, aria singing, and anthem singing.

No consistent group differences in relative displacements were noted across the singing activities. Differences observed were idiosyncratic, as, for example, for subject JD, who demonstrated a lesser rib cage contribution for many of his slow-singing breath groups than for other singing activities.

Superimposed on the general displacement patterns were marked changes in relative contributions. These differed in kind, some involving shifts from essentially all rib cage contribution to all abdominal contribution, or vice versa, and some involving paradoxical movement of either the rib cage or the abdomen. Examples of such changes can be seen in the fast-singing data for subject TA and in the slow-singing and anthem-singing data for subject JD. Most often, marked changes in relative contributions were associated with abrupt changes within the musical passages. For example, changes to marked inward abdominal displacement with paradoxical outward displacement of the rib cage were associated with increases in loudness, stress, or high-note performance (see the left-most tracing for subject PW's fast singing when he was performing a loud, high note). For another example, changes to marked inward rib cage displacement with paradoxical outward displacement of the abdomen (i.e., downward and rightward on the charts) often were associated with utterance segments involving high flows, as in the case of voiceless fricative elements.

SEPARATE VOLUMES OF THE RIB CAGE AND ABDOMEN. Singing activities were performed over a wide range of rib cage and abdominal volumes, including some outside the ranges associated with relaxation between TLC and RV. Rib cage volumes extended from well above those for relaxation at TLC to approximately those obtained during relaxation at RV. The majority of breath groups were initiated within the range of rib cage volumes associated with relaxation between 100% and 80% VC. Subjects TA, DM, WL, and JD often initiated breath groups at rib cage volumes equal to those for relaxed

TLC, whereas subjects WL and JD initiated some breath groups at even greater rib cage volumes. Exceptions on the low side of the 100% to 80% VC rib cage volume initiation range were confined mainly to subject SF, who occasionally started breath groups at rib cage volumes as low as those associated with relaxation at 60% VC (see his fast-singing and anthem-singing data). Starting level differences in rib cage volume did not differ systematically for the subject group across activities, although three subjects (TA, DM, and WL) showed a tendency for aria singing to involve higher starting volumes than other activities.

Most singing breath groups were terminated within the range of rib cage volumes associated with relaxation between 80% VC and FRC. Exceptions at the lower end of this range were confined mainly to subject SF, who occasionally used rib cage volumes as low as those associated with relaxation at 10% VC. Exceptions at the higher end of the range were primarily for subject DM, especially his aria singing (see Fig. 10–4).

Typical rib cage excursions for singing were on the order of 55% to 15% VC changes in relaxed rib cage volume through the vital capacity midrange. Subjects WL and JD were exceptions above the high end of this range on occasion (see data for JD's aria and anthem singing). Frequent exceptions below the lower end of the same range were subjects TA and DM (see DM's aria data).

It can be seen in Figures 10–3 to 10–8 that, during singing activities, abdominal volume ranged from magnitudes as great as those associated with relaxation at 75% VC to magnitudes much smaller than those obtained during relaxation at RV. Most breath groups were initiated at abdominal volumes within the range associated with relaxation between 60% and 15% VC. Exceptions at the lower end of this range were confined mainly to subjects TA and DM (see TA's data for fast singing and aria singing), whereas exceptions at the upper end of the same range were confined mainly to the same two subjects and to subject WL (see his aria data). Subjects differed widely in the variation of abdominal volume starting levels. For example, subjects TA and DM demonstrated a large range of starting volumes (usually between volumes comparable to those for relaxation between 75% and 0% VC), whereas subjects PW and JD initiated breath groups from abdominal volumes confined to a very small range (usually between volumes comparable to those for relaxation between 45% and 35% VC).

Singing breath groups were terminated over a substantial range of abdominal volumes, but almost invariably at volumes equal to or less than those associated with relaxation at 10% VC. Subjects frequently ended breath groups at abdominal volumes much smaller than those obtained during relaxation at RV, as can be seen in the data charts for TA, DM, and JD.

Abdominal volume excursions varied greatly in magnitude among breath groups for singing. Subjects DM, WL, and JD typically used abdominal excursions encompassing more than the equivalent of 50% of the abdominal volume range between relaxed TLC and relaxed RV. At times, these three subjects generated breath groups that far exceeded 100% of the relaxed abdominal volume range (see their aria data for excursions as great as 165%, 135%, and 145%, respectively). Subjects PW and SF, by contrast, typically performed with excursions involving magnitudes the equivalent of <50% of the relaxed TLC to relaxed RV range of abdominal volumes (see PW's slow-singing data). Subject TA showed a mixture of the two trends mentioned, with some of his excursions being less and some being more than the same 50% value separating the other subjects. Differences across singing activities were idiosyncratic as, for example, in subject DM, who typically used greater excursions for aria singing than for the other singing activities (see Fig. 10–4).

When the separate volume data for the rib cage and abdomen are considered relative to those for the subjects' relative volume relaxation characteristics, it is apparent that singing took place to the left of the relaxation configurations of the chest wall in each chart in Figures 10–3 to 10–8. Thus, the rib cage was relatively more and the abdomen was relatively less expanded than they were in the relaxed state at the same lung volume. In many instances, the descriptions of *relatively more expanded* and *relatively less expanded* represented near maximum departure from relaxation volumes.

RESPIRATORY PHASE TRANSITIONS. To this juncture, consideration has been given to those parts of the singing respiration cycle associated with inspiration and the utterance portion of expiration. Although these two represent the bulk of the cycle, transitions between them must be considered to complete the picture of singing function for certain subjects.

Inspiration-expiration transitions occurred in two forms. For both of these, lung volume remained constant but volume was displaced between the two parts of the chest wall in a manner similar to that associated with the performance of a limited, unidirectional, isovolume shape change. Most often observed was a transition form in which volume was shifted quickly from the abdomen to the rib cage. This adjustment, illustrated by the dashed tracing in the upper left chart in Figure 10–9, occurred frequently for subject WL, less often for subject TA, and on occasion for subjects DM and JD (see subject WL's slow-singing data). The other inspiration-expiration transition form, observed less often, was one in which volume was shifted quickly from the rib cage to the abdomen. This adjustment, illustrated by the dashed tracing in the lower left chart in Figure 10–9, was confined to subjects PW and SF but most often was associated with the singing of subject SF, particularly slow singing and anthem singing. For the two forms observed, the magnitudes of the volume shifts between the two parts of the chest wall differed considerably within and between subjects. On some occasions the adjustments involved were relatively small, whereas on other occasions they were considerable, involving rib cage and abdominal excursions equivalent to major portions of the ranges of excursions associated with relaxation between TLC and RV.

RESPIRATORY PHASE TRANSITIONS

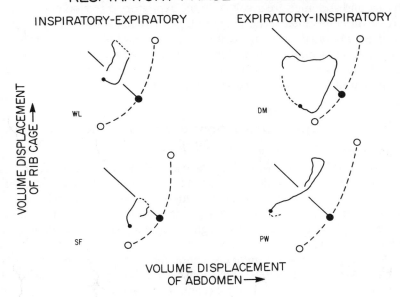

FIGURE 10-9. Respiratory phase transitions associated with singing.

Expiration-inspiration transitions also occurred in two forms. Both of these involved quick decrements in lung volume and most often preceded inspirations of relatively marked quickness. The magnitude of the lung volume decrease involved varied considerably within and between subjects and singing activities. Subjects TA, DM, WL, and JD demonstrated decrements ranging mostly between 5% and 10% VC, although TA and DM occasionally showed lung volume decreases of as much as 15% to 20% VC. Subjects PW and SF routinely showed decrements of about 5% VC. The most frequently observed form of expiration-inspiration transition was that in which the lung volume decrement involved a substantial decrease in rib cage volume accompanied by a lesser increase in abdominal volume. Such an adjustment is illustrated by the dashed tracing in the upper right data chart in Figure 10-9. The decrement in rib cage volume charted there actually exceeds that of the lungs by an amount equal to the paradoxical inspiratory (outward) displacement of the abdomen. This form of transition occurred most often in subjects TA, DM, WL, and JD. The other expiration-inspiration transition form, occurring less frequently, was one in which the adjustment usually was associated with a decrease in abdominal volume accompanied by a lesser decrease or no decrease in rib cage volume. This transition form was characteristic of the adjustments of subjects PW and SF and is illustrated by the dashed tracing in the lower right chart in Figure 10–9. In the example shown for subject PW, both the rib cage and abdomen are involved in the expiratory direction during the first part of the adjustment. The magnitudes of excursions of the rib cage and abdomen differed considerably within and between subjects for the two types of expiration-inspiration transitions observed. For the most part, however, rib cage displacements predominated for the first transition form, whereas abdominal displacements predominated for the second.

Subjects' Descriptions of Their Respiration for Singing

Table 10–2 presents verbatim what each subject wrote in response to the request to write separate descriptions of how he inspired and expired during classical singing. As seen in the table, written accounts differed widely among the subjects. Many structural elements were referred to by the subjects, including the chest, rib cage, diaphragm, abdomen, back, sides, mouth, nose, trachea, and lungs.

Regarding the mechanism of inspiration for singing, the subjects presented a broad spectrum of beliefs. Three subjects, TA, DM, and WL, wrote of their use of an elevated and expanded rib cage configuration for inspiration. Subject TA wrote of his belief that his diaphragm descended during inspiration as a result of air entering the lungs. Subjects DM and PW wrote of their sensations of a downward and outward expansion of the abdominal area, whereas subject WL wrote of an expansion and contraction of his abdomen. Subject JD described his sensation of low expansive breaths with outward movements of his lower back and sides, and subject SF wrote of air flowing through his body. Several subjects, TA, DM, and WL, wrote statements indicating their belief that inspiratory flow was a passive event, as reflected, respectively, in the following: "allows air to enter," "I do not draw in the air," and "letting the air 'fall into the lungs' rather than frantically sucking in air." Subject WL stated that he tried to breathe in the same manner for both singing and speaking. And subject DM made indirect reference to the depth of inspiration taken for singing by describing the creation of a "huge tub."

Concerning the mechanism of expiration for singing, the subjects again presented a broad spectrum of beliefs. Three subjects, TA, PW, and WL, wrote that they used an elevated and expanded rib cage position and did not allow the rib cage (chest) to collapse. Subject TA wrote of his diaphragm lifting and pushing air out of his lungs, whereas subjects PW and WL wrote of their abdomen moving inward. Subject DM, in contrast to PW and WL, wrote of his lower abdominal wall expanding outward. Subject JD described his attempt to keep an "expansive feeling" and to fight his impulse of "caving in," whereas subject SF again wrote, as for inspiration, of using a consistent flow of air through his whole body. Two subjects, DM and WL, wrote in a manner suggesting a belief that the expiratory phase of classical singing was relatively

Table 10-2. *Verbatim Written Descriptions of How Each Subject Believed He Inspired and Expired During Classical Singing*

Subject	Inspiration Description	Expiration Description
TA	Keeping rib cage elevated and expanded allows air to enter lungs causing diaphragm to sink.	Keeping rib cage elevated and expanded allows diaphragm to lift and push air out of lungs.
DM	I feel and/or imagine the bottom of my abdominal area open down and outward creating a huge tub. The air comes in through the mouth and nose, travels down a long pipe (about one inch in diameter), and begins to fill the tub. As the tub fills from bottom to top with air, the tub bottom continues to expand until the tub completely fills with air. I do not draw in the air. Rather, I simply open my body, and the air rushes in of its own volition— much as air or water outside a vacuum container would rush into the container when the seal is broken. The chest is kept high, though not rigidly, so that there is no interference with the expansion of the lungs.	The breath pours out of the mouth as if I were sighing, but is measured or metered out according to the length of the musical phrase, so that no air is wasted. As the breath pours out of the mouth, the lower abdominal wall (at the pelvic base) continues to expand down and outward.
PW	I attempt to feel a release and then a feeling of downward and outward expansion.	I try to keep the chest high and not let it collapse, while allowing the abdomen to press inward and upward.
WL	I try to breathe in the same manner whether singing or speaking. The body must remain relaxed and flexible throughout inspiration. Breathing is accomplished by letting the air "fall into the lungs" rather than frantically sucking in air. During singing the chest is normally somewhat expanded, so as breathing takes place the abdomen expands and contracts to a much greater degree than does the chest.	When one expires during singing the upper body (i.e., the chest) does not collapse, but remains in an expanded state as the abdomen narrows and allows the air to escape. The air is not forced from the body, but is released.
JD	I take low, expansive breaths, trying to feel an outward movement through my lower back and sides.	As I start to sing, I try not to think of my expiration. Instead, I try to direct my attention to keeping an expansive feeling. I try to fight the impulse of "caving in" as I run out of air by keeping an erect posture and by using more support.
SF	My process of breathing during the act of inspiration involves a consistent flow of air flowing through my whole body.	The act of expiration can be explained very simply. It involves the same flow of air as in inspiration but is regulated very closely in the amount of air that is allowed to flow into the phrase, while utilizing the consistent flow of air throughout the whole body.

passive from a respiration viewpoint. Subject DM wrote that "the breath pours out of the mouth as if I were sighing," whereas subject WL wrote that "the air is not forced from the body, but is released."

DISCUSSION

Findings are discussed with regard to the following topics: respiratory adjustments in speaking, respiratory adjustments in singing, subjects' beliefs about their respiratory adjustments for singing versus the actual adjustments used, and implications for the training of singers.

Respiratory Adjustments in Speaking

The kinematic data generated by the present subjects for various speaking activities are highly similar to those obtained from vocally untrained normal men studied previously (see Chapters 3 and 8). Only the occasional use of slightly higher lung volumes and rib cage volumes separates the present subjects from untrained subjects, a difference that most likely is attributable to the present subjects' tendency toward somewhat "more dramatic" speaking in comparison to untrained subjects.

Direct measurements of the muscular forces generated by different parts of the chest wall during speaking have been made (see Chapter 4)—in fact, made on some of the same subjects included in the untrained group just mentioned (see Chapter 3). Accordingly, it can be stated with relative certainty what muscular mechanisms prevailed during speaking activities performed by the present subjects. Presumably, they were as follows. For the expiratory portion of the breathing cycle, the rib cage and abdomen exerted expiratory forces that drove the chest wall at a speech-specific configuration dictated largely by a predominant activity of the abdomen. This combination of forces was the same but heightened for loud speaking. When inspiration was called for during speaking activities, the rib cage reduced its expiratory force to zero, or nearly so, while the abdomen continued to exert a major effort. From off the general background configuration set by the abdomen, the diaphragm was activated and worked against the relatively taut abdomen to elevate the relaxed (or nearly so) rib cage. The powerful inspiratory activity of the diaphragm thus restored the respiratory apparatus to a higher lung volume, rib cage volume, and abdominal volume by lifting the rib cage and overpowering the active abdomen, forcing it outward despite its continued expiratory effort.

Respiratory Adjustments in Singing

Kinematic data of the type gathered in the present investigation on respiratory adjustments in singing have been available previously only for the performance of *The Star Spangled Banner* by vocally untrained subjects (see Chapter 3). Such data reveal that untrained subjects use respiratory adjustments in singing that are similar to those they use for either normal or loud speaking. The present subjects, whose speaking performances were essentially identical to those for these untrained subjects, performed *The Star Spangled Banner* in strikingly different manners than did their untrained counterparts.

Singing of the present subjects was characterized by essentially continuous adjustments in lung volume, rib cage volume, and abdominal volume. Changes in lung volume were extensive, with individual breath groups typically beginning at relatively high lung volumes and continuing through a major portion of the vital capacity, often ending at relatively low lung volumes. In using such large volume strokes, the present subjects departed in a major way from their usual tidal breathing volumes. Because work was often involved against high relaxation pressures at the volume extremes, the overall muscular costs of the subjects' singing performances had to be high, and much more so than were the costs of their companion speaking performances. The choice of initiating singing breath groups from high lung volumes most likely had two bases. One was the potential to capitalize on the high respiratory recoil forces available at such volumes, because singing, as loud as it was, required relatively high driving pressures (Bouhuys, Proctor, and Mead, 1966). The other was the need to provide a sufficient reserve potential in lung volume to fulfill the prolonged expiration demands associated with musical phrases of extended length, such as are characteristic of classical singing. The volumes expired by the subjects varied from one singing breath group to another. Several factors were undoubtedly sources of this variation, including the linguistic content of the sung utterances; the manner in which the singing activities were artistically interpreted by the performers; differences in average flow, as for example, in association with different laryngeal adjustments involved with different loudnesses, pitches, and qualities; and the musical phrasing within and between singing activities.

Changes in lung volume during singing were accomplished by the present subjects through a great range of relative volume contributions by the rib cage and abdomen. Variations in contributions were of two general natures, one involving relatively gradual background shifts in relative contributions and one involving relatively abrupt shifts in contributions in association with rapid adjustments of one form or another within the performance content of the passage being sung. Overall patterns differed a great deal across subjects, revealing a variety of individual styles of chest wall displacement for singing. Why individual subjects performed so differently with regard to relative contributions is uncertain. Clearly there are a number of degrees of freedom of performance in using the respiratory apparatus for singing purposes. The strategy employed by a subject and the manner in which its patterning becomes neurally ingrained may depend in part on how the subject has learned on his own to use his muscular system most effectively against the passive mechanical properties of his respiratory apparatus. The strategy a subject used also may have been conditioned by the extensive instruction given in one form or another to the present subjects on how to use the respiratory apparatus for classical singing. How such instruction translates into differences in the data from the present subjects is unknown but may be relevant considering that subject differences in relative contributions for singing far exceeded those for speaking. In this regard, it is interesting that the untrained subjects in the investigation described in Chapter 3 showed kinematic patterns for singing similar to those associated with either their normal or loud speaking. Variation associated with instruction would not, of course, have been a factor in the case of such untrained singers.

The chest wall was distorted continuously from its relaxed configurations during singing by the present subjects, meaning that muscular forces were continuously in operation. The rib cage was found always to be maintained in a more expanded state and the abdomen always to be maintained in a less expanded state than they were when relaxed at corresponding lung volumes. The general nature of the distortion of the chest wall for singing was similar to that for speaking, although singing, in contrast to speaking, usually involved far greater deformation of the chest wall from relaxation and very different volume histories for the rib cage and the abdomen (i.e., very different pathways on the data charts).

For the expiratory, or breath group, phase of the respiratory cycle for singing, the general background task for the present subjects presumably was to exert increasingly more positive chest wall efforts (i.e., either less inspiratory or more expiratory) as lung volume decreased. For those breath groups begun at high lung volumes or involving soft singing, or both, the first part of this background task undoubtedly involved the generation of negative muscular pressures to offset partially the high positive relaxation pressures that prevailed.[1] Later in these breath groups, positive muscular pressures were required from the chest wall to supplement the increasingly less positive (i.e., either less expiratory or more inspiratory) relaxation pressures. For those breath groups begun at mid or low lung volumes, the background task presumably was analogous to that involved in the later portions of breath groups begun at high lung volumes. That is, positive muscular pressures were called for.

Under high lung volume or soft singing conditions, or both, the mechanism most likely operating generally would entail increasingly less negative efforts by the rib cage and increasingly more positive efforts by the abdomen.[2] The possibility of significant diaphragm activity seems remote,

---

[1]Determinations of the sign and magnitude of muscular pressure demands are based on estimates of the approximate alveolar pressures required for different activities and knowledge of the typical recoil pressures available at the prevailing lung volumes for normal adult male subjects (see Chapters 3 and 4 and Agostoni and Mead, 1964; Bouhuys et al., 1966).

---

[2]Muscular mechanisms underlying the activities performed by the present subjects can be inferred from consideration of the possible muscular forces that could account for observed instantaneous chest wall configuration and its history. Interpretations depend largely on comparisons

given that previous research (see Chapter 4 and Bouhuys et al., 1966) has revealed the diaphragm to be inactive, or minimally active, during speaking, singing, and the sustaining of vowels through the high lung volume range. Implication of the rib cage in the proposed mechanism is supported by the very high rib cage volumes used by the present subjects through the high lung volume range. Such high rib cage volumes are consistent with those observed in investigations on upright subjects in which it has been found that negative chest wall efforts against high positive relaxation pressures invariably are generated with inspiratory muscles of the rib cage (see Chapter 4 and Bouhuys et al., 1966; Draper, Ladefoged, and Whitteridge, 1959). Presumably, use of the rib cage, and not the diaphragm, to generate negative muscular pressures under the conditions described has to do with several advantages the rib cage offers to the singer. First, the rib cage is in contact with a far greater portion of the surface of the lungs (about three fourths) than is the diaphragm (about one fourth). This means that movements of the rib cage need to be far less extensive than those of the diaphragm to effect the same changes in alveolar pressure. Second, the inspiratory muscles of the rib cage are smaller in size, faster acting, greater in number, and more richly endowed proprioceptively than those of the diaphragm. This affords the rib cage a finer graded control over inspiratory efforts than is possible through use of the diaphragm. Third, the rib cage is able, in the upright body position, to supplant the need for contraction of the diaphragm during inspiratory efforts by virtue of its influence on the hydraulic forces exerted through the abdominal contents (see Chapter 4 and Bouhuys et al., 1966). This permits net inspiratory control of the respiratory apparatus through the high lung volume range via recourse to the use of only one inspiratory part of the chest wall.

Implication of the abdomen in the proposed mechanism for the high lung volume range is supported by the general abdominal volume decrease and frequent rib cage volume increase demonstrated by the present subjects through the high lung volume range. Active abdominal involvement under the circumstances that prevailed is consistent with the abdominal action observed in investigations on upright subjects, in which it has been found that significant expiratory efforts by the abdomen usually accompany negative rib cage efforts produced in the face of high positive relaxation pressures at high lung volumes (see Chapter 4 and Eblen, 1963). Initially, it may seem counterintuitive that the abdomen, a positive muscular generator only, would be operating at high lung volumes at which inspiratory chest wall efforts are required and are being provided by inspiratory efforts of the rib cage. There

---

of chest wall configuration during activities and relaxation, with departures from the relaxed configuration at corresponding lung volumes being ascribed to a small number of possible combinations of muscular actions of the chest wall. It can be reasoned as to the more likely of these possible combinations by taking into account the probable sign and magnitude of the chest wall effort required for the activity being performed (see Footnote 1). For detailed descriptive and graphic considerations, see Chapters 3 and 6.

is, however, an important efficiency gain to be had for the singer through significant activation of the abdomen under such circumstances. That gain is that the active abdomen provides an opposing member in the parallel arrangement of the chest wall (rib cage and abdomen) against which the rib cage can develop pressure. This means that the increasingly less negative efforts by the rib cage can be resolved economically into alveolar pressure rather than into chest wall shape change (principally an outward moving abdomen) that would partially offset the decreasing force adjustment of the rib cage. The inferred generation of an increasingly more forceful abdominal effort as the breath group proceeds through the high lung volume range is consistent with the desirability of providing an increasingly firm and less distant opposing member for the rib cage to work against as it delivers increasingly less negative efforts.

It seems probable that an additional efficiency gain from abdominal activity, albeit one not having to do with the expiratory breath group, per se, relates to the influence of the abdomen on the diaphragm. Expiratory displacement of the abdomen forces the diaphragm headward, increasing the length of its fibers and its radius of curvature. These consequences on the diaphragm are relevant to inspirations called for at the ends of short breath groups within the high lung volume range because the configurations imposed on the diaphragm mechanically tune it to be able to function quickly and powerfully as a force generator. In this regard, it is noteworthy that previous research (see Chapters 3 and 4) involving utterances produced throughout most of the vital capacity on single breaths did not show the major abdominal volume decrease and frequent rib cage volume increase often demonstrated by the present subjects through the high lung volume range. Perhaps the certainty of not having to inspire quickly during the course of such utterances allows the individual the freedom of using less effortful abdominal activity at high lung volumes. Unfortunately, the present subjects were not required to produce utterances throughout most of the vital capacity on single breaths so that a strategy comparison cannot be made between high lung volume activities with and without potential inspiratory requirements.

Under mid or low lung volume conditions, the mechanism most likely operating involved expiratory rib cage efforts and abdominal efforts of increasing magnitudes. Implication of both the rib cage and the abdomen in the suggested mechanism is supported by (1) the general rib cage volume and abdominal volume decreases demonstrated by the present subjects through the mid and low lung volume ranges and (2) the frequent changes in relative volume contributions of the rib cage and abdomen observed for the subjects through these ranges. Use of such presumed rib cage and abdominal expiratory efforts is consistent with the actions observed for these two structures in investigations on upright subjects in which data reveal that expiratory rib cage and abdominal muscle activities are generated to supplement prevailing relaxation pressures (see Chapter 4 and Eblen, 1963; Hoit-Dalgaard, Lansing, Plassman, and Hixon, 1983).

Rib cage activity during the generation of positive muscular pressures at mid and low lung volumes takes advantage of rib cage assets for expiratory efforts that are analogous to two of those mentioned earlier for inspiratory efforts: first, the structure's large surface contact with the lungs; and second, the structure's capability for fine graded control of muscular pressure. Abdominal activity during the generation of positive muscular pressures at mid and low lung volumes takes advantage of the efficiency gains just mentioned for abdominal activity through the high lung volume range: first, the structure's provision of an opposing member for the rib cage to work against; and second, the structure's mechanical tuning of the diaphragm. Abdominal activity under such conditions also involves an additional efficiency gain in the form of a mechanical tuning of the rib cage. Expiratory activity of the abdomen exceeded that of the rib cage at mid and low lung volumes, as evidenced by the continuous distortion of the chest wall toward a larger rib cage volume and a smaller abdominal volume than those that would have existed during relaxation at prevailing lung volumes. Predominant activity of the abdomen delivers an upward lifting force to the rib cage that elevates the structure, increases its volume, and places its expiratory muscles at greater and more optimal lengths for generating quick, forceful pressure changes.

The abdominal component of chest wall distortion reflected in much of the singing data generated by the subject group often was substantially more than that associated with the group's speaking data. This difference may be related to the large pressure swings involved in singing as compared to speaking—swings that would require that a firmer opposing member be provided by the abdomen for the rib cage for singing than for speaking.

Inspirations of the subject group for singing usually were very quick, involved large volume excursions of the lungs, rib cage, and abdomen, and were accomplished using a wide range of relative volume contributions by the two chest wall parts. As with the expiratory phase of the respiratory cycle, subjects demonstrated a variety of chest wall displacement styles for inspiration, the determinants of which are unknown but probably are the same as those mentioned earlier for expiratory styles—self-preference for what seems effective and instruction on how to inspire while singing.

Of the styles observed for inspiration, the most prevalent involved rib cage and abdominal volume increases. Such increases traced pathways on data charts that tended to be concave toward the Y axis of the display and that, when unequal for the two parts, usually showed a predominant abdominal volume increase followed by a predominant rib cage volume increase. Unlike inspirations for speaking, inspirations for singing often involved changes in rib cage and abdominal volumes that were outside the confines of volumes associated with relaxation. Like inspirations for speaking, however, inspirations for singing showed a generalized distortion of the chest wall from its relaxed configuration toward a more expanded rib cage volume and a less expanded abdominal volume.

During inspiration, the general background task for the present subjects presumably was to exert rapidly increasing negative chest wall efforts. The mechanism most likely functioning at such times would involve increasingly negative efforts by the diaphragm and decreasingly positive efforts by the abdomen. Inspiratory effort by the rib cage does not seem a likely possibility, given the relative volume contributions observed for the present subjects and given that previous research (see Chapter 4) has shown the rib cage to be inactive or minimally active in the expiratory direction during inspirations associated with speaking and singing. Implication of the diaphragm as the prime inspiratory driver is supported by the large outward movements of the abdomen during inspirations, often particularly in association with the first part of the incremental excursion. Such movements are consistent, as is their presumed underlying cause, with observations by Bouhuys and colleagues (1966) and Proctor (1968) on singers showing large changes in transdiaphragmatic pressure reflective of vigorous diaphragmatic contraction. Proctor, in fact, presented data showing forceful diaphragmatic actions during the inspirations associated with a trained singer's performance of the same aria as performed by present subject WL.

Use of the diaphragm, not the rib cage, to generate negative muscular pressures for inspiration may have certain system advantages. First, the diaphragm is the most powerful of inspiratory muscles and through its contraction can displace both parts of the chest wall in the inspiratory direction—the abdomen because of a component of movement resolved footwardly and the rib cage because of a component of movement resolved headwardly. Second, use of the diaphragm as the sole inspiratory driver leaves the rib cage free of inspiratory assignment and, therefore, able to engage instantly in continued expiratory activity for singing once diaphragmatic activity is terminated. Third, the diaphragm can be continuously mechanically tuned by the abdomen for inspiratory action regardless of the lung volume, whereas such a tuning of the rib cage would run counter to the desirability of tuning the rib cage for expiratory function in singing.

Implication of the abdomen in the inspiratory mechanism suggested is supported by the observation that, throughout the inspirations of the present subjects, the volume of the abdomen was smaller, and often appreciably so, than the volumes associated with relaxation at corresponding lung volumes. The continued exertion of a positive abdominal effort during inspiration presumably provided a mechanical fulcrum for the diaphragm to work from in its action to elevate the rib cage and inflate the lungs. At times when inspiratory movements showed only moderate increases in abdominal volume, the level of abdominal effort probably was high in opposition to footward displacement of the diaphragm, whereas at times of substantial increases in abdominal volume the activity of the abdomen probably was less. Active abdominal involvement under the inspiratory circumstances described here appears to be similar to that inferred (see Chapter 3) and measured directly (see Chapter 4) during the speaking and singing of untrained subjects. The different patterns of inspiratory style demonstrated among the present subjects probably are related to the particular abdominal control strategy chosen by different subjects, not to significant differences in diaphragmatic function.

Inspiration-expiration transitions for the present subjects' classical singing involved the displacement of volume from one chest wall part to the other under isovolume conditions for the lungs. The most often observed of these transitions entailed a quick shift of volume from the abdomen to the rib cage. The probable mechanism underlying this adjustment would appear to be a forceful incremental activation of the abdomen, which served to "set up" the chest wall for operation during the ensuing breath group. The use of this mechanism, although a distinct phase of the expiratory process in certain subjects, also may have had a modified representation in breath groups, in which large inward abdominal movements occurred coincident with the initial moments of utterance. Chest wall function of the general nature inferred seems analogous to that observed for the initiation of connected speaking and singing in studies of untrained subjects (see Chapters 3 and 4, and Baken, Cavallo, and Weissman, 1979) and represents a form of preferred posturing of the chest wall, probably for reasons of mechanical advantage.

A quick shift of volume from the rib cage to the abdomen was an inspiration-expiration transition occasionally observed during the singing of a few of the present subjects. The mechanism operating for this adjustment would seem likely to be an incremental activation of the rib cage in the expiratory direction simultaneous with the maintenance of continued expiratory activation of the abdomen. The latter is inferred because the abdomen was maintained at sizes smaller than what it would assume during relaxation at the prevailing lung volume despite its enlargement during the transition. Again, chest wall set-up is involved, but of a type probably related to the preceding inspiration and its departure from the form for the majority of the inspiration-expiration transition patterns.

Expiration-inspiration transitions also constituted an important part of the respiratory cycle for singing. These involved rapid decreases in lung volume, sometimes the result of rib cage volume decreases and abdominal volume increases, and less often the result of abdominal volume decreases accompanied by a lesser or no decrease in rib cage volume. Rapid decreases in lung volume at the end of singing breath groups may be seen in the published records of other investigations of singing (Bouhuys et al., 1966; Proctor, 1968), although neither such decreases nor their role in mechanism have been discussed.

Unlike speaking, in which driving pressure usually trails off gradually near the end of the breath group, singing generally requires a continuation of alveolar pressurization of great magnitude to the very end of the phrase. In fact, in many circumstances, singing requires even more stringent pressure demands at the very end of the breath group than earlier, as for example in the case of dramatic endings of phrases or the hitting of so-called "money notes" of high intensity and high frequency. Breath group termination takes several forms but most often involves either an abrupt laryngeal release of a tracheal overpressure, resulting in a loud glottal aspiration, as in association with vowel phrase-endings, or an abrupt articulatory release (of a closure or constriction) of an oral overpressure, resulting in a loud upper airway frication, as in association with consonant phrase-endings. For most of the present subjects, expiration-inspiration transitions involved decreases in rib cage volume and paradoxical increases in abdominal volume. Most likely this adjustment is of active muscular origin and reflects a combined continuation of rib cage expiratory drive and reduction of abdominal drive. Continuation of rib cage expiratory drive under such circumstances would tend to force the abdomen outward paradoxically until contraction of the diaphragm would prevail and begin the inspiratory excursion. Such rib cage drive is consistent with a preference for making lung volume increase an abdominal event foremost during the first part of inspiration.

But what of those fewer expiration-inspiration transitions that were of a form characterized by somewhat further expiratory movement of the abdomen? It seems likely that the mechanism underlying such an adjustment involved a further stiffening of the abdomen so that diaphragmatic action would resolve initially into a lifting of the rib cage followed by a lesser outward movement of the abdominal wall. Such abdominal action is consistent with a preference for making rib cage displacement an early component of the inspiratory excursion.

Is there any significance to the singer in the differences between the two expiration-inspiration forms observed, their mechanisms, and their ensuing different inspiration forms? The answer may be affirmative and is addressed with some anecdotal considerations under the last heading here.

In summary, the present data for singing suggest a role for the abdomen that is mainly one of posturing the chest wall in a manner that aids both the rib cage and diaphragm in their primary functions. This role involves the configuration of the chest wall and extends across both phases of the respiratory cycle for singing. Pressurization of the pulmonary system for singing, by contrast, appears to be the major role of the rib cage during the expiratory side of the respiratory cycle as that structure functions to generate aeromechanical events of importance to the demands of the singing program. Finally, the diaphragm has as its assignment the inspiratory side of the respiratory cycle, its role being to inflate the pulmonary system quickly so the singing program can proceed.

Subjects' Beliefs About Their Respiratory Adjustments for Singing Versus the Actual Adjustments Used

Many teachers of singing and singers themselves often refer to the importance of "being in touch with the vocal instrument," of knowing how it works and how subtle adjustments in it influence singing performance. Along these lines, much attention often is focused on what singing teachers and singers believe are "correct" or "best" or "preferred" ways of breathing during singing as well as various "imageries" to be associated with these ways of breathing. It would seem probable that the more training a singer has had and the more extensive his or her performance experience, the more likely it is that he or she would be correct in beliefs about the mechanisms involved in his or her singing performance. Furthermore, it might be assumed that highly trained singers, in particular, would be in touch with what they are doing with their respiratory apparatus during singing. The present investigation generally fails to support either of these expectations. To the contrary, it demonstrates that singers who are highly trained, and in some cases have been recognized through success in competitions, generally do not have accurate knowledge of the mechanisms associated with their singing performance.

It is of interest to attempt to sort out why the present subjects' beliefs usually bore little or no correspondence to the respiratory events associated with their actual performance. It cannot be traced to their knowledge of respiratory anatomy, for by and large the present subjects demonstrated, through their written descriptions, that they had a reasonably good working knowledge of the structures of the respiratory apparatus.

Part of the incongruity can be traced to the present subjects' lacking a full understanding of the function of certain respiratory apparatus parts. For example, one subject referred to how he used his diaphragm to lift and push air out of the lungs, which, of course, cannot occur because the diaphragm is a muscle capable of delivering inspiratory force only. Part of the incongruity also can be traced to misconceptions of the present subjects concerning physical principles, some involving cause and effect, associated with respiratory physiology and mechanics. For example, one subject wrote of how air entered the lungs causing the diaphragm to sink, when it is descent of the diaphragm that causes air to enter the lungs. For another example, one subject wrote of his respiratory apparatus as a huge tub that fills from bottom to top, whereas the distribution of flow to the lungs, of course, does not demonstrate such a gradient. A further discrepancy between beliefs and actual events can be traced to misconceptions the present subjects had with regard to the function of the respiratory apparatus as a system. For example, subject statements such as "I do not draw in the air" and "Breathing is accomplished by letting the air 'fall into the lungs' " indicate that these subjects were not aware that the respiratory apparatus is a negative pressure pump that sucks air into the pulmonary system. For another example, subject descriptions such as "The air is not forced from the body, but is released" and "The breath pours out of the mouth as if I were sighing" suggest that their authors did not understand that the expiratory phase of the breathing act during singing is under constant muscular control that literally drives air from the respiratory apparatus. Thus, it can be seen that the present singers' beliefs about mechanism and actual mechanism did not coincide for multiple reasons, most of which are related to misunderstandings of certain biomechanical aspects of respiratory behavior. The singing folklore is rich in misconceptions concerning the transform between body biomechanics and artistic performance, and the outcome here should not be surprising. The myth of singing from the diaphragm, for example, has persisted for about as long as has the history of vocal performance (Hixon, 1975). The present data suggest that it and some other myths are alive in even highly trained singers, one consequence being that subjects who sing in relatively similar manners can come to conceptualize their performances in dramatically different ways.

Implications for the Training of Singers

What of significance for the training of singers can be derived from the results of this investigation?

A striking finding of the present investigation was the discrepancy between how subjects thought they breathed during classical singing and how they actually breathed. This finding suggests the need for additional emphasis in educating singers with regard to the workings of the respiratory apparatus and how such workings translate into performance. It seems reasonable to suppose that singers who have accurate conceptualizations about respiratory function would be in a better position to influence their performance product and use the respiratory apparatus more efficiently in performance.

As reviewed by Hixon and Hoffman (1979), many different teaching strategies currently are used in training classical singing students. The polar positions among these strategies place a great deal of emphasis on the positioning of the abdominal wall in the singing act. The findings of the present investigation on highly trained singers reveal that all of them employed the so-called "belly in" strategy for singing. Unanimous use of this strategy by the subject group suggests that it may have a collection of advantages for the singer toward which he or she naturally migrates with performance experience.

Even within the general "belly in" strategy used by the present subjects there were functional differences in kind. Certain patterns of chest wall adjustment occurred more often than others. Perhaps most notable were the differences observed among the subjects in patterns of inspiration during singing. The majority of inspirations involved predominant abdominal displacement followed by predominant rib cage displacement. This inspiratory pattern seemed to be preferred under most singing circumstances to the less occurring pattern of predominant rib cage displacement followed by predominant abdominal displacement. One of the present subjects, PW, who routinely used the less preferred pattern of the subject group, attempted to retrain his inspiratory patterning while observing his kinematic data "live" in chart form on the oscilloscope. In only a few minutes, he was able to train himself to the preferred pattern and routinely to incorporate its use in a new breathing style for singing. Although his report is anecdotal, nevertheless, he reported a clear preference for the "preferred" pattern of the subject group over his original pattern, stating that the preferred pattern made it much easier for him to take quick inspirations during singing. This is an encouraging note relative to the ease of use and instructive power of kinematic displays in reinstructing certain uses of the respiratory apparatus for singing. Perhaps the use of only verbal instruction, visual example, and imagery in training singers should be discontinued. That is, it may be that in the case of respiratory function, at least, there is a useful role to be played by instrumentation of the type used in this investigation.

ACKNOWLEDGMENT

The preparation of this manuscript was supported by grants from the National Institute of Neurological and Communicative Disorders and Stroke. Ms. Cynthia Hoffman of the Manhattan School of Music, New York, consulted on matters pertaining to classical singing.

REFERENCES

Agostoni, E., and Mead, J. (1964). Statics of the respiratory system. *In* W. Fenn and H. Rahn (Eds.): *Handbook of physiology. Respiration 1, Sect. 3.* Washington, DC: American Physiological Society.

Baken, R., Cavallo, S., and Weissman, K. (1979). Chest wall movements prior to phonation. *Journal of Speech and Hearing Research, 22,* 862–872.

Bouhuys, A., Proctor, D., and Mead, J. (1966). Kinetic aspects of singing. *Journal of Applied Physiology, 21,* 483–496.

Draper, M., Ladefoged, P., and Whitteridge, D. (1959). Respiratory muscles in speech. *Journal of Speech and Hearing Research, 2,* 16–27.

Eblen, R. (1963). Limitations of the use of surface electromyography in studies of speech breathing. *Journal of Speech*

and Hearing Research, 6, 3–18.

Hixon, T. (1975). *Respiratory function in speech and singing: Myth and reality.* Paper presented at the Voice Foundation Annual Symposium on Care of the Professional Voice, New York.

Hixon, T., and Hoffman C. (1979). Chest wall shape in singing. *In* V. Lawrence (Ed.): *Transcripts of the Seventh Symposium on Care of the Professional Voice, Part I: The Scientific Papers.* New York: The Voice Foundation.

Hoit-Dalgaard, J., Lansing, R., Plassman, B., and Hixon, T. (1983). *Abdominal EMG activity during speech.* Paper presented at the Annual Meeting of the Society for Neuroscience, Boston.

Proctor, D. (1968). The physiologic basis of voice training. *Annals of the New York Academy of Science, 155,* 208–228.

APPENDIX A

Years of Singing Training, Performance Experience, and Competition Awards of the Subjects Studied

Subject TA had studied classical singing for 20 years and was completing a Doctor of Musical Arts degree in choral conducting, with a minor in vocal performance. His performance experience included two major roles with the Denver Opera Company, four major roles with the Arizona Opera Company, one major role with an opera company in Greeley, one major role with an opera company in El Paso, and 10 major roles in university or college productions. He also was Artist in Residence with the Arizona Opera Company. TA had performed 10 oratorio roles with civic music organizations and had performed four graduate recitals. He had won or placed in the following competitions: regional finalist in the Metropolitan Opera Auditions; first-place winner in the graduate men's division of the Colorado-Wyoming National Association of Teachers of Singing Contest; vocal division winner of the University of Arizona President's Contest Competition; and first-place winner in the graduate division of the Northern Colorado Symphony Orchestra's Concerto Contest.

Subject DM had studied classical singing for 12 years and had completed a Doctor of Musical Arts degree in vocal performance. His performance experience included eight major roles with the Arizona Opera Company, two major roles in civic opera productions, and twelve major roles in university or college productions. He also had been a soloist with the Pittsburgh Symphony Orchestra. DM had performed five graduate recitals and was twice a district winner in the Metropolitan Opera Auditions. In addition, he was a winner in the San Francisco Opera Auditions and had participated in the San Francisco Merola Program.

Subject PW had studied classical singing for 10 years and had completed a Master of Music degree in vocal performance. His performance experience included one major role with a civic opera production and five major roles in university or college productions. PW had been a soloist in a university production of an oratorio, and had completed two graduate recitals.

Subject WL had studied classical singing for 10 years and was completing a Doctor of Musical Arts degree in choral conducting. His performance experience included two major roles in university productions. He also had been a soloist in one civic music organization's production of an oratorio.

Subjects are listed in order of decreasing years of training.

Subject JD had studied classical singing for 6 years and was completing a Master of Music degree in vocal performance. His performance experience included one major role with the Albuquerque Opera Theater and two major roles in university or college productions. He had been a soloist for one university production of an oratorio.

Subject SF had studied classical singing for 5 years and was completing a Master of Music degree in vocal performance. He had performed three major operatic roles in university or college productions. SF also had completed one graduate recital.

APPENDIX B

Information on the Arias Performed by the Subjects Studied

Subject: **TA**
Title: "Avant de Quitter"
Source: Faust
Composer: Gounod
Language: French
Key: E^b major
Range: C$_3$–C$_C$
Musical Characteristics: One section sustained with a high tessitura and one section declarative with vigorous singing.

Subject: **DM**
Title: "Pierrot's Tanzlied"
Source: Die Tote Stadt
Composer: Korngold
Language: German
Key: D^b major
Range: D$^b_3$–G$^b_4$
Musical Characteristics: Slow and sustained with a high tessitura and high pianissimo singing.

Subject: **PW**
Title: "Avant de Quitter"
Source: Faust
Composer: Gounod
Language: French
Key: D^b major
Range: B$^b_2$–F$_4$
Musical Characteristics: Same as described for Subject TA above.

Subject: WL
Title: "But Who May Abide the Day of His Coming"
Source: The Messiah
Composer: Handel
Language: English
Key: D minor
Range: G_2–E_4
Musical Characteristics: One section slow and sustained and one section vigorous and florid.

Subject: JD
Title: "Deh Vieni Alla Finestra"
Source: Don Giovanni
Composer: Mozart
Language: Italian
Key: D major
Range: D_3–E_4
Musical Characteristics: Primarily legato singing.

Subject: SF
Title: "Eri tu che Macchiavi"
Source: Un Ballo in Maschera
Composer: Verdi
Language: Italian
Key: F major
Range: C_3–G_4
Musical Characteristics: Sustained and dramatic with a high tessitura.

CHAPTER 11

Respiratory Kinematics in Classical (Shakespearean) Actors

Thomas J. Hixon
Peter J. Watson
Mary Z. Maher

To breathe or not to breathe—
that is the question.

Anonymous

A cting involves simulated behaviors, pretenses, that most often are thought of in terms of their dramatic progression and emotional content. These, however, are not the only levels at which it is important to examine the performance features of acting. Another has to do with the biomechanical manifestations of acting. Although it may seem novel to consider acting from such a perspective, forceful arguments can be made that the manner in which an actor uses the speech apparatus is fundamental to much of what dramatic progression and emotional content are all about. Furthermore, the effective and efficient use of the speech apparatus undoubtedly is one of the keys to a successful and sustained acting career.

To know how experienced, premier actors use the speech apparatus during performance would be valuable to students learning to act and to individuals wishing to refine their acting skills through performance modeling of those at the top of the acting craft. As with the biomechanical process underlying singing (see Chapter 10), substantial folklore surrounds the biomechanical bases of acting and what constitutes appropriate use of the production apparatus. When attempting to assess various viewpoints about appropriate use of the speech apparatus in acting, it is found that there is a paucity of biomechanical data on acting performance.

In an attempt to meet part of the need for information in this area, the present investigation sought to provide data on the function of one subsystem of the actor's speech production apparatus, namely, the respiratory apparatus. Actors with a wide range of performance capabilities and especially renowned for classical drama were chosen for study. Classical drama, the drama of the Greeks and of Shakespeare, is believed by many to constitute the highest challenge to an actor. Its performance is among the most physically demanding, having, in many regards, parallels to the types of performance demands often required of classical singers. Like classical singers (see Chapter 10), classical actors usually perform without amplification, go on for prolonged periods, and tax essentially the full range of vocal ability. And, like classical singers and their position atop the technical hierarchy of singing, classical actors, most would agree, are at the top of the technical hierarchy of their craft.

The approach chosen for this investigation was the kinematic method of Hixon, Goldman, and Mead (see Chapter 3). This method is noninvasive and requires little experimental sophistication on the part of those being studied (see Chapters 5 and 10). As shown by examples in Chapters 3 through 10, previous investigations have demonstrated that comprehensive accounts of respiratory function can be developed using this method and that accurate determinations can be made of the inherent and volitional forces involved in the respiratory activities considered.

METHOD

Subjects

Four normal adults, three men and one woman, served as subjects. Data on certain of their physical characteristics are presented in Table 11–1. All subjects had extensive dramatic training and performance experience and were earning their livelihoods as professional actors. All were members of the Royal Shakespeare Company and of Britain's Classical Company at the National Theatre in London. In addition, each subject had substantial experience in acting for motion pictures and television. Performance experience of each subject is summarized briefly in Appendix A. By all criteria, the subject group would be considered to consist of world-class professional actors.

Table 11-1. *Data on Certain Physical Characteristics of the Subjects Studied*

Subject (ID)	Age (yr)	Height (cm)	Weight (kg)	Vital Capacity (L)
JG	50	188.0	78.5	4.3
JB	52	172.7	67.6	4.4
DR	36	182.9	72.6	4.9
SA	53	170.2	61.3	3.0

Subjects JG, JB, and DR are men. Subject SA is a woman.

Performance Conditions

Observations were made in a lecture hall having a small stage raised off the main floor and a raked-type seating arrangement. The acoustical characteristics of the hall were judged by both the investigators and the subjects to be adequate for the purposes of the performances.

Each subject stood toward the front and in the center of the stage and faced out toward the seats of the lecture hall. Male subjects performed bare-chested. The female subject performed while wearing a loose-fitting hospital gown over a bathing suit. Subjects were instructed to avoid raising their arms or shifting their posture during recordings.

The audience consisted of the three investigators, a video equipment operator, and, on occasion, one or more of the subjects who already had participated in the investigation. In an attempt to put a live performance "edge" on the subjects, they were told that audio-video and audio tape-recordings of their performances would be made available to student actors and other professionals concerned with acting and the voice.

Procedure

Five days before the observations were made, each subject was given a copy of a poem and told that he or she would be asked to perform a dramatic reading of it during the investigation proper. Each subject was told to practice reading the poem until comfortable with it, but not to memorize it for the performance. Each subject also was asked to come to the observation session prepared to perform a monologue of choice from any play by William Shakespeare. The only restrictions imposed were that the monologue of choice had to be committed to memory and, in the subject's judgment, best display his or her classical acting ability. Finally, subjects were asked to write out descriptions of how they believed they breathed during classical acting performances.

Three types of observations were made during the investigation: audio-video recordings, audio recordings, and recordings of the kinematic behavior of the chest wall (see Fig. 11–1).

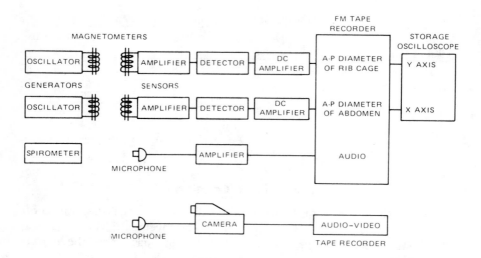

FIGURE 11–1. Diagram of the equipment used.

For audio-video recordings, the acoustic signal was sensed by an air microphone, and the video signal was sensed by a color video camera.

A second air microphone was used to sense the acoustic signal, to enable synchronization of speech audio events with the kinematic behavior of the chest wall and to assist in the correlation of audio-video events and kinematic behavior. The output of this second microphone was amplified and fed to a direct-record channel of an FM tape recorder.

Respiratory data were obtained using a streamlined form of the kinematic method of Hixon and colleagues (see Chapter 3). This method treats the chest wall as a two-part system consisting of the rib cage and the abdomen. Each part displaces volume as it moves, and together they displace a volume equal to that displaced by the lungs. Volume changes of the rib cage and abdomen are related linearly to changes in their respective anteroposterior diameters. Therefore, only diameter changes need to be determined to obtain measures of the volumes displaced by these individual parts and the lungs.

For this investigation, diameter changes were sensed using linearized magnetometers (GMG Scientific Inc., 1980). These devices include electromagnetic coil pairs that provide a voltage analog of the distance between them. Two such pairs were used, one for the rib cage and one for the abdomen. A generator coil in each pair was attached to the front of the torso at the midline, that for the rib cage at sternal midlength and that for the abdomen slightly above the navel. A sensor coil in each pair was attached to the back of the torso at the midline and at the same axial level as its generator mate. Output signals from the two sensor coils were processed electronically and recorded on two channels of an FM tape recorder.

The streamlined method required that subjects perform several respiratory activities. These included vital capacity maneuvers, isovolume shape changes of the respiratory apparatus at the resting tidal end-expiratory level (i.e., at the functional residual capacity, FRC), and momentary breath holding at 1 L above FRC. Three vital capacity maneuvers were performed. For each, the subject (wearing a noseclip) inspired fully, and then expired fully through a mouthpiece attached to a spirometer. The largest of the three measured expiratory excursions was taken as the subject's vital capacity (VC). Isovolume shape changes were performed several times at the end of resting tidal breaths. For these, each subject fixed the lung volume, closed the larynx, and slowly displaced volume back and forth between the rib cage and abdomen by alternately moving the abdominal wall inward and outward. For the momentary breath holding activity, each subject (wearing a noseclip) was instructed to stop breathing at the resting tidal end-expiratory level, inspire to 1 L above this level through a mouthpiece coupled to a spirometer, and once again momentarily stop breathing until signaled to recommence by an investigator.

Each subject performed four speaking activities. For the first, the subject engaged in approximately 3 minutes of spontaneous conversational discourse with one of the investigators. The second speaking activity involved reading aloud a declarative paragraph, "The Rainbow Passage" by Fairbanks (1960), in what the subject judged to be a typical conversational manner. None of the subjects had knowledge of this declarative paragraph prior to being asked to read it. The third speaking activity involved the dramatic reading of a poem, "The Hand that Signed the Paper Felled a City," by Dylan Thomas (1946). This was the poem that the subjects had been given five days earlier and told to practice reading. The fourth and final speaking activity was the subject's performance of his or her monologue of choice from a play by Shakespeare. Appendix B provides information on the monologues performed by the subjects.

Data Charts

Data charts were formed in which the anteroposterior diameter of the rib cage, increasing upward on the Y axis, was displayed against the anteroposterior diameter of the abdomen, increasing rightward on the X axis (see Fig. 11–2). To facilitate direct reading of such charts, their axes were converted from diameters to displacements. This was done by adjusting the amplifier gains on the Y and X channels of the display oscilloscope during playback of each subject's performance of isovolume shape changes at FRC until the resulting isovolume line on the screen had a slope of -1. In conjunction with the conversion of the Y and X axes of the charts, a third axis also was added. This axis displayed the volume displacement of the lungs, which is the sum of the rib cage volume and abdominal volume represented

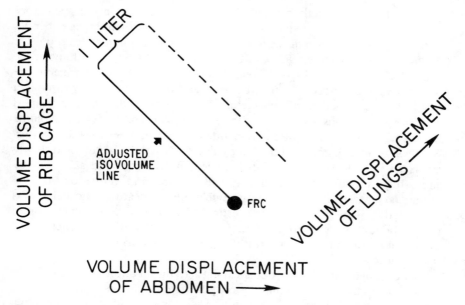

FIGURE 11–2. Relative volume chart with isovolume lines at FRC (functional residual capacity) and at 1 L above FRC.

by each point on the chart. On this axis, running at a 45-degree diagonal, lung volume increases upward and rightward. With the data charts so formed, it was possible to read them directly for (1) the volumes of the rib cage and the abdomen, given by position along their respective axes, (2) the relative volume displacement of the two parts, given by the slope of any pathway formed, and (3) the volume displacement of the lungs, given by the distance between any two points parallel to the third axis of the charts. The solid isovolume line depicted in Figure 11–2 represents that generated during the actual isovolume maneuvers and corrected from diameters-to-displacements upon playback of the data. The dashed line running above and parallel to the actual isovolume line is a line representing isovolume at 1 L above the actual FRC isovolume line. This line is an extension from the chest wall configuration attained by the subject during breath holding at 1 L above the resting tidal end-expiratory level (at FRC) and is constructed under the assumption that an actual isovolume line generated at this lung volume would parallel the isovolume line produced by the subject at FRC.

RESULTS

Figure 11–3 presents kinematic data from the four subjects studied.

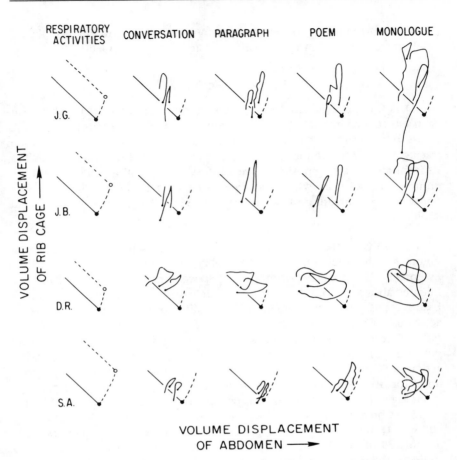

FIGURE 11–3. Kinematic data for the four subjects studied. See text for explanation.

Respiratory Activities

Data generated from respiratory maneuvers were used to construct the left-most data chart shown for each subject. The solid isovolume line in each chart in Figure 11–3 is at FRC, whereas the dashed isovolume line is at 1 L above FRC. The filled and open circles at the righthand ends of the solid and dashed isovolume lines suggest the relative volumes that would have been obtained were the subjects to have relaxed completely at FRC and at 1 L above FRC, respectively. These circles and the dashed line that interconnects them are estimations based on relaxation characteristic data generated by other normal adult subjects (see Chapters 3 and 4). The actual isovolume lines generated by the subjects at FRC were flat loops or single lines, each being linear or approximately so. Selected portions of the left-most charts in Figure 11–3 are reproduced in the remaining charts for each subject.

Speaking Activities

Data for speaking activities are shown in the right-most four charts for each subject in Figure 11–3. Representative data tracings are portrayed in the charts, but only a few tracings are shown to avoid cluttering the displays. Each tracing is for a single respiratory cycle. The dotted end of each tracing specifies its inspiratory starting position. The discussion that follows is based on the entire data pool from which the tracings have been drawn. This data pool consists of 386 breath groups and includes 82 to 121 tracings for individual subjects.

LUNG VOLUME.   For the most part, speaking activities took place at lung volumes within the midrange of the vital capacity (i.e., the middle 50% VC). Essentially all expiratory portions of the speech breathing cycles (98%) were initiated above FRC. Of these, approximately 85% were begun between 1.25 L above FRC and FRC. Initiation levels differed across the four speaking activities for the different subjects, but differently so for each subject. The only discernible group trend was that initiation levels for monologue performance frequently were higher than those for the other three speaking activities. This was most strikingly the case for subject JG, whose expiratory limbs (breath groups) typically were initiated an average of 1.0 L higher for monologue than for conversation, paragraph reading, and poem reading.

Most breath groups (83%) ended between 0.5 L above FRC and 0.6 L below FRC. Within this range, approximately one third of the expiratory limbs terminated above FRC. Termination levels differed across activities and subjects, the only group trend being relatively similar termination levels for the subjects on the paragraph reading activity (roughly 50% ending above FRC and 50% ending below FRC for each subject). Subjects JG and DR demonstrated a significant dissimilarity to general group trends for monologue performance. Both frequently ended breath groups for such performance well below FRC, sometimes as much as 1.5 L or more into the expiratory reserve volume.

Lung volume excursions ranged considerably among the breath groups generated by the subjects. Approximately 80% of such excursions were between 0.25 and 1.5 L in magnitude. Excursion magnitude revealed a tendency to increase across the four speaking activities for the subject group (i.e., from conversation to paragraph reading to poem reading to monologue performance). The contrast between the monologue data and those for the other three activities was particularly striking. Excursions of 1.5 to 2.0 L were common, with those for subject JG frequently ranging between approximately 2.0 and 3.0 L.

RELATIVE VOLUME DISPLACEMENTS OF THE RIB CAGE AND ABDOMEN. Lung volume change for the four speaking activities resulted from a wide variety of relative displacements of the rib cage and abdomen.

Data tracings indicated that the findings were mixed across the subject group with regard to relative contributions of the rib cage and abdomen during the inspiratory phase of the respiratory cycle. For subjects JG and JB, the volume contribution of the rib cage exceeded that of the abdomen throughout the inspiratory phase in 53% of the respiratory cycles. In another 44% of such cycles, these same two subjects demonstrated equal rib cage and abdominal displacements throughout the inspiratory phase, or inspiratory displacements that shifted from rib cage predominance to equal rib cage and abdominal contributions, or the converse. Subject SA demonstrated a range of relative volume displacements of the rib cage and abdomen during her inspirations. For about 85% of her inspiratory phases she used some form of rib cage predominance or equal contributions of the rib cage and abdomen. However, for about 15% of her inspirations (always involving poem or monologue performances), she began her inspirations with a predominant abdominal displacement followed by a predominant rib cage displacement. Subject DR showed inspiratory excursions that were characterized by mixed relative contributions of the rib cage and abdomen from cycle to cycle, but which primarily involved a predominant abdominal displacement followed by equal rib cage and abdominal displacements (i.e., in 53% of his respiratory cycles) or by predominant rib cage displacement (see sample monologue tracings for DR).

For portions of some (about 4%) of the inspirations of the subjects as a group, paradoxical displacement of the abdomen was demonstrated. That is, although the volume displacement of the lungs was in the inspiratory direction, the displacement of the abdomen was in the expiratory direction. Subject DR also demonstrated paradoxical displacement of the rib cage during portions of some of his inspiratory phases. In such instances, the volume displacement of the lungs was in the inspiratory direction, while that of the rib cage was in the expiratory direction. For his poem reading and monologue performance, for example, approximately half of DR's respiratory cycles revealed moments of paradoxical rib cage displacement during inspiration (see Fig. 11–3 for examples).

For the expiratory phase of the respiratory cycle, the data tracings also indicated findings, both across the subject group and from activity to activity for individual subjects, that were mixed with regard to relative contributions of the rib cage and abdomen. The range of relative contributions extended from marked predominance of the rib cage to marked predominance of the abdomen, with the two extremes being manifested by subjects JG and DR, respectively (e.g., see the sample tracings for their poem readings). Subjects JG, JB, and SA demonstrated either rib cage predominance or equal rib cage and abdominal contributions in 70% of the expiratory limbs associated with their conversational discourse, paragraph reading, and poem reading activities. When engaged in monologue performance, however, these same three subjects tended to shift toward patterning that involved abdominal predominance followed by rib cage predominance. This latter patterning of relative contributions was displayed with great frequency for all of the speaking activities by subject DR (i.e., in about 60% of his breath groups), as were other patterns involving predominant abdominal contributions (in another approximately 20% of his breath groups). Thus, a relatively consistent group trend was observed in varying degrees for relative volume displacements by all of the subjects for the monologue performance. This entailed an initial predominant displacement of the abdomen followed by a predominant displacement of the rib cage as the expiratory excursion proceeded.

For portions of some (about 15%) of the expiratory limbs of the subject group, paradoxical displacement of the abdomen was observed. That is, although the volume displacement of the lungs was in the expiratory direction, the displacement of the abdomen was in the inspiratory direction (e.g., see JG's monologue data). Likewise, for portions of some (approximately 20%) of the expiratory limbs generated, especially those for monologue performance by subjects JG, JB, and SA, and for the performance of activities in general by subject DR, paradoxical displacement of the rib cage was observed. In this case, the change in lung volume was in the expiratory direction, whereas the displacement of the rib cage was in the inspiratory direction. In some cases (approximately 25% of all expiratory limbs) for subject DR, in fact, this paradoxing prevailed throughout the entire expiratory limb (e.g., see paragraph reading) such that the rib cage continuously increased in size as utterance proceeded.

Superimposed on the general displacement patterns that have been described were occasional rapid, marked changes in the relative contributions of the rib cage and abdomen. These differed in kind, some involving shifts from essentially all rib cage contribution to all abdominal contribution, or the converse, and some involving abrupt paradoxical displacements of either the rib cage or the abdomen. Contrasting examples can be seen in the poem reading data in Figure 11–3 for subjects JG and SA. Most often, these changes were associated with abrupt changes in the spoken material itself. For example, changes to marked inward abdominal displacement with paradoxical outward displacement of the rib cage were associated with increases in loudness or linguistic stress (see JG's poem data). For another example, changes to marked inward rib cage displacement with paradoxical outward displacement of the abdomen (i.e., downward and rightward on the charts) often were associated with linguistic segments involving high flows, as in the case of voiceless fricative elements.

SEPARATE VOLUMES OF THE RIB CAGE AND ABDOMEN. Essentially all expiratory limbs (breath groups) were initiated at rib cage volumes larger than those associated with the resting tidal end-expiratory level. Of these, approximately 75% were initiated between 2.0 and 0.5 L above this resting landmark. Initiation levels differed across speaking activities in ways that were idiosyncratic to individual subjects. Only in the case of monologue performance was a group trend apparent; the average rib cage starting volumes for breath groups were higher for monologue performance than for the other three speaking activities, for all of the subjects. The largest difference was observed for subject JG, whose expiratory limbs were sometimes initiated more than 1.0 L higher in rib cage volume for monologue performance than for conversation, paragraph reading, and poem reading. In relation to JG's rib cage volume at the resting tidal end-expiratory level, some of his rib cage initiation levels for monologue performance were as much as 3.0 L higher in rib cage volume.

Approximately 80% of the expiratory limbs were terminated at rib cage volumes ranging between 1.0 L above and 0.5 L below the rib cage volume associated with the resting tidal end-expiratory level. Of these, approximately three fourths were terminated at rib cage volumes in excess of those at the resting end-expiratory level. No discernible group trends characterized the termination levels across the four speaking activities. Each subject demonstrated a different data pattern across activities. Subject DR was a notable exception to the general rib cage volume termination range employed by the subjects as a group. In his case, rib cage volume at the end of expiratory limbs often (i.e., for approximately 55% of the breath groups) was greater than the 1.0 L upper limit for the subject group in general. As noted earlier, for approximately 25% of DR's expiratory limbs, rib cage volume increased continuously. This means that his rib cage volume at breath group termination actually was higher than the volume that prevailed at breath group initiation.

Rib cage excursions ranged from zero to 1.5 L for the bulk of the expiratory limbs (86%). Excursions in excess of 1.5 L were confined mainly to subjects JB and JG, especially for monologue performance. The subjects demonstrated a tendency to generate greater rib cage excursions for monologue performance than for the other three speaking activities. It is further noteworthy that in those instances for which subject DR's rib cage volume was greater at the end than at the beginning of an expiratory limb, his net rib cage excursion was actually inspiratory. This means that the expiratory displacement of the abdomen actually exceeded the expiratory displacement of the lungs by an amount equal to the inspiratory displacement (i.e., excursion) of the rib cage.

Most expiratory limbs (about 80%) were initiated at abdominal volumes between 0.4 L larger and 0.6 L smaller than the abdominal volume associated with the resting tidal end-expiratory level. Subjects JG, JB, and DR tended to start expiratory limbs at abdominal volumes equal to or smaller than the abdominal volumes at resting tidal end-expiratory level. By contrast, subject SA began approximately half of her expiratory limbs at abdominal volumes larger than that associated with her resting end-expiratory level. No group trends were discernible across the four speaking activities involved.

For the most part, termination volumes of the abdomen ranged between the abdominal volume at the resting tidal end-expiratory level and 1.0 L smaller than this reference level. Subject DR proved an exception for paragraph reading, poem reading, and monologue performance in that his abdominal termination levels usually were in excess of 1.0 L smaller than that at his resting tidal end-expiratory level. A group trend was observed for lower abdominal volume terminations for monologue performance than for the other three speaking activities. Otherwise, data patterns across the speaking activities were different from subject to subject.

Volume excursions of the abdomen ranged from zero to 0.5 L for approximately 90% of the breath groups generated by subjects JG, JB, and SA. In sharp contrast to the data for these three subjects, subject DR showed abdominal excursions that were routinely in excess of 0.5 L for paragraph reading, poem reading, and monologue performance. For some breath groups, DR's abdominal excursions encompassed magnitudes in excess of 2.0 L.

Considering the separate volume data for speaking activities relative to those for the subjects' presumed relaxation characteristics, it is found that respiratory cycles took place to the left of the relaxation configurations of the chest wall in each panel in Figure 11–3. This means that the rib cage was relatively more and the abdomen was relatively less expanded during speaking activities than they would be in the relaxed state at corresponding lung volumes.

RESPIRATORY PHASE TRANSITIONS. To this point, consideration has been given to those parts of the respiratory cycle associated with inspiration and the utterance portion of expiration. Phase transitions between these two also occurred and warrant consideration.

Inspiration-expiration transitions took two forms. For each of these, lung volume remained constant but volume was shifted between the two parts of the chest wall in a manner similar to that involved in the performance of a limited, unidirectional isovolume shape change. Most often observed was a transition in which volume was shifted abruptly from the abdomen to the rib cage. This adjustment was limited almost exclusively to respiratory cycles associated with monologue performance. The other form of inspiration-expiration transition involved an abrupt shift of volume from the rib cage to the abdomen. This adjustment was used by subject SA and was most often associated with monologue performance. For both inspiration-expiration transition forms observed, the magnitude of the volume shifts between the two chest wall parts was relatively small (i.e., a maximum of 0.05 L).

Expiration-inspiration transitions also occurred in two forms. Both of these involved abrupt decreases in lung volume. Each form most often preceded relatively quick inspirations. The most frequently observed form of expiration-inspiration transition was that in which the decrease in lung volume involved a substantial decrease in rib cage volume and a lesser increase in abdominal volume. This form of transition occurred most often during monologue performance for the subject group, however, for subject DR, it was a prominent feature of many of his respiratory cycles for all the speaking activities. The magnitude of lung volume and rib cage volume decrements associated with this form of transition occasionally reached as high as 0.5 L. The other expiration-inspiration transition form occurred only during monologue performance, and most prominently so for subject JG. In this form of transition, both the rib cage and abdomen were involved in the expiratory direction during the adjustment, with the lung volume decreases attaining magnitudes as great as 0.8 L on some occasions. In almost all instances, abdominal displacement predominated over that of the rib cage during the transition.

The reader interested in graphic illustrations of the transition forms just discussed should consult Figure 10–9. The transitions shown in that figure for classical singers, although usually most extensive in terms of rib cage, abdominal, and lung volume displacements, are quite similar in kind to those observed for the present subjects.

Subjects' Descriptions of Their Speech Breathing During Classical Acting

Table 11–2 presents a written description of how each subject believed he or she used the respiratory apparatus during classical acting. Descriptions are verbatim. As seen in the table, written accounts differed markedly among the subjects.

Several structural elements were referred to by the subjects, including, the diaphragm, rib cage, lungs, shoulders, upper chest, intercostal muscles, chest cavity, lower regions of the back, stomach, neck, rib areas, throat, and resonator cavities of the chest, mouth, and head.

With regard to mechanism on the inspiratory side of the respiratory cycle, the subjects presented a broad spectrum of beliefs. Subjects JG, DR, and SA wrote of their beliefs about regional action in the respiratory apparatus during inspiration. Subject JG described inspiration as a process in which activation of the diaphragm is followed by activation of the rib cage. Subject DR wrote of "breathing low" and diaphragmatically and of using the intercostal muscles to expand the rib cage. Subject SA wrote of allowing the lungs to fill in the lower regions of the back and stomach (i.e., presumably the abdomen). Subjects also made reference to different levels of awareness with regard to inspiratory action in relation to performance. For example, subject JB wrote that he did "not employ anything approximating to a conscious technique"

Table 11-2. *Written Descriptions of How Each Subject Believed He or She Used the Respiratory Apparatus During Classical Acting*

Subject	Description
JG	I inhale by muscular contraction of the diaphragm followed by that of the rib cage. I breathe in by expanding my rib cage, which creates a vacuum in my lungs when air is drawn in. I breathe out using a reverse procedure.
JB	I do not employ anything approximating to a conscious technique. Occasionally, I will be aware that there is a sequence of two or three lines that I wish to deliver on one breath, so to avoid pausing I will find a point where I can take a larger breath or a snatched one to sustain these particular lines.
DR	I was taught to relax the shoulders and to breathe not with the upper chest but diaphragmatically, and I think that some of this teaching sunk in. Certainly, I'm aware of a necessity to take in more air to "support" the voice during a performance and have an experience of "breathing low." I was also taught "rib reserve" technique, which involves using the intercostal muscles to expand the rib cage on the in-breath and to keep them expanded during difficult or demanding passages. The theory is that this (a) enlarges the chest cavity and gives more resonance, particularly to lower notes, and (b) gives you a reserve of air in case you run short on a long phrase—i.e., you may have shoved out all the air you have with the diaphragm, but you can then collapse the rib cage and can find the air to end the sentence. I think it works, and do to some extent use it, although many voice teachers condemn the technique as "unnatural."
SA	How on earth do I breathe? This takes some working out, because by now what my teachers were instilling into me at 16 has become automatic. It's basically learning to allow the lungs to fill in the lower regions of the back, and even stomach. Not in the neck or rib areas, because this will create tension around the neck and throat causing stress, and also it will limit the resonator cavities of the chest, mouth, and head. Once you have the air inside you, you have to learn to relax and trust it is there and will serve you. Your mind then has to be freed, like the wind, to roam where it will, and you have to learn to let the breath go with it. All I know is, I see a piece of prose, and I inhale and unconsciously know how to use it.

except on occasion when he needed to take "a larger breath or a snatched one." Subject DR wrote of his awareness "of a necessity to take in more air to 'support' the voice during a performance." And subject SA wrote of her belief that at this stage in her career what she had learned had become "automatic."

Concerning the expiratory side of the respiratory cycle, subjects again presented a broad spectrum of beliefs. Subject JG wrote that he expired "using a reverse procedure" of that which prevailed during the inspiratory side of the respiratory cycle. Subject DR described how he was taught to keep the rib cage "expanded during difficult or demanding passages" to give him a "reserve of air" for long phrases. He gave as an example of the relevance of this strategy the notion that "you may have shoved out all the air you have with the diaphragm, but you can then collapse the rib cage and can find the air to end the sentence." Finally, subject SA indicated that the expiratory side of the speech breathing cycle was not something to which she gave much concern. She wrote as follows: "Once you have the air inside you, you have to learn to relax and trust it is there and will serve you. Your mind then has to be freed, like the wind, to roam where it will and you have to learn to let the breath go with it. All I know is, I see a piece of prose, and I inhale and unconsciously know how to use it."

DISCUSSION

Findings are discussed under the following headings: respiratory adjustments in conversation, paragraph reading, poem reading, and monologue performance; subjects' beliefs about their respiratory adjustments and the actual adjustments used; and implications for the training of actors.

Respiratory Adjustments in Conversation, Paragraph Reading, Poem Reading, and Monologue Performance

The kinematic data generated by three of the present subjects (JG, JB, and SA) for spontaneous conversational discourse, reading of a declarative paragraph, and dramatic reading of a poem are relatively similar to those obtained for analogous speaking activities from vocally untrained normal men (see Chapters 3 and 8) and women (Hodge, Hixon, and Putnam, 1982). They also are relatively similar to data obtained for such speaking activities from highly trained classical singers (see Chapter 10). Taken collectively, these present and past data reveal conversation and reading to be generated through respiratory adjustments that (1) occur mainly within the midrange of the vital capacity, (2) involve general chest wall deformations toward larger rib cage volumes and smaller abdominal volumes than those associated with relaxation at corresponding lung volumes, and (3) include relative volume contributions that range from all rib cage displacement to all abdominal displacement.

Past research involving direct measurements of chest wall dynamics has documented the muscular mechanisms involved in respiratory control for conversation and reading (see Chapter 4). Based on the kinematic similarities between data obtained in that research and in the present investigation, it seems reasonable to assume that the muscular mechanisms underlying the conversation, paragraph reading, and poem reading of the present subjects were as follows. Presumably, for the expiratory phase of the respiratory cycle, the rib cage and abdomen exerted expiratory forces that drove the chest wall at a configuration determined mainly by a predominant activity of the abdomen. For inspirations associated with the three speaking activities of concern, the rib cage presumably decreased its expiratory effort to zero (or nearly so) while the abdomen continued to exert a major effort. From off the background configuration maintained by the abdomen, the diaphragm functioned against the opposing taut abdomen to elevate the passive (or nearly so) rib cage. The strong inspiratory activity of the diaphragm restored the respiratory apparatus to a higher lung volume, rib cage volume, and abdominal volume by elevating the rib cage axially and forcing the active abdomen outward in counteraction to its continued expiratory effort.

The kinematic data generated by subject DR for conversation, paragraph reading, and poem reading are quite different from those generated for these activities by the other three subjects studied. Furthermore, subject DR's data for these activities are quite different in important regards from those generated for analogous activities by all normal subjects previously studied with the kinematic method (e.g., see Chapters 3, 4, 6, 7, 8, 10, and 12; and Mead, Hixon, and Goldman, 1974). As noted earlier, subject DR often showed rib cage paradoxing throughout extended portions of both phases of the respiratory cycles associated with his conversation and reading activities. In the case of his expiratory phases, in fact, such paradoxing often continued throughout the entire expiratory limb (i.e., abdominal displacements continuously exceeded those of the lungs, and the volume of the rib cage actually increased from the beginning to the end of the breath group). Previously studied normal subjects have not shown extended rib cage paradoxing of the types characteristic of much of subject DR's data. Thus, much of his data are unique with regard to both the inspiratory and expiratory phases of the speech breathing cycles associated with conversation and reading.

Presumably, the mechanism underlying DR's use of the chest wall for the three speaking activities of concern involved simultaneous expiratory efforts by the rib cage and abdomen, but with the latter predominating to such a great extent that the rib cage was forced more and more axially headward during a major part or all of each expiratory limb. This means that DR not only used his abdomen to set the background configuration of the chest wall for the expiratory phase of the cycle, but also that he used it in relation to the rib cage in such a fashion that the expiratory drive of the rib cage was more than counteracted by the drive from the abdomen. For inspirations associated with DR's conversation and reading, the rib cage presumably decreased its expiratory effort to zero (or nearly so) while the abdomen substantially decreased its powerful expiratory effort. Concomitant with these actions, the diaphragm functioned to elevate the rib cage and force the abdominal wall outward in counteraction to its continued expiratory effort. The paradoxical rib cage displacement during DR's inspirations presumably was related to the rapid, powerful contraction of the diaphragm, which abruptly and substantially lowered pleural pressure and sucked the rib cage inward. The durations of subject DR's inspirations for conversation and reading were, on the average, less than half those for the other three subjects in the present investigation.

Across all activities the average was 0.32 seconds for DR, versus 0.65 seconds for the other three subjects. Why are subject DR's overall kinematic patterns and underlying mechanisms unique? An answer will be suggested after consideration of the monologue data for the subject group.

Before leaving the topic of conversation and reading, one additional area warrants consideration. The kinematic data obtained for conversational discourse, paragraph reading, and poem reading proved to be relatively similar within individual subjects. However, in replaying the audio and audio-video recordings made during the investigation, it became apparent that each subject's dramatic reading of the poem involved substantially louder speech and greater "carrying power" than did the same subject's conversation and paragraph reading. This observation was further validated by two judges who, using direct magnitude estimation procedures, scaled the loudness of each subject's speaking activities relative to the loudness of his or her conversational discourse. Dramatic reading of the poem always was rated to be at least twice as loud as conversational discourse and substantially louder than paragraph reading.

Past research on vocally untrained subjects (see Chapters 3 and 4) has shown them generally to produce louder-than-normal speech from higher lung volumes. With louder speech demanding a higher driving pressure, the shift to higher lung volumes for such speech apparently takes advantage of the higher respiratory recoil forces available at such lung volumes. In the case of the present classical actors, they did not go to higher lung volumes during their dramatic reading of the poem, despite the fact that this reading was judged to be substantially louder than conversation and paragraph reading. It may be that their solution to providing a higher driving pressure was to apply a higher muscular pressure to the respiratory apparatus without changing the range of lung volumes involved. Interestingly, study of classical singers (see Chapter 10) has shown half of them to follow the loudness-increase strategy of vocally untrained subjects (see Chapters 3 and 4) and half to follow the strategy of the present world-class classical actors.

What is it about vocal training that would cause the present subjects and many classical singers to adopt strategies different from those of untrained persons? Although it is conjecture, it may be worth considering such findings from the perspective of upper airway adjustments rather than from the perspective of solely respiratory adjustments. Classical singers are known to produce a special "singing formant" or "ring" within the voice, a form of localized acoustical resonance that increases the carrying power of the voice and enhances its "projection" (Sundberg, 1974; Leeper, 1984). Perhaps the difference between normal reading and dramatic reading is accomplished by the highly trained classical actor through the use of a similar mechanism. That is, there may well be a "ring" to the dramatic speaking voice that is the result of upper airway adjustments and that would be sufficient to achieve the desired difference between normal and dramatic reading while not requiring major adjustments in respiratory drive. Perhaps the fact that half of the classical singers that have been studied showed respiratory adjustments similar to vocally untrained subjects and half showed adjustments similar to highly trained classical actors indicates that some highly trained singers applied their "ring" strategy to loud speaking as well as to singing. There is clearly a need for further study that would focus on the acoustical characteristics of the voices of classical actors.

Next to be discussed is the monologue performance of the present subjects. The kinematic data generated by the subjects for such performance were different in several ways from those they generated for the other three speaking activities. Considered in general terms, these differences were that monologue performance tended to involve (1) higher lung volume initiation levels, (2) lower lung volume termination levels, (3) larger lung volume excursions, (4) higher rib cage volume initiation levels, (5) larger rib cage excursions, (6) lower abdominal volume termination levels, (7) larger abdominal excursions, (8) patterns of predominant abdominal displacement followed by predominant rib cage displacement, and (9) frequently occurring patterns of inspiration-expiration and expiration-inspiration phase transitions.

As noted earlier, the only restrictions imposed on each subject's choice of a monologue to perform was that it be committed to memory and that it best display the subject's acting ability. All of the subjects chose monologues whose dramatic characteristics called for a strongly emotional presentation, and all met this call through very forceful and loud vocal performances. In fact, when the loudness of the monologue performances was scaled relative to that for spontaneous conversational discourse (in the manner discussed earlier), each subject's monologue performance was judged to be several times louder than conversational discourse and substantially louder than dramatic poem reading.

All of the kinematic differences noted between monologue performance and the other three speaking activities are consistent with the major difference noted between them in loudness. Although the loudness increase between conversational discourse and dramatic reading of a poem could be accomplished by the present subjects without major kinematic adjustments in the respiratory apparatus, it appears that the much greater loudness increase for monologue performance could not be so accomplished. That is, the subjects had to make changes in their respiratory control strategies that were clearly manifested in their kinematic data. Speech of the type needed for a forceful and emotional monologue presentation required a different participation by the respiratory apparatus than that for the other types of speaking activities studied.

Taken collectively, the differences noted between the data for monologue performance and the other three speaking activities of the present subjects show a striking resemblance to the differences noted between the data for singing performance and speaking activities of most classical singers studied. Because of this congruity, it seems reasonable to consider the mechanisms underlying forceful vocal activity in monologue performance as being similar to those mechanisms underlying forceful vocal activity in singing performance, such as that characteristic of a vigorous aria. These mechanisms have been elucidated in considerable detail in Chapter 10 (pp. 360–368). As is summarized there, the data suggest a role for the abdomen that is mainly one of posturing the chest wall in a manner that aids both the rib cage and diaphragm in their primary functions. This role involves the configuration of the chest wall and extends across both phases of the respiratory cycle. Pressurization of the pulmonary system, by contrast, appears to be the major role of the rib cage during the expiratory side of the respiratory cycle as that structure functions to generate aeromechanical events of importance to the demands of vocalization. Finally, the diaphragm has as its assignment the inspiratory side of the respiratory cycle, its role being to inflate the pulmonary system quickly so that vocalization can proceed.

The suggestion of probable common mechanisms in monologue performance and singing performance is not meant to imply that the two types of performance involve identical respiratory activities. It is intended to suggest that classical acting and classical singing lie close to one another along a continuum of respiratory behaviors, and that they are at least similar in kind. Their seemingly qualitative similarity in respiratory behavior may be shared by other activities as well. For example, tasks involving high oral pressures, such as oboe playing and trumpet playing, have been found to involve respiratory kinematic patterns of the type observed for classical actors and classical singers (Dr. Thomas J. Hixon, personal communication, April, 1986). It may well be that the similarity observed between certain respiratory behaviors of the present subjects and classical singers is representative of a general class of kinematic patterns observed whenever the respiratory task involves an alternation between prolonged high alveolar driving pressures against high resistive loads and extremely rapid reinflations of the respiratory apparatus. To pursue this notion, it would be instructive to study artists who perform in more than one of the areas suspected of fitting the general class of kinematic patterns mentioned (e.g., someone who is both a classical singer and a trumpet player).

Finally, there remains the question of why subject DR demonstrated kinematic patterns of respiratory function and inferred underlying mechanisms that are unique for conversation and reading among all subjects studied to date. The answer may be tied to the fact that, of all the present subjects, only DR's respiratory behavior closely fits what he described it to be before the investigation. DR seems to have been strongly affected by what in his description appears to have been a strategy taught to him of speaking while holding the rib cage in an elevated position (i.e., his so-called rib reserve technique), providing the major drive with his abdominal wall (his "breathing low" experience), and ending long expiratory breath groups with a drive from his rib cage (his "collapse the rib cage . . . to end the sentence" technique). In a few words, subject DR seems to have performed faithfully in the manner of his formal instruction. In the present investigation, he performed qualitatively similarly for all of the activities studied. That is, despite instructions to converse and read in a "non-performing" manner, subject DR appears to have carried out these activities in his "performance mode." A review of his FM tape recording tended to confirm this suspicion. When caught "off guard" telling a joke to one of the investigators, DR's kinematic data were quite unlike those generated during the investigation proper. They were, in fact, similar to those that have been observed in other subjects during spontaneous conversational discourse.

Subjects' Beliefs About Their Respiratory Adjustments and the Actual Adjustments Used

Acting pedagogy abounds with different viewpoints about how the actor should use the respiratory apparatus during performance. As do teachers of singing (see Chapter 10), teachers of acting often espouse what they consider to be "preferred" or "correct" or "best" ways of breathing during acting. Also, as with teachers of singing, teachers of acting tend to favor various "imageries" in association with the respiratory methods they teach. To a considerable degree, the findings here for world-class actors bear close correspondence to those obtained for highly trained classical singers. That is, the verbatim statements provided by the present classical actors and those provided by highly trained classical singers are quite similar. In fact, when edited to delete the special lexicons of each of these two groups of performing artists, the resulting descriptions are indistinguishable from one another.[1] Thus, the present investigation generally (excepting subject DR) fails to support expectations that professional actors might be fully "in touch" with the manner in which they use the respiratory apparatus during performance or that they might be fully correct in their beliefs about the mechanisms involved in control of the speech apparatus for dramatic performance. It is clear that subjects who

---

[1]Such indistinguishability was tested on ten judges who were asked to categorize edited single paragraph descriptions as being written by either a classical actor or a classical singer. For the present subjects, only the description written by subject JB was identified correctly above chance as having been written by a classical actor. Subject DR was identified incorrectly as a classical singer by all ten judges. Of the six subjects who were classical singers (see Chapter 10), only one (subject JD) was identified correctly as a classical singer above chance by the group of judges. Eight of the ten judges incorrectly categorized subject PW as a classical actor.

use the respiratory apparatus in relatively similar manners during classical acting can come to conceptualize their respiratory behaviors in quite different ways.

It is of interest that at least a portion of the training of each of the present subjects was from the same institution, the Royal Academy of Dramatic Art in London. Post hoc questioning of the subjects revealed that the instruction each had received at this academy was basically the same with regard to how best to use the respiratory apparatus for acting. However, the subjects did not all use the respiratory apparatus similarly for acting in this investigation, nor did they all conceptualize respiratory function for acting similarly. It seems likely that a common training would differently influence different subjects, depending on when it occurred within the skills development of a given actor and depending on what breathing strategies already had been acquired naturally or were instilled by earlier formal training. Many variables probably influenced the outcomes here, thus making it difficult to provide unequivocal explanations for the incongruities between how the present subjects believed they used the respiratory apparatus during performance and the actual adjustments used.

Implications for the Training of Actors

The results of the present investigation warrant consideration with regard to their potential impact on the training of other classical actors. It seems clear from this investigation that different highly trained professional actors can achieve desired speech products through different respiratory means. This finding speaks to the degrees of freedom of motor performance available to the actor and argues that what the actor comes to use and consider the "best" respiratory control strategy for him or her may be conditioned by various factors. One such factor, for example, may be the actor's body type (see Chapter 12). Body type has been shown to have an impact on what might be the most efficient or effective control strategy for using the respiratory apparatus during speech production. It seems probable that there may not be a single "best" set of respiratory adjustments for all actors or singers (see Chapter 10). Rather, there may be different "best" strategies for individuals of different body types. It is interesting to ponder whether or not the strategies espoused by different teachers of acting and singing, and which they claim work for them, are those most efficient and effective for their own particular body types. Perhaps some of the "best-way-of-doing-things" controversies among different teachers of acting and singing would tend to resolve were the morphology and composition of the respiratory apparatuses of these same teachers taken into account. This notion is intriguing and one that seems not to have been addressed previously in the literature. It would be useful to know if part of the incongruity between what actors and singers believe they do with the respiratory apparatus during performance and what they actually do is related to their natural adoption of strategies that are "best" for them despite what they are taught or what they conceptualize from that teaching.

There are important commonalities among the data of the present subjects. All of the subjects employed a chest wall control strategy that is analogous to the "belly in" strategy used by highly trained classical singers (see Chapter 10). Unanimous use of this strategy by world-class actors and highly trained classical singers suggests that there may be a collection of advantages to using such a strategy as opposed to other strategies. These advantages have been outlined in considerable detail elsewhere (Hixon and Hoffman, 1974) and have been discussed in the context of classical singing (Chapter 10).

There is, of course, the obvious question of how the present subjects would compare to novice classical actors and whether or not any differences, if they existed, would provide insights into training. Fortunately, this question can be addressed directly by comparing the present data to data obtained from a recent investigation of a group of novice classical actors (Mr. Peter J. Watson, personal communication, May, 1986). In this recent investigation, four novice actors were subjected to the same protocol as was used in the present investigation. All of these individuals were undergraduate drama majors at the University of Arizona. With regard to spontaneous conversational discourse, declarative paragraph reading, and dramatic reading of a poem, the data obtained from these four novice actors were similar to those for subjects JG, JB, and SA.

Findings for the novice actors and the world-class actors regarding monologue performance were quite different in several respects, however. Figure 11–4 shows data from the monologue performance of one of the novice actors studied. These data are representative of those for all four novice performers. As a group, the novice actors used much less abdominal displacement during monologue performance than did the world-class actors. The novice actors also showed much less variation in respiratory patterning during monologue performance than did their more accomplished counterparts. This included far fewer of the rapid, marked changes in relative contributions of the rib cage and abdomen that the world-class actors superimposed on the general background displacement patterns of the respiratory apparatus. And rarely during monologue performance did the novice actors use the mechanically efficient respiratory phase transitions that characterized the monologue performance of the world-class actors. In this latter regard, there was a clear trend for novice actors to make slower respiratory adjustments during the non-utterance portions of the speech breathing cycle. For example, the average inspiratory durations for the novice and professional actors were 0.74 and 0.56 sec, respectively. That there are differences between the respiratory events associated with monologue performances by world-class and novice classical actors is clear. How to apply knowledge of these differences directly to the training of novice actors is not

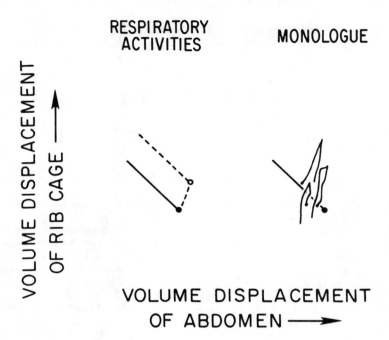

FIGURE 11-4. Kinematic data for monologue performance by a novice actor. See text for explanation.

so clear. Perhaps the ease of use and instructive power of kinematic biofeedback in retraining singers in certain uses of the respiratory apparatus for singing (see Chapter 10) also would apply to acting. That is, equipment of the type used in this investigation may be useful in the training of actors.

As noted earlier in the discussion of subjects' beliefs about their breathing, classical actors and classical singers have many overlapping notions about how they use the respiratory apparatus for vocal performance. The same impression emerges from the teachings of many instructors of classical acting and classical singing. For example, the pedagogical literature directed at these two different groups of performing artists more often than not is quite similar with regard to its advice about how to use the respiratory apparatus during performance. To the extent that the previously discussed similarities between monologue performance and singing performance are representative of other salient performance comparisons between the groups, similarities in pedagogical literature for the two groups of artists should not be surprising.

This chapter opened with the statement, "To breathe or not to breathe— that is the question." Clearly, to breathe or not to breathe is only a part of the question. The larger part of the question is "How to breathe and how not to breathe." This investigation represents an initial step toward answering this question.

ACKNOWLEDGMENT

The preparation of this manuscript was supported by grants from the National Institute of Neurological and Communicative Disorders and Stroke.

REFERENCES

Fairbanks, G. (1960). *Voice and articulation drillbook* (2nd ed.). New York: Harper and Row.

GMG Scientific Inc. (1980). *Operation manual for linearized magnetometers.* Burlington, MA: GMG Scientific.

Hixon, T., and Hoffman, C. (1979). Chest wall shape in singing. *In* V. Lawrence (Ed.): *Transcripts of the Seventh Symposium on Care of the Professional Voice, Part I: The Scientific Papers.* New York: The Voice Foundation.

Hodge, M., Hixon, T., and Putnam, A. (1982). *Respiratory kinematics in adult female speakers.* Paper presented at the Annual Convention of the Canadian Speech-Language-Hearing Association, Vancouver, British Columbia.

Leeper, A. (1984). Respiro-laryngeal contributions to vocal loudness and projec-

tion. *In* V. Lawrence (Ed.): *Transcripts of the Thirteenth Symposium on Care of the Professional Voice, Part I: The Scientific Papers.* New York: The Voice Foundation.

Mead, J., Hixon, T., and Goldman, M. (1974). The configuration of the chest wall during speech. *In* B. Wyke (Ed.): *Ventilatory and phonatory control systems.* London: Oxford University Press.

Sundberg, J. (1974). Articulatory interpretation of the "singing formant." *Journal of the Acoustical Society of America, 55,* 838–844.

Thomas, D. (1946). The hand that signed the paper felled a city. *In: The selected writings of Dylan Thomas.* New York: New Directions Publishers.

APPENDIX A

Performance Experience of the Subjects Studied

Subject JG was trained at the Royal Academy of Dramatic Art in London. He has had an extensive career as a classical actor. His Shakespearean roles, about 20 altogether, include Macbeth in *Macbeth* at the Bristol Old Vic, and Claudius in the 1980 *Hamlet* which opened at the London Old Vic and then went on world tour. His stage acting career encompasses a number of major and minor roles in Britain with the Royal Shakespeare Company, the Old Vic and Prospect Companies, and the National Theatre in London. JG has had an equally extensive film career with a dozen roles in such films as *Tom Jones, The Adding Machine, Star Wars*, and a major role in the James Bond film, *For Your Eyes Only*. He has done over 25 television roles, which include British series and docudrama work such as *Nancy Astor, Q.E.D., Henry VIII, Dombey and Son*, and most recently, the role of the father in *By the Sword Divided*. He has appeared in several American television detective series as well.

Subject JB trained at the Royal Academy of Dramatic Art and has performed as a classical actor in approximately 20 Shakespearean roles including Pistol in *Henry IV, Part II*, and Duke Frederick in *As You Like It*. His non-Shakespearean roles number many more and were performed primarily at the Royal Shakespeare Company as well as at other London theaters. JB's television credits include roles in the BBC's *The Shakespeare Plays* series and other video work at BBC-TV, ITV, and Thames TV. JB has appeared in movies as well, including *Give My Regards to Broad Street* and *Sakharov*.

Subject DR trained at the Royal Academy of Dramatic Art and Edinburgh University and has performed in approximately a dozen Shakespearean roles, including Demetrius in *A Midsummer Night's Dream* at the National Theatre, and Prince Hal in *Henry IV, Parts I and II*, at the Royal Shakespeare Company. His non-Shakespearean roles number over 20 and were presented at regional theaters in Britain and a number of London theaters. He has many television, radio and film credits, but probably is best known to American audiences via his role of Mr. Darcy in the BBC's version of *Pride and Prejudice*.

Subject SA was trained at the Royal Academy of Dramatic Art in London. After working in regional theater in Bristol and Birmingham, she worked mainly with the Royal Shakespeare Company in Stratford and London. Her Shakespearean roles, some dozen and a half, include Lady Percy in *Henry IV, Parts I and II*, Goneril in *King Lear*, Queen Constance in *King John*, and Portia in *Merchant of Venice*. Her film and television credits, approximately 20 to date, include the roles of Mrs. Pethwick-Lawrence in *Shoulder to Shoulder* and Jocasta in *King Oedipus*. SA also has performed in theater in New York and has taught at the Lee Strasberg Theatre Institute as well as at the London Academy of Dramatic Art, the Royal Academy of Dramatic Art, and the Guildhall School.

APPENDIX B

Information on the Shakespearean Monologues Performed by the Subjects Studied

Subject: JG
Source: King Lear
Character: Lear
Passage: ACT III, scene ii
Dramatic Characteristics: The character cries out in an explosive curse of anger and grief, for here the storm on the heath equals the encroaching madness within his mind.

Subject: JB
Source: King Lear
Character: Kent
Passage: ACT II, scene ii
Dramatic Characteristics: The character expresses bitter contempt as he reprimands one who has treated his master badly.

Subject: DR
Source: King Lear
Character: Edmund
Passage: ACT I, scene ii
Dramatic Characteristics: The character loudly and cynically challenges the gods by expressing his darker purpose within the play.

Subject: SA
Source: Henry IV, Part II
Character: Lady Percy
Passage: ACT II, scene ii
Dramatic Characteristics: The character severely chastises all who would make war in this outburst of grief and anger at her father.

CHAPTER **12**

Body Type and Speech Breathing

Jeannette D. Hoit
Thomas J. Hixon

I nvestigation of breathing kinematics during connected speech production
has shown that normal subjects use relatively similar lung volumes and chest
wall configurations but quite different relative volume contributions of the
rib cage and abdomen (see Chapter 3). For speech produced in the upright
body position, for example, normal subjects use relative volume contributions
that range from all rib cage displacement to all abdominal displacement. Hixon
and colleagues indicated that they were unable to account for such differences
and that their bases were open to speculation (Chapter 3). They offered that
the "motion strategy chosen by a subject and the manner in which its
patterning becomes neurologically ingrained probably depend largely on how
the subject has learned to use the muscular system most effectively against

Reprinted by permission of the publisher from the *Journal of Speech and Hearing Research*,
29, 313–324. © 1986, American Speech-Language-Hearing Association, Rockville, MD.

the passive mechanical properties of the respiratory apparatus." Although this suggestion seems reasonable, it lacks explanatory power with regard to mechanism.

Recognizing this problem, Hixon (1983) later suggested that differences in speech breathing among normal subjects may be related, in part, to morphological differences among them. The basis of his suggestion was the notion that the structure and form of the bony framework and musculature of the breathing apparatus and the geometric distribution of its constituents may condition its function. Hixon pointed out that many of the salient morphological characteristics of the breathing apparatus are manifested in the surface configuration of the torso and that body type may be one factor contributing to subject differences in kinematic behavior during speech breathing. Hixon did not directly postulate the existence of specific relations between body type and subject performance. He indicated that knowledge is limited with regard to how body configuration might affect breathing function in general (Grassino, 1974) and that it is premature to hypothesize about body type and speech breathing without exploratory study.

The investigation reported in this chapter was designed to meet this exploratory need through the study of three markedly different groups of subjects. Each group was characterized by a prominence on one of three components of body type—fatness, musculoskeletal development, or linearity. It was reasoned that if components of body type were relevant to subject performance, the study of markedly different groups of subjects would place such relevance in bold relief for subsequent hypothesis testing.

METHOD

Subjects

Twelve healthy adult male subjects were studied. They ranged in age from approximately 18 to 23 years. Those chosen to participate were included because, on the basis of ratings obtained using a standardized method (see subsequent description), they fit one of three different body-type categories. Four subjects were assigned to each of three groups, hereafter referred to as endomorphs (high in relative fatness), mesomorphs (high in relative musculoskeletal development), and ectomorphs (high in relative linearity). Selected physical characteristics of the subjects are given in Table 12–1.

In addition to meeting body-type criteria, subjects also had the following characteristics. All were white, were American English speakers, and had normal speech, language, and hearing. Each was free of respiratory disease. None had a history of surgery involving the speech apparatus. Finally, none had received formal training in singing, public speaking, or wind instrument playing.

Table 12-1. *Selected Physical Characteristics of the Subjects*

	Body-Type Rating			Age	Height	Weight	Vital Capacity
	Endo	Meso	Ecto	(yr:mo)	(cm)	(kg)	(L)
Endomorphs							
PD	9	8	½	22:2	180.6	126.4	5.6
ES	6½	5	1	20:7	170.1	82.7	4.7
MK	8	6½	½	21:2	182.6	106.4	5.1
RM	6	5½	½	20:10	166.3	85.5	5.0
Mesomorphs							
MM	2	5½	2½	20:0	185.9	79.5	5.7
CG	1	7	1½	18:1	187.1	94.5	5.9
JK	5½	10	½	21:4	178.6	109.1	4.0
MG	3	7½	½	20:8	176.1	99.5	5.4
Ectomorphs							
PP	½	2	6½	22:10	186.5	60.9	5.3
JJ	2	2½	5½	20:11	195.0	73.2	5.2
JD	1	2½	5½	18:10	187.5	66.4	4.8
NS	1	2½	5½	19:6	174.0	52.7	4.3

Note. Endo = endomorphy; Meso = mesomorphy; Ecto = ectomorphy. See text for explanation of body-type categories and ratings.

Body Typing

Subjects were categorized into body-type groups on the basis of the rating they obtained when evaluated by the *Heath-Carter Somatotype Method* (Carter, 1980). This method is an offshoot of experimental modifications by Heath (1963) and Heath and Carter (1967) of the work of Sheldon, Stevens, and Tucker (1940). In brief, it provides a standardized description of physical morphology and composition in the form of a three-numeral rating of body type. Each numeral is derived from a relatively independent physical component.[1] Components include endomorphy (relative fatness), mesomorphy (relative musculoskeletal development), and ectomorphy (relative linearity). Endomorphy ratings are derived from measurements of skinfold thickness of the triceps and of the subscapular and suprailiac regions. Mesomorphy ratings are based on measurements of bone diameters (humerus and femur) and muscle girths (biceps and calf) in relation to height. Ectomorphy ratings are derived from the calculation of height/$\sqrt[3]{\text{weight}}$. Instruments

---

[1]The *Heath-Carter Somatotype Method* includes two different sets of procedures for assigning a body-type rating, one photoscopic and one anthropometric. Photoscopic rating is based on visual judgments of photographs of front, side, and back views of a subject. Anthropometric rating is based on physical measurements of a subject. The anthropometric procedure was used in this investigation because it has been shown to be more reliable and less subjective than the photoscopic procedure (Carter, 1980).

used in making these measurements include a skinfold caliper, an anthropometer, a cloth measuring tape, and a standard weight scale. In practice, ratings are assigned to the nearest half point with the lowest rating on any component being $\frac{1}{2}$. Generally, the highest rating given is 14 for endomorphy, 10 for mesomorphy, and 9 for ectomorphy. Ratings of $\frac{1}{2}$ through $2\frac{1}{2}$ are regarded as low, 3 through 5 as average, $5\frac{1}{2}$ through 7 as high, and above 7 as extremely high. The ratings assigned to the three components, which together constitute the overall body-type rating, are reported as a sequence of numbers with the endomorphy rating first, mesomorphy second, and ectomorphy third. For example, a body-type rating of 1-4-8 describes an individual who is low in endomorphy, average in mesomorphy, and extremely high in ectomorphy.

For this investigation, categorization into body-type groups was predicated on criteria developed in consultation with Dr. J. E. Lindsay Carter (personal communication, March, 1984), codeveloper of the *Heath-Carter Somatotype Method*. It was reasoned that the exploratory needs of the present investigation could best be met through the selection of subjects who were markedly different in body type. For this reason, subject selection criteria were designed to yield groups that displayed prominence on one component of body type. On the basis of the normal distribution of body-type components in young, white, adult, male subjects (e.g., the study of 2,420 such subjects by Bailey, Carter, and Mirwald, 1982), the following prominence criteria were believed to generate sufficiently diverse subject groups for the purpose of this investigation. Prominence for the mesomorphic and ectomorphic components were defined as a rating of at least 3 points higher on either of them as primary component than on the other two components rated. Prominence for the endomorphic component was defined as a rating of at least one half point higher on endomorphy as primary component than on the other two components rated. A more lenient criterion for endomorphic prominence was required because of the difficulty in finding individuals with a high endomorphy rating accompanied by a relatively low mesomorphy rating. That is, in the young adult group of interest, most subject candidates who are high in relative fatness are correspondingly high in relative musculoskeletal development.

Kinematic Recordings

Kinematic recordings were made in accordance with the theoretical framework of Konno and Mead (1967). The chest wall was treated as a two-part system consisting of the rib cage and abdomen. Each part displaces volume as it moves, and the sum of their displacements is equal to the volume displaced by the lungs. Changes in the anteroposterior diameters of the rib cage and abdomen are related linearly to their respective volume displacements.

Therefore, diameter changes can be used to estimate directly the volumes displaced by the individual parts.[2]

Changes in the anteroposterior diameters of the rib cage and abdomen were sensed with linearized magnetometers (GMG Scientific Inc., 1980). Two generator–sensor coil pairs were used, one for the rib cage and one for the abdomen (see Chapter 3). The generator coil in each pair was attached to the front of the torso at the midline, that for the rib cage was attached just above the nipples, and that for the abdomen was placed just above the navel. The sensor coil in each pair was attached to the back of the torso at the midline and at the same axial level as its generator mate. Output signals from the two sensors were processed electronically and recorded on an FM tape system. Recorded signals were played back into a storage oscilloscope, where they were displayed and traced onto translucent paper.

All recordings were made with subjects in an upright body position. Each participant stood on a footplate attached to a tilt table oriented approximately 15 degrees off vertical toward supine (see Chapter 3). With his head and neck supported by a pillow, the subject leaned backward against the table, which was covered with a thick polyurethane pad. The segment of the pad supporting the torso had a rectangular indentation running vertically at the midline to provide a space within which the coils on the subject's back were free to move. The off-vertical position was selected because it was more comfortable than free standing for long periods and because it was an easier task than free standing for maintaining a constant degree of extension of the vertebral column. Subjects were told to avoid raising their arms, moving their hands, and shifting their posture during recordings.

The speech audio signal was sensed by an air microphone, amplified, and recorded on a direct-record channel of the FM tape system. This signal provided a record of the subject's speech, a banter channel for the investigators, and a means of synchronizing speech performance with breathing behavior.

Performance Tasks

CHEST WALL MANEUVERS. Two chest wall maneuvers were performed several times by each subject: isovolume adjustments and relaxation of the

---

[2]To ensure that body type did not have a differential influence on the degrees of freedom of the rib cage or abdomen, three subjects, one chosen randomly from each body-type category, were subjected to multiple diameter analysis according to the method and the sites used by Konno and Mead (1967) and at various transverse sites. Results indicated that, for the types of activities performed by the subjects in this investigation, the assumption of a single degree of freedom for the rib cage and abdomen was met satisfactorily.

chest wall musculature. Isovolume adjustments involved having the subject close his larynx and slowly displace volume back and forth between his abdomen and rib cage. Two such adustments were performed, one at functional residual capacity (FRC) and one at 1 L above FRC as measured by a spirometer. Isovolume data permitted subsequent calibration of data charts (see later description).

Relaxation of the chest wall musculature involved having the subject completely relax his breathing apparatus against a closed larynx at FRC. Data from this maneuver allowed subsequent landmarking of data charts in a manner that facilitated inferences with regard to muscular forces acting on the breathing apparatus.

RESTING TIDAL BREATHING. The resting tidal breathing task required that the subject stand quietly and breathe through his nose for 5 min. The data obtained provided information on a common breathing behavior not associated with speech and a reference to which speech production data could be compared.

SPEECH PRODUCTION ACTIVITIES. Three speech production activities were performed at least twice by each subject: conversational speaking, reading aloud a long paragraph, and reading aloud a short paragraph.

The conversational speaking activity consisted of 3 to 5 min of spontaneous discourse between the subject and an investigator. During this time, the investigator sat on a tall stool facing the subject so that the latter could maintain eye contact without shifting posture.

Reading activities involved paragraphs that the subject had practiced reading aloud. An investigator held the reading material at the subject's eye level so that the latter would not need to move his arms or shift his posture. The long paragraph, a descriptive passage concerning geographic characteristics of California, consisted of 15 sentences ranging in length from 7 to 53 syllables and differing substantially in grammatical structure. This paragraph was written specifically for this investigation for the purpose of eliciting a large number of breath groups of various lengths. The short paragraph, the first paragraph of "The Rainbow Passage" by Fairbanks (1960), consisted of five sentences ranging in length from 10 to 30 syllables. This paragraph has been used in previous studies of speech breathing kinematics and was included to provide a basis for comparing the present data with other available data.

RESULTS
The Relative Volume Chart and Its Interpretation

Figure 12–1 is a relative volume chart illustrative of those used to display the kinematic data. Volume of the rib cage is shown on the vertical axis, increasing upward, and volume of the abdomen is indicated on the horizontal axis, increasing rightward. Volume of the lungs is portrayed on a diagonal axis,

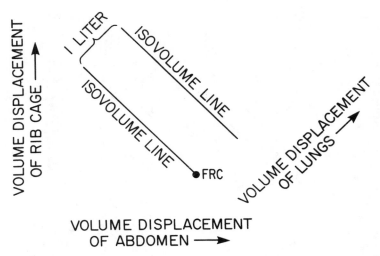

FIGURE 12-1. A relative volume chart (rib cage versus abdomen) illustrative of those constructed for data display. FRC = Functional residual capacity.

increasing upward and rightward. The two isovolume lines in the chart represent pathways traced during the shifting of volume back and forth between the abdomen and rib cage at fixed lung volumes. The lower line is located at FRC and the upper line is positioned at 1 L above FRC. The isovolume lines are adjusted to a slope of − 1 to show equal volume changes for recorded diameter changes of the rib cage and abdomen, thus permitting direct reading of the chart for volume events. The filled circle at the right end of the lower isovolume line depicts the position associated with relaxation of the chest wall musculature at FRC.

As configured, the chart can be used to determine the following: (1) changes in lung volume, given by the distance perpendicular to the isovolume lines; (2) relative volume contributions of the rib cage and abdomen, given by the slope of any line; and (3) separate volumes of the rib cage and abdomen (i.e., chest wall configuration), given by position along the chart axes. The chart also can be used to make inferences about certain aspects of muscular mechanism. Such inferences depend on comparisons of chest wall configuration during relaxation at FRC with departures from this configuration during activities. Mechanism is inferred by considering the forces that could operate to bring about any combination or series of combinations of rib cage and abdominal volumes (see Chapter 3 for further details).

Kinematic Data

Kinematic data for the subjects are presented in Figures 12–2 to 12–4. Subject groupings within the three figures are based on body-type prominence.

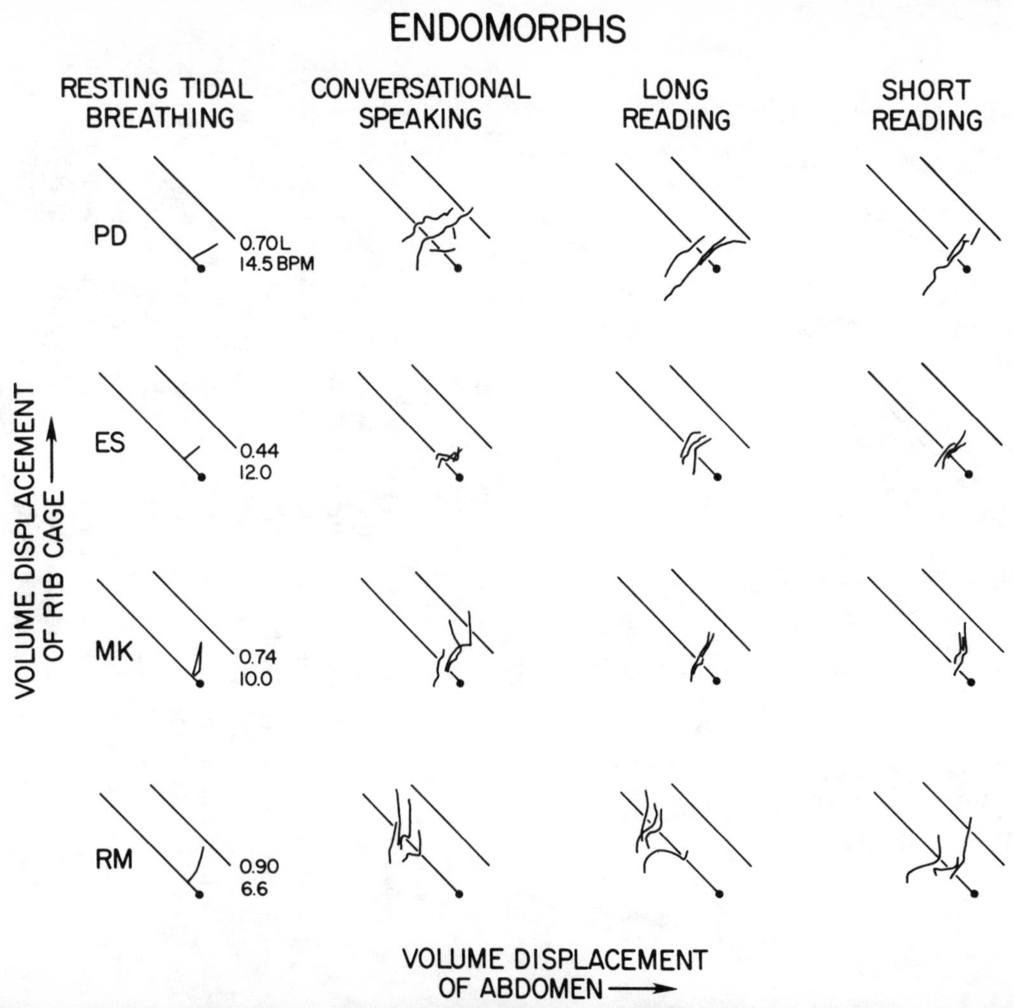

ENDOMORPHS

SHORT READING · LONG READING · CONVERSATIONAL SPEAKING · RESTING TIDAL BREATHING

PD 0.70L 14.5BPM
ES 0.44 12.0
MK 0.74 10.0
RM 0.90 6.6

VOLUME DISPLACEMENT OF RIB CAGE ⟵

VOLUME DISPLACEMENT OF ABDOMEN ⟶

Contained in the figures are relative volume charts for resting tidal breathing, conversational speaking, reading aloud a long paragraph, and reading aloud a short paragraph. Data from chest wall maneuvers are represented in each of the four charts for each subject. These representations show isovolume pathways as straight lines. Isovolume tracings actually were single lines or flat loops, each being linear or approximately so.

RESTING TIDAL BREATHING. Resting tidal breathing tracings are representative of what was judged to be each subject's most stable cycling behavior during the middle 3 min of his 5 min of quiet breathing.

Tidal Volume and Breathing Rate. Tidal volume (in L) and breathing rate (in BPM) are indicated next to each subject's representative tracing. Values reported are averages for consecutive breathing cycles for 3 min running for all subjects except NS, in whose case values are averages for 1 min running. As can be seen, tidal volume ranged from 0.44 to 0.9 L and breathing rate ranged from 6.6 to 20 BPM. For the entire group of subjects, tidal volume averaged 0.59 L and breathing rate averaged 15.2 BPM.

When the tidal volume and breathing rate data are examined in relation to body type, those for the endomorphic group stand out. Endomorphic subjects demonstrated the three largest tidal volumes (Endomorphs PD, MK, and RM)[3] and the three lowest breathing rates (Endomorphs ES, MK, and RM) of all the subjects. In addition, the average tidal volumes for the endomorphic subjects (0.7 L) are substantially higher than those for the mesomorphic and ectomorphic subjects (0.55 and 0.51 L, respectively), and the average breathing rates for the endomorphic subjects (10.8 BPM) are substantially lower than those for the mesomorphic and ectomorphic subjects (17.3 and 17.7 BPM, respectively). No differences are apparent between the mesomorphic and ectomorphic groups.

Relative Volume Contributions of the Rib Cage and Abdomen. Relative contributions of the rib cage and abdomen differed considerably across subjects and from moment to moment during the tidal excursions of most subjects. Seven subjects (Endomorphs MK and RM; Mesomorphs JK and MG; Ectomorphs PP, JJ and JD) showed relative contributions that generally involved a predominance of rib cage displacement, ranging from all rib cage (Endomorph MK) to slightly more rib cage than abdomen (Mesomorph MG).

---

[3]Because reference to body type might be relevant to the consideration of data, hereafter each subject's initials often will be preceded by a designation of his body type (e.g., Endomorph PD; or Ectomorphs PP, JJ, and JD).

FIGURE 12–2. Relative volume charts containing representative data for the endomorphic subjects. Tidal volume (L) and breathing rate (BPM) are noted adjacent to the relative volume charts for resting tidal breathing.

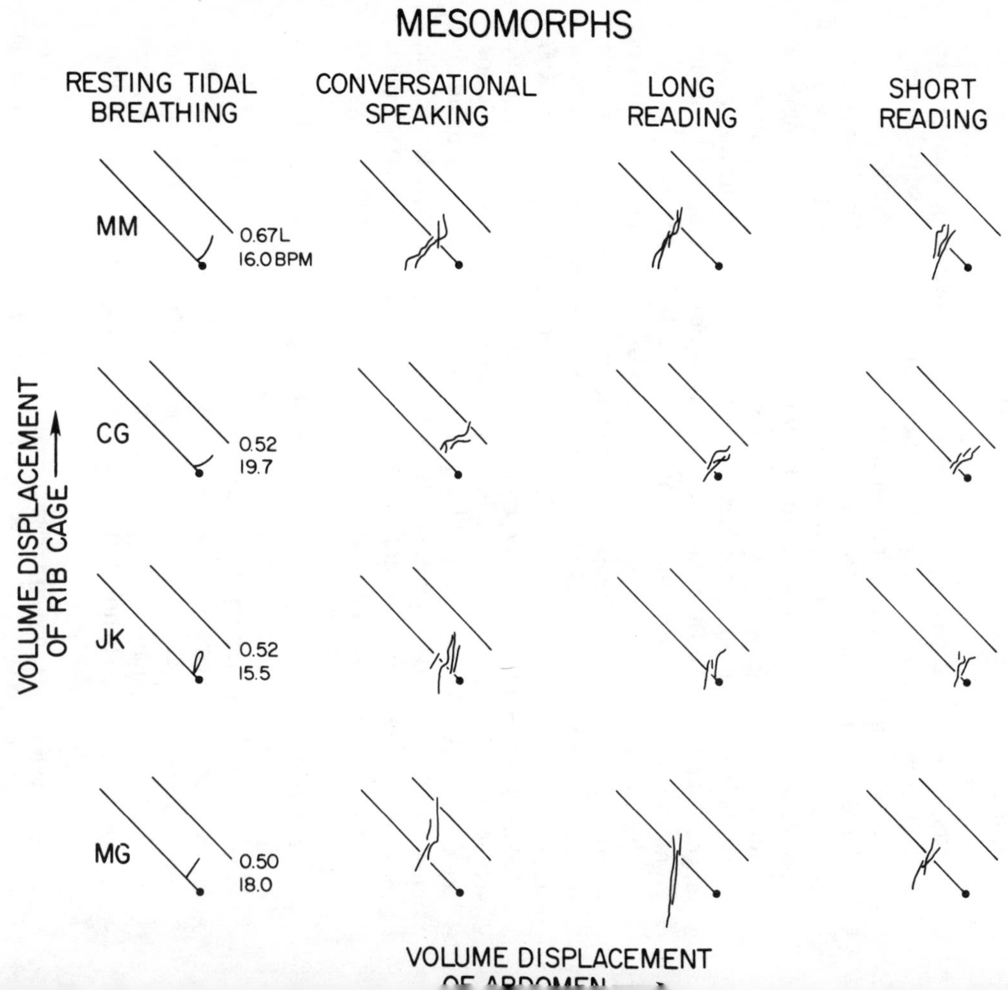

MESOMORPHS

RESTING TIDAL BREATHING · CONVERSATIONAL SPEAKING · LONG READING · SHORT READING

MM — 0.67L 16.0 BPM

CG — 0.52 19.7

JK — 0.52 15.5

MG — 0.50 18.0

VOLUME DISPLACEMENT OF RIB CAGE

VOLUME DISPLACEMENT OF ABDOMEN

Two subjects (Endomorphs PD and ES) demonstrated relative contributions that involved a predominance of abdominal displacement, one to a moderate degree (PD) and one to a slight degree (ES). Three subjects (Mesomorphs MM and CG; Ectomorph NS) showed relative contributions that alternated between rib cage and abdominal predominance.

When all aspects of the relative contribution data are considered, no trends are discernible in relation to body type. In fact, essentially the full range of relative contribution findings for the 12 subjects of the investigation are included in the data generated by the endomorphic group of subjects.

Separate Volumes of the Rib Cage and Abdomen: Chest Wall Configuration. For all subjects, resting tidal breathing occurred at configurations relatively similar to those recorded during relaxation of the chest wall musculature at FRC. That is, tidal breathing occurred with the abdomen far outward along its potential range of positions and the rib cage about midway along its potential range of positions. For 10 subjects, the end-expiratory configuration of the chest wall involved a larger rib cage volume and a smaller abdominal volume than those associated with a relaxed chest wall, whereas for two subjects (Ectomorphs PP and JD), the end-expiratory configuration was identical to the relaxed configuration of the chest wall at FRC.

When the configuration data are considered with regard to body type, those for the endomorphic subjects generally are found to be different from those for the mesomorphic and ectomorphic subjects. This difference is in the form of a greater deformation of the chest wall at the tidal end-expiratory level from its relaxed configuration in three of the four endomorphic subjects (PD, ES, and RM) than is characteristic of all other subjects (except Mesomorph MG). That is, as a group, the endomorphic subjects tended to breathe from a resting tidal end-expiratory configuration that was associated with a relatively smaller abdomen and a larger rib cage in relation to the relaxed FRC configuration than those employed by the other groups of subjects.

SPEECH PRODUCTION ACTIVITIES. Data charts for speech production activities include multiple tracings. Each tracing represents an individual breath group (i.e., the expiratory limb of a speech breathing cycle). Tracings shown were judged to be representative of the data pool for a particular activity. Only a few expiratory limbs are displayed for each activity to avoid cluttering the charts. The discussion that follows, however, is based on the entire data pool from which the tracings have been drawn. This data pool consists of 715 tracings and includes 46 to 75 tracings for individual subjects.

The data generally were similar across the three speech production activities (conversational speaking, reading aloud a long paragraph, and reading

FIGURE 12-3. Relative volume charts containing representative data for the mesomorphic subjects.

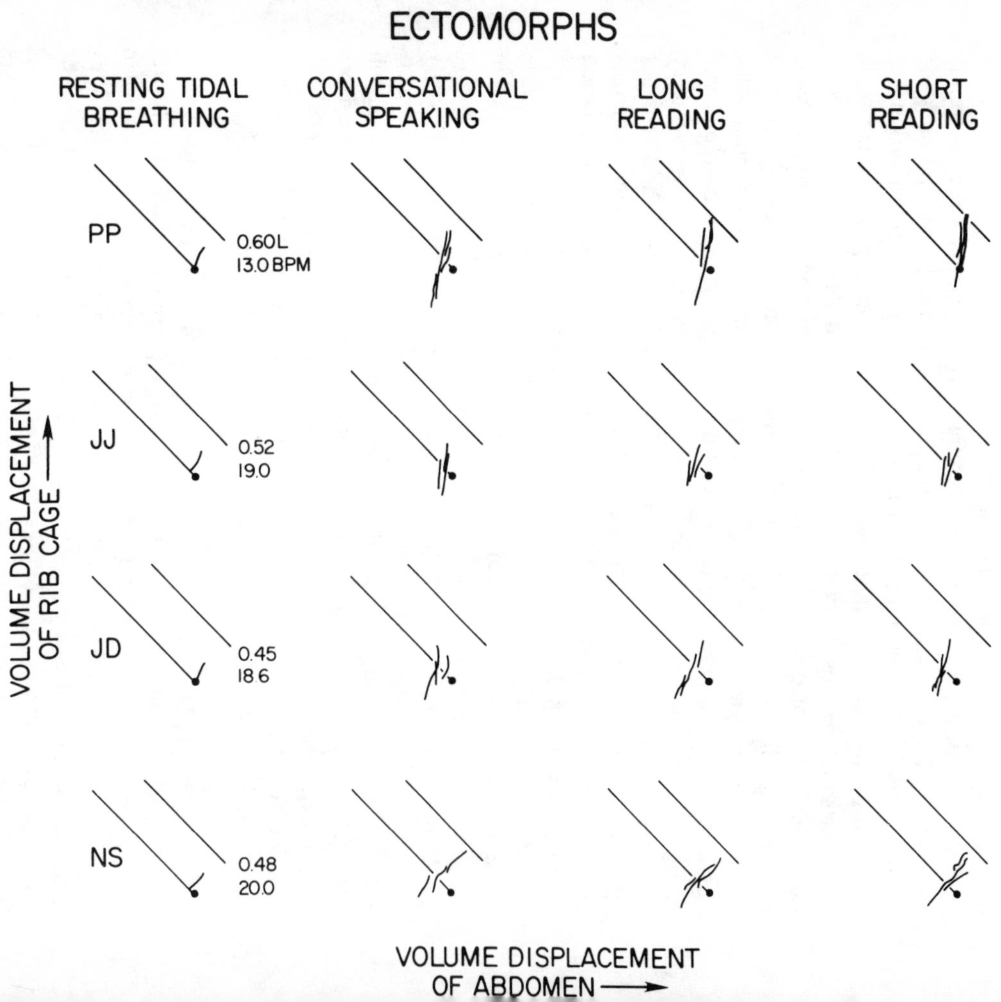

ECTOMORPHS

SHORT READING

LONG READING

CONVERSATIONAL SPEAKING

RESTING TIDAL BREATHING

PP 0.60 L 13.0 BPM

JJ 0.52 19.0

JD 0.45 18.6

NS 0.48 20.0

VOLUME DISPLACEMENT OF RIB CAGE

VOLUME DISPLACEMENT OF ABDOMEN

aloud a short paragraph) for the subjects. When activity-related differences were observed, those differences were slight and involved idiosyncratic patterns for a few subjects. Therefore, unless otherwise indicated, data from the three speech production activities are considered collectively in the discussion that follows.

Lung Volume. Most breath groups (86%) were initiated between 1 L above FRC and FRC. Of these, approximately half were begun from within the resting tidal volume range. Those begun below FRC generally were limited to four subjects (Mesomorph MM; Ectomorphs PP, JD, and NS) and involved 10% to 15% of their initiations.

Most breath groups (88%) ended between 0.4 L above FRC and 0.8 L below FRC. Within this range, about two thirds of the termination levels fell below FRC. Four subjects (Endomorph PD; Mesomorphs MM and MG; Ectomorph PP) terminated about 10% of their breath groups more than 1 L below FRC. Almost all breath groups terminating above FRC ended within the tidal breathing range. Although termination levels did not differ substantially across the speech production activities, there was a tendency in five subjects (Endomorph MK; Mesomorph MM; Ectomorphs PP, JD, and NS) for lower breath group terminations to be associated with the reading of the long paragraph and conversational speaking than with the reading of the short paragraph.

Lung volume excursions varied considerably. The smallest excursion was between 0.1 and 0.3 L for each subject. The largest excursion was 1 L for three subjects (Endomorph ES; Mesomorph JK; Ectomorph JJ), 1.5 L for five subjects (Endomorphs MK and RM; Mesomorph MG; Ectomorphs JD and NS), and in excess of 2 L for four subjects (Endomorph PD; Mesomorphs MM and MG; Ectomorph PP).

Only one group-related trend was apparent in the lung volume data. That trend involved a generally higher proportion of breath group initiations below FRC for the ectomorphic subjects (10%) than for the endomorphic and mesomorphic subjects (3% and 5%, respectively).

Relative Volume Contributions of the Rib Cage and Abdomen. About 70% of the breath groups were characterized by various degrees of rib cage predominance, ranging from marked (e.g., long reading for Mesomorph MG and all activities for Ectomorph PP) to moderate (e.g., reading activities for Mesomorph MM). Some breath groups (12%) involved generally equal volume contributions of the rib cage and abdomen (e.g., all activities for Ectomorph NS) and a small number (5%) showed an abdominal predominance (e.g., conversational speaking for Endomorph PD). Some breath groups (13%) were not easily characterized as being only predominantly rib cage or abdomen

FIGURE 12-4. Relative volume charts containing representative data for the ectomorphic subjects.

(e.g., all activities for Endomorph RM). Three subjects (Endomorphs PD and ES; Mesomorph MM) tended to use a lesser rib cage or greater abdominal contribution for conversational speaking than for reading activities. These subjects also demonstrated a wider range of relative volume contributions for conversational speaking than for reading.

Relative volume contributions changed in various ways within breath groups. Some changes involved a decrease in the contribution of the rib cage as utterance proceeded (e.g., conversational speaking for Ectomorph JD). Others involved alternating decreases and increases in the relative contributions of the two chest wall parts (e.g., data for Endomorph RM).

Paradoxing, wherein either the rib cage or abdomen moved in the inspiratory direction during speech production, was demonstrated by all subjects. Abdominal paradoxing most often occurred above FRC during the initial part of breath groups. It was demonstrated almost twice as frequently as rib cage paradoxing (35% and 19%, respectively) and was especially prevalent in the data of three subjects—Endomorph MK (conversational speaking and short reading), Endomorph RM (all activities), and Ectomorph JD (conversational speaking)—all of whom demonstrated outward movement of the abdomen in over half of their breath groups for the activities indicated. Of the remaining subjects, five (Endomorph PD; Mesomorphs MM, JK, and MG; Ectomorph PP) showed abdominal paradoxing during roughly one third of their breath groups, whereas four (Endomorph ES; Mesomorph CG; Ectomorphs JJ and NS) demonstrated such paradoxing during one fifth or fewer of their breath groups. Rib cage paradoxing most often occurred slightly above FRC midway through breath groups. It most commonly was demonstrated by six subjects: Endomorph PD (conversational speaking and long reading), Endomorph ES (conversational speaking), Endomorph MK (short reading), Endomorph RM (conversational speaking), Mesomorph MM (all activities), and Mesomorph CG (all activities). The remaining six subjects rarely or never demonstrated rib cage paradoxing.

When relative volume contributions are considered with regard to body type, several trends are apparent. All of the endomorphic subjects demonstrated a predominant abdominal contribution during portions of many of their breath groups (about 60% for the group). Subjects from the endomorphic group also tended to use a greater variety of relative volume contributions than subjects from the other two groups, particularly with regard to conversational speaking. Most of the subjects in the ectomorphic group (PP, JJ, and JD) demonstrated a relatively marked rib cage contribution throughout individual breath groups. Furthermore, in contrast to the other two groups of subjects, the ectomorphic subjects generally showed only a small amount of change in the relative volume contributions of the rib cage and abdomen during the course of their breath groups. Subjects in the ectomorphic category also demonstrated much less breath group variation within and across activities than the other subjects. Finally, the ectomorphic subjects showed essentially no rib cage paradoxing during speech production, a sharp contrast to the findings for the endomorphic and mesomorphic subject groups, which demonstrated rib cage paradoxing on 28% and 27% of their breath groups, respectively.

Separate Volumes of the Rib Cage and Abdomen: Chest Wall Configuration. Essentially all breath groups were initiated at rib cage volumes larger than those associated with relaxation at FRC. Most (at least 90%) were initiated at rib cage volumes between 1 L above relaxed FRC and relaxed FRC for five subjects (Mesomorphs CG and JK; Ectomorphs JJ, JD, and NS), between 1.6 and 0.4 L above relaxed FRC for six subjects (Endomorphs PD, ES, and MK; Mesomorphs MM and MG; Ectomorph PP), and between 2.8 and 1 L above relaxed FRC for one subject (Endomorph RM).

For 10 subjects, almost all (97%) breath groups were terminated at rib cage volumes ranging between 0.7 L above and 0.6 L below the relaxed FRC rib cage volume. The remaining two subjects used rib cage termination volumes in the range of 1.3 to 0.2 L above relaxed FRC (Endomorph RM) and 1.4 L above to 0.8 L below relaxed FRC (Mesomorph MG).

Rib cage excursions ranged from 0.1 to 1.5 L for nearly all (94%) of the breath groups. Rib cage excursions for Mesomorph MG and Ectomorph PP occasionally (13% and 23%, respectively) were larger than 1.5 L.

For eight subjects, breath groups were initiated at abdominal volumes between 0.4 L larger and 0.6 L smaller than the abdominal volume at relaxed FRC. For three of the remaining subjects (Endomorph RM; Mesomorphs MM and MG), most (at least 90%) abdominal initiation volumes fell between the relaxed abdominal volume at FRC and 1.6 L smaller than the relaxed FRC volume. Endomorph PD initiated breath groups at abdominal volumes ranging from 0.9 L larger to 0.8 L smaller than his relaxed FRC abdominal volume.

For eight subjects, termination volumes of the abdomen ranged between the relaxed abdominal volume at FRC and 1 L smaller than the relaxed FRC abdominal volume. For two subjects (Mesomorphs MM and MG), essentially all breath groups were terminated at abdominal volumes ranging from 0.4 to 0.7 L smaller than the relaxed abdominal volume at FRC. In contrast, Endomorph PD used a wider range of abdominal termination volumes (95% were between relaxed FRC and 1.8 L smaller than relaxed FRC) and Endomorph RM used generally smaller abdominal termination volumes (85% were between 1.4 and 2.1 L smaller than relaxed FRC) than the overall subject group.

Volume excursions of the abdomen ranged from zero to almost 2 L. Six subjects (Endomorphs ES, MK, and RM; Mesomorphs MM and CG; Ectomorph NS) used abdominal excursions between zero and 0.8 L for most (at least 90%) of their breath groups. Five subjects (Mesomorphs JK and MG; Ectomorphs PP, JJ and JD) used a more limited range of abdominal excursions (zero to

0.4 L) for most (at least 90%) of their breath groups. One subject (Endomorph PD) demonstrated a particularly wide range of abdominal excursions extending from zero to 1.9 L.

Most speech was produced with a background chest wall configuration characterized by larger rib cage volumes and smaller abdominal volumes than those associated with relaxation at FRC. The extent to which the chest wall was deformed from its relaxation configuration differed from subject to subject, ranging from slight (Ectomorph PP) to marked (Endomorph RM). Five subjects (Mesomorphs CG and JK; Ectomorphs JJ, JD, and NS) showed chest wall deformations that tended to be relatively small. Another five subjects (Endomorphs PD, ES, and MK; Mesomorphs MM and MG) demonstrated relatively large deformations from the relaxation configuration of the chest wall. Certain subjects (Endomorphs PD, ES, and RM; Mesomorphs JK and MG) demonstrated gradual shifts in the general background configuration of the chest wall during the course of speech production. These shifts occurred during the first few breath groups of an activity and were of a form in which the volume of the rib cage progressively increased while that of the abdomen decreased. Accordingly, there was a tendency for the deformation of the chest wall to increase in magnitude for a few breath groups until the general deformation became relatively stable. This general adjustment was most pronounced in the speech performance of Endomorph RM.

Finally, when the separate volumes of the rib cage and abdomen are considered in relation to body type, differences among the three groups of subjects are apparent with regard to general background chest wall deformations and abdominal excursions. The endomorphic subjects demonstrated significant general deformations of the chest wall during speech production in contrast to the ectomorphic subjects, who showed little general deformation of the chest wall from relaxation. The mesomorphic subjects demonstrated chest wall deformations of various magnitudes that generally ranged between those observed for the other two groups of subjects. With regard to abdominal excursions, the ectomorphic subjects (with the exception of NS) showed substantially smaller displacements than did most of the subjects in the other body-type groups.

DISCUSSION
Resting Tidal Breathing

The resting tidal breathing data generated by the present subjects resemble those reported for comparable subjects with regard to tidal volume (see Chapter 3 and Bergofsky, 1964; Mead and Agostoni, 1964; Needham, Rogan, and McDonald, 1954), breathing rate (Harris, 1975; Mead, 1960), relative volume contributions of the rib cage and abdomen (see Chapter 3 and Fugl-Meyer, 1974), and general background configuration of the chest wall (see Chapter 3 and Mead, 1974).

Considering the present data with regard to body type, the differences observed between subjects categorized as endomorphic and those categorized as mesomorphic and ectomorphic are striking. In general, the endomorphic subjects demonstrated the largest tidal volumes, lowest breathing rates, and greatest chest wall deformations from relaxation at end-expiration. These group trends most likely have mechanical roots. Both the depth and rate of tidal breathing are known to be conditioned in considerable measure by the most effective strategy for achieving the least costly muscular force demands and the minimal amount of work for breathing (Mead, 1960; Younes and Remmers, 1981). The most effective and least costly strategy for the present endomorphic subjects apparently involved moving the breathing apparatus relatively slowly and over relatively large excursions. The large chest wall deformations generally used by the present endomorphic subjects involved a significant volume shift from the abdomen to the rib cage at the tidal end-expiratory level. It seems reasonable to assume that such a shift was brought about through an expiratory adjustment of the abdomen that lifted the rib cage in the inspiratory direction. The mechanical importance of this adjustment probably resided in the influence it had on the diaphragm. Inward positioning of the abdomen tends to tune the diaphragm mechanically by increasing the length of its costal fibers, an effect that renders diaphragmatic function more efficient (see Chapter 4 and Goldman, 1974). For the present endomorphic subjects, a significant inward positioning of the abdomen is consistent with major activity in the abdominal musculature that serves to counteract the gravitational pull placed on the diaphragm by footward displacement of the large abdominal mass. Were substantial abdominal activity not used, the diaphragm would be flattened somewhat, thereby decreasing its effectiveness in moving the rib cage in the inspiratory direction during tidal breathing.

Presumably, the diaphragm was the prime inspiratory driver off the platform provided by abdominal tautness in 10 of the 12 subjects. Such an interpretation is consistent with the present data, which show both rib cage and abdominal volumes to increase during the inspiratory phase of tidal breathing. It also is consistent with volume-pressure studies of resting tidal breathing (Goldman, 1974; Mead, 1974). For those two subjects who breathed from an end-expiratory configuration that was identical to that for relaxation at FRC, it seems reasonable to assume that abdominal platforming was not involved but that, as in the other subjects, the diaphragm alone was responsible for inspiratory chest wall displacement in tidal breathing.

Speech Production Activities

The speech production data generated by the present subjects generally are of a nature consistent with those reported by previous investigators (see Chapters 3, 4, 8, and 10). One noteworthy difference is the placement of lung volume events within the vital capacity. Specifically, many of the present subjects tended to initiate and terminate their breath groups at slightly lower lung volumes (about 5% to 10% of the vital capacity) than did previously studied subjects. This difference may be related to the fact that the present subjects were substantially younger than subjects in earlier investigations. This suggestion is highly speculative, however, because the influence of age on speech breathing is unknown.

When the present speech production data are considered with regard to body type, support is found for the notion that body type and speech breathing kinematics are linked. Body type accounted, in part, for differences observed in relative volume contributions of the rib cage and abdomen during speech production in different subjects. Furthermore, several other kinematic behaviors were found to differ in subjects with different body types. The most striking contrasts in speech breathing function involved the endomorphic and ectomorphic subject groups. In a broad sense, speech production was associated with a high degree of abdominal participation in the endomorphic subjects and a high degree of rib cage participation in the ectomorphic subjects. This general conclusion is based on several kinematic findings: (1) the endomorphic subjects frequently demonstrated a relative volume predominance of the abdomen over the rib cage, whereas the ectomorphic subjects usually demonstrated a rib cage predominance over the abdomen; (2) the endomorphic subjects used large abdominal excursions, whereas the ectomorphic subjects used small abdominal excursions; (3) the endomorphic subjects often demonstrated rib cage paradoxing, whereas the ectomorphic subjects never demonstrated such paradoxing; and (4) the endomorphic subjects demonstrated large chest wall deformations from relaxation, whereas the ectomorphic subjects showed small deformations. Against this contrastive backdrop, the data for the mesomorphic subjects generally fell somewhere between the extremes demonstrated by the endomorphic and ectomorphic subjects. In fact, the data for the mesomorphic subjects generally represented a mixture of the characteristics of the other two subject groups.

It can be assumed from past research that for each of the present subjects the relative volume relaxation characteristic would pass through the right-most extreme of the lower isovolume line shown in each chart, that is, through the relaxed FRC configuration(see Chapters 3 and 4). Speech production data for the present subjects lie to the left of the presumed relaxation characteristic on their relative volume charts. This means that during utterance the rib cage was larger and the abdomen was smaller than they would have been were the subjects relaxed at the prevailing lung volumes. Muscular activities that could bring about distortion of this nature include the following: (1) net inspiratory forces operating on the rib cage; (2) expiratory forces operating on the abdomen; (3) a combination of 1 and 2; and (4) a combination of expiratory forces operating on both the rib cage (net) and abdomen, but with the latter predominating.

It can be speculated as to which alternative was most likely to have been operating on the basis of the presumed sign and magnitude of the muscular pressure needed and the relaxation pressure available at the prevailing lung volumes (see Chapters 3 and 4). Alveolar pressures used by the subjects probably were similar in magnitude to those used by other normal-speaking subjects (see Chapters 3 and 4), and the probable relaxation pressure available at each lung volume can be predicted with reasonable accuracy from existing data on healthy, normal subjects (Agostoni and Mead, 1964).

It seems reasonable to assume that the present subjects' speech production activities involved the generation of continuous positive muscular pressure and that this pressure increased with decreases in lung volume. Given that utterances generally took place through the midrange of the vital capacity, alternative 4 listed earlier seems most likely to account for the speech production observations on the present subjects. Alternatives 1 and 3 probably can be discounted because each includes inspiratory forces that usually are characteristic of only high lung volume segments or very soft speech (see Chapter 3). Alternative 2 seems unlikely because of the predominant rib cage contribution associated with chest wall configuration change. Not only is alternative 4 the most consistent with the present observations, it also is consistent with what is known to be the muscular mechanism operating during the same type of speech production activities in subjects studied through the use of volume-pressure methodology and for which muscular mechanisms have been determined empirically (see Chapter 4 and Mead, Hixon, and Goldman, 1974).

For the present endomorphic subjects, the configuration of the chest wall during speech production involved a relatively greater deformation of the abdomen in the expiratory direction than was characteristic of most of the other subjects. Presumably the muscular mechanism underlying such deformation involved a greater muscular pressure contribution from the abdomen. And, in the case of those subjects who demonstrated a gradually increasing inward displacement of the abdomen in successive breath groups, it seems probable that a gradually increasing muscular pressure from the abdomen was responsible for changing the general background configuration of the chest wall.

Of final interest with regard to muscular mechanism are the frequent changes in pathway slope that were demonstrated in the charts of many of the subjects. These can be accounted for only by muscular pressure adjustments of the rib cage and abdomen that are superimposed on the major background adjustment of the chest wall just considered. That is, leftward jogs on the relative volume charts probably were the result of relatively greater increases in abdominal drive during utterance, whereas rightward jogs on the charts probably were the result of relatively lesser decreases or greater increases in rib cage drive.

Pursuing the Body Type–Kinematic Behavior Link

The impetus for this investigation was the suggestion that differences in body type might account for differences in speech breathing behavior among normal subjects (Hixon, 1983). Indeed, body type has been found in this investigation to have an appreciable effect on chest wall behavior in resting tidal breathing and selected speech production activities. Subjects categorized by relative prominence on three components of body type have been shown to demonstrate certain subsets of kinematic behaviors that generally differentiate them from one or both of two other groups of subjects with prominence on other components.

Although a body-type effect is borne out empirically by the present data, there remains the problem that body type, as defined in this investigation, did not account for all the differences observed in resting tidal breathing and speech breathing among the subjects studied. General trends on certain kinematic aspects of function were a common feature of certain body-type categories, whereas other aspects were not unique to a category and were characteristic of two or all three of the categories studied. This is not to say, however, that body type might not account for even more variability in performance across subjects were its components combined in some weighted fashion yet to be determined. The present subjects were categorized along three standard components of physical morphology and composition but were not themselves identical in the relative weighting of these components within their designated body-type categories. To have done this through subject screening would have required an unwieldy and time-consuming selection process to find subjects who were perfectly matched within body-type groups. The subject-selection compromise made in this investigation was to categorize subjects according to a major prominence on one of the three components of body type—relative fatness, relative musculoskeletal development, or relative linearity.

It also is open to question whether or not some of the variability in performance across subjects that is not accounted for by body type is related to the criteria used to group the subjects. That is, there may be features of body type that are significant but are not represented in the measurements involved in the body typing method used here. To the extent that the *Heath-Carter Somatotype Method* (Carter, 1980) does not include all conceivable measurements of body type features, its use in the categorization of subjects could account for some of the unexplained variability in speech breathing performance.

Perhaps a relevant consideration of the body type-speech breathing link could be made through the study of twins of identical body type in whom even other elements of variance might be minimized in making between-subject comparisons. Short of having such data available, a fortuitous, albeit limited, inquiry of performance in different subjects matched perfectly for body-type components according to the *Heath-Carter Somatotype Method* is actually contained within the present data. That is, ectomorphic subjects JD and NS happened by chance to have identical ratings on body-type components: $1-2\frac{1}{2}-5\frac{1}{2}$ (for endomorphy, mesomorphy, and ectomorphy). When compared on kinematic data, however, these two subjects are not identical. For resting tidal breathing, they demonstrated similar tidal volumes, breathing rates, and background chest wall configurations but different relative contributions of the rib cage and abdomen. For speech breathing, they showed similar lung volume events and background chest wall configurations but different general relative contributions of the rib cage and abdomen, different relative frequencies of abdominal paradoxing, and different magnitudes of abdominal excursions for breath groups. Thus, within one body-type category, two subjects rated identically on a standardized measure of physical morphology and composition are found to differ significantly in several aspects of resting tidal breathing and speech breathing kinematics.

Further consideration of these two subjects may offer insight into other physical characteristics that may be related to the differences between them in breathing performance. Although these two subjects were rated identically in body type and were sized only about 10% differently with regard to height, weight, and vital capacity (see Table 12–1), they differed substantially from one another in certain torso characteristics. Detailed measurements were made on the following dimensions of each subject at his resting tidal end-expiratory level: (1) torso length (suprasternal notch to symphysion); (2) shoulder breadth (at acromion processes); (3) rib cage anteroposterior diameter, transverse diameter, and circumference (at fourth costosternal articulation); (4) abdomen anteroposterior diameter, transverse diameter, and circumference (at top of iliac crest); and (5) waist circumference (between xyphoid and navel). On the basis of these measurements, subject JD was found to be larger than subject NS in rib cage transverse diameter (10%), abdomen transverse diameter (18%), abdomen circumference (13%), and waist circumference (8%). Considering the measurements for the two subjects, it was apparent that the two differed considerably in torso form, with JD showing a much more elliptical rib cage and abdomen configuration (long axis transversely) and a larger upper abdomen circumference (waist) than subject NS. It seems possible that differences of such a nature may contribute to different mechanical advantages in the musculoskeletal components of the breathing apparatus and, therefore, different resultant kinematic behaviors during tidal breathing and speech production. Knowledge of how such torso configuration factors might affect breathing function is meager. Thus, it is difficult to speculate rationally about the mechanical consequences such subject differences might have on kinematic behaviors.

What seems pertinent here, however, is the fact that two subjects, identical in standard body-type ratings but different in some important breathing kinematic aspects, also differ in their torso characteristics. This suggests that some form of torso-type data might be even more powerful than body-type data in attempting to account for the variability in kinematic performances among subjects. Unfortunately, standard torso-typing methods are not available currently (Dr. Walter H. Birkby, personal communication, May, 1985). Perhaps it would be fruitful to develop a torso-typing method that would include physical measurements of the kind just mentioned as well as pertinent measures of torso composition and musculoskeletal development.

At an intuitive level, the possibility of individuals with identical body types (by standard measurement methods) demonstrating different torso types that could influence breathing kinematics is appealing. It might be reasoned that, although a body type-kinematic behavior link is supported by the findings of this investigation, the underlying relation may not be a direct cause-and-effect one. Rather, body type may be related to torso type, which, in turn, is the primary determiner of differences among subjects in breathing kinematics. The need for research into the relationship between body type and torso type is obvious.

Clinical Implications

What can be taken from this investigation to improve the evaluation and management of persons with speech breathing disorders? First, it is now clear that any conceptualization of normal speech breathing behavior, at least in kinematic terms, must be modified by knowledge of the influence of body type on function. It has been learned that subjects of different body types perform somewhat differently in speech breathing. Obviously this knowledge must be taken into account when comparing abnormal function to a presumed normal standard of function. For example, the clinician confronted with two clients, one highly endomorphic (fat) and one highly ectomorphic (lank), might reach very different clinical decisions with respect to the two were they both to demonstrate essentially all rib cage displacement during their conversational speech production in the upright body position. Such displacement for the endomorphic client might reflect abnormal function, whereas it would be consistent with normal function for the ectomorphic client. For another example, the clinician confronted with two clients, one highly ectomorphic and one highly endomorphic, might reach very different clinical decisions with respect to the two were they both to demonstrate frequent rib cage paradoxing while reading aloud in the upright body position. Such paradoxing for the ectomorphic client might reflect abnormal function, whereas it would reflect normal function for the endomorphic client.

Second, it would appear from the results of this investigation that there may be a need to consider the effect of body type on chest wall configuration when deciding on the extent to which the abdomen should be positioned inward when being managed for paresis or paralysis (see Chapter 7 and Hixon, 1975). Binding or corsetting the abdomen to an identical relative degree in two clients, one highly endomorphic and one highly ectomorphic, might effect different clinical results, assuming the two clients were otherwise comparably impaired. Specifically, it might be necessary to bind or corset an endomorphic client to a greater relative degree than an ectomorphic client to achieve the large deformation of the chest wall from relaxation that is characteristic of the normal endomorphic individual.

Finally, the present results reveal that the pattern of rib cage and abdominal displacement for resting tidal breathing generally is not predictive of the pattern of rib cage and abdominal displacement for speech production. The implication of this distinct difference between these two activities is that the clinician interested in evaluating speech breathing function should not generalize from observations of nonspeech breathing activities. This is the case regardless of body type and is consistent with the viewpoint of von Euler (1982) that it is "meaningless to attempt to infer much about the control of the breathing activity during speech from studies of automatic respiration" (p. 97).

ACKNOWLEDGMENT

The preparation of this manuscript was supported by a grant from the Graduate Student Program Development Fund of the University of Arizona and a grant from the National Institute of Neurological and Communicative Disorders and Stroke (NS-21574). The consultations of Dr. J. E. Lindsay Carter, Professor of Physical Education, San Diego State University, and Dr. Walter H. Birkby, Professor of Physical Anthropology and Director of the Human Identification Laboratory, University of Arizona, are gratefully acknowledged.

REFERENCES

Agostoni, E., and Mead, J. (1964). Statics of the respiratory system (pp. 387–409). In W. Fenn and H. Rahn (Eds.): Handbook of physiology. Respiration 1, Sect. 3. Washington, DC: American Physiological Society.

Bailey, D., Carter, J., and Mirwald, R. (1982). Somatotypes of Canadian men and women. Human Biology, 54, 813–828.

Bergofsky, E. (1964). Relative contributions of the rib cage and diaphragm to ventilation in man. Journal of Applied Physiology, 19, 698–706.

Carter, J. (1980). The Heath-Carter somatotype method (3rd ed.). San Diego: San Diego State University Press.

Euler, C. von (1982). Some aspects of speech breathing physiology (pp. 95–103). In S. Grillner, B. Lindblom, J.

Lubker, and A. Persson (Eds.): *Speech motor control*. Oxford: Pergamon Press.

Fairbanks, G. (1960). *Voice and articulation drillbook* (2nd ed.). New York: Harper and Row.

Fugl-Meyer, A. (1974). Relative respiratory contribution of the rib cage and abdomen in males and females with special regard to posture. *Respiration*, 31, 240–251.

GMG Scientific Inc. (1980). *Operation manual for linearized magnetometers*. Burlington, MA: GMG Scientific Inc.

Goldman, M. (1974). The mechanical coupling of the diaphragm and rib cage (pp. 50–63). *In* L. Pengelly, A. Rebuck, and E. Campbell (Eds.): *Loaded breathing*. London: Churchill Livingstone.

Grassino, A. (1974). Influence of chest wall configuration on the static and dynamic characteristics of the contracting diaphragm (pp. 64–72). *In* L. Pengelly, A. Rebuck, and E. Campbell (Eds.): *Loaded breathing*. London: Churchill Livingstone.

Harris, L. (1975). *Clinical respiratory physiology*. Bristol: John Wright & Sons, Ltd.

Heath, B. (1963). Need for modification of somatotype methodology. *American Journal of Physical Anthropology*, 21, 227–233.

Heath, B., and Carter, J. (1967). A modified somatotype method. *American Journal of Physical Anthropology*, 27, 57–74.

Hixon, T. (1975). *Respiratory-laryngeal evaluation*. Paper presented at the Veterans Administration Workshop on Motor Speech Disorders, Madison, WI.

Hixon, T. (1983). *Respiratory control in speech and singing*. Paper presented at the Voice Foundation Annual Symposium on Care of the Professional Voice, New York.

Konno, K., and Mead, J. (1967). Measurement of the separate volume changes of rib cage and abdomen during breathing. *Journal of Applied Physiology*, 22, 407–422.

Mead, J. (1960). Control of respiratory frequency. *Journal of Applied Physiology*, 15, 325–336.

Mead, J. (1974). Mechanics of the chest wall (pp. 35–49). *In* L. Pengelly, A. Rebuck, and E. Campbell (Eds.): *Loaded breathing*. London: Churchill Livingstone.

Mead, J., and Agostoni, E. (1964). Dynamics of breathing (pp. 411–427). *In* W. Fenn and H. Rahn (Eds.): *Handbook of physiology. Respiration 1, Sect. 3*. Washington, DC: American Physiological Society.

Mead, J., Hixon, T., and Goldman, M. (1974). The configuration of the chest wall during speech (pp. 58–66). *In* B. Wyke (Ed.): *Ventilatory and phonatory control systems*. London: Oxford University Press.

Needham, C., Rogan, M., and McDonald, I. (1954). Normal standards for lung volumes, intrapulmonary gas-mixing, and maximum breathing capacity. *Thorax*, 9, 313–325.

Sheldon, W., Stevens, S., and Tucker, W. (1940). *The varieties of human physique*. New York: Harper.

Younes, M., and Remmers, J. (1981). Control of tidal volume and respiratory frequency (pp. 621–671). *In* T. Hornbein (Ed.): *Regulation of breathing. Part 1, Volume 17*. New York: Dekker.

Author Index

Subject Index

BACK TALK

" . . . and so there ain't nothing more to write about, and I am rotten glad of it, because if I'd a knowed what a trouble it was to make a book I wouldn't a tackled it and ain't agoing to no more."

Mark Twain

" . . . at least not 'till I get me in a new batch of them floppin' disks and a few days a golfin'."

Thomas J. Hixon

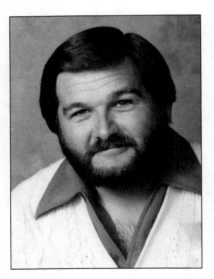

Thomas J. Hixon is a professor in the Department of Speech and Hearing Sciences and a member of the Multidisciplinary Committees on Neurobiology and Motor Control at the University of Arizona. He received his M.A. and Ph.D. degrees in speech pathology from the University of Iowa and did postdoctoral work in physiology at Harvard University. Dr. Hixon is a fellow of the American Speech-Language-Hearing Association, holds its Certificate of Clinical Competence in Speech-Language Pathology, and is a former editor of its *Journal of Speech and Hearing Research*. His professional interests center around normal and abnormal speech production.

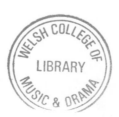